74

USHERNED

THE SOCIOLOGY
OF HEALTH AND HEALING

THE SOCIOLOGY OF HEALTH AND HEALING

A Textbook

MARGARET STACEY

University of Warwick

London and New York

First published in 1988 by Unwin Hyman Ltd
Third impression 1990

Reprinted 1991
by Routledge
11 New Fetter Lane, London EC4P 4EE

Simultaneously published in the USA and Canada
by Routledge
a division of Routledge, Chapman and Hall Inc.
29 West 35th Street, New York, NY 10001

© Margaret Stacey 1988

Printed and bound in Great Britain by Biddles Ltd, Guildford
and King's Lynn

British Library Cataloguing in Publication Data
Stacey, Margaret, 1922–
  The sociology of health and healing: a textbook.
1. Social medicine
I. Title
362.1′042   RA418

Library of Congress Cataloging in Publication Data
Stacey, Margaret.
  The sociology of health and healing
Bibliography: p.
Includes index.
1. Social medicine.   2. Social medicine – Great Britain.
I. Title.
RA418.S76   1988   306.4   88–1145

ISBN 0–415–07872–5

For Jennifer

Contents

x   *Contents*

Figures

Preface

This book has been developed out of lectures delivered over a period of years to third-year students at Warwick University and before that at Swansea University College; as importantly, it has come from the associated seminars where problems not well tackled in any medical sociology text were thrashed out. Some of the difficulties of writing the book have come from the need in a textbook to articulate, rather more precisely than a group can do in an hour's seminar, the relationship between conventional and less conventional sources.

The theoretical and para-theoretical framework which has been used is discussed in Chapter 1. There are two features which I would like to mention in advance, however. The first is that in writing this text I write as a woman and as a feminist. In writing I have tried to represent reasonably all points of view, including when I disagree, and to draw attention to texts where students may find fuller expositions. At the same time I have tried to avoid a mode of writing, in which I was brought up, which treats women as the other. In common with women of my generation I learned (rather than being consciously taught) to write in what I can now describe only as a masculinist mode. After long years I all too often find myself writing still in that way. It seems comfortable, for after all it is the dominant mode. To counteract this tendency I have used the word 'us' rather than 'them' when talking of women, particularly in the later chapters when matters of contemporary dispute are under discussion. This may read uncomfortably to those used to the more conventional mode; I hope they will accept my usage. No science can be value free; that which so appears is invariably unchallenging of current or dominant values. Each of us has to work – be we woman or man – from our own social situation and from our own values. This should, however, not prevent us from balanced exposition.

What I have tried to write is sociology which is informed by feminist thinking, which seeks to revise the conventional understandings in the light of feminist theory and feminist empirical research; to bring together the work done in the tradition of the founding fathers with the more recent feminist critiques.

The use of 'us' in context to mean 'us women' may be found difficult by some. Another stylistic foible may also annoy. It arises from the way I have thought about readers as I have been writing and have tried to go through a journey with them. The use of 'we' in the text, unless the context clearly indicates otherwise, implies 'you, the readers, and me'. It is not intended as a royal 'we'. Where I mean 'I think so-and-so' I have used the first person. Many of the topics discussed have no definitive answers; throughout the book, we (you and I and people in our society) are on a voyage of discovery.

The second main point is the use I have made of history. I am not a historian. I read sociology from my undergraduate days. I did, however, have the great privilege of hearing H. L. Beales lecture; from him I first really began to grasp the relevance of history to the understanding of contemporary society. Since I am not a historian, there is a qualitative difference between the chapters of Part One and Part Two of this book. Part One is taken entirely from secondary sources; while this is also true of much of Part Two, I have done a good deal of hands-on health-care research – and still do. Also, all of the anthropological kinds of work that I have done, I have done in the UK, although not all of it in England; anthropologists will no doubt perceive weaknesses in Chapter 2 analogous to those which historians will find in Chapters 3–8.

As a fieldworker I am acutely aware of the misinterpretations that may be made by those who have not immersed themselves in the field. The same goes for historical periods and historical sequences. Yet it seemed to me to be better to try to analyse from secondary sources what the developments were over time in some detail. The alternative appears to be to rely on brief broad sweeps, commonly linked with a particular school of sociological thought, sweeps which by their very generality must conceal more than they reveal. However, readers should note that Part One is not anthropology or history. Rather, it is an attempt to use some of the excellent work which anthropologists and historians have done to illuminate the analysis of health and illness, healing and health care in contemporary society – to set the issues of our own society today in its context as a small part of time and space. In contrast with the brief summary or broad sweep, this approach does at least make plain whose data I have been using to develop my arguments.

Acknowledgements

It is impossible to acknowledge all the people who have helped me write this book. They include colleagues in at the universities of Swansea and Warwick as well as all those I have taught and with whom I have researched in both those places; they are not confined to those who were studying medical sociology, although these have been particularly influential. Special mention must be made of the Warwick Formation of postgraduates and researchers who were such fun, so supportive and who did such good work in the late 1970s and early 1980s; they were dispersed all too soon by restrictions on research funding. Special thanks, too, to Virginia Olesen for opening new horizons for me and for her unfailing academic and personal support, her well-trained fieldwork and her analytical skills.

It is bound to be the case towards the end of a long academic life that one has forgotten exactly where and from whom one came by ideas or revealing fragments of data. I trust that failures to acknowledge of that kind may be forgiven and perhaps taken as part of the generalized academic exchanges which we all enjoy.

I owe a special debt of thanks to those who read part or all of the draft typescript; they must be named. Frederick Kaona read and criticized Chapter 2 with the experienced eye of an African health worker well versed in sociological research in health care; Ivan Waddington's critique of Chapter 6 was valuable and also encouraging to one who had ventured untrained into the historical arena; here my debt to Margaret Pelling, who read all the historical chapters, is even greater. The way sociologists use and misuse history is enough to make any historian wince. Margaret Pelling's own work pays infinite attention to detail and eschews any dubious inferential leap. This being so, I am particularly grateful to her for her patience in ploughing through an earlier draft and not only pointing out obvious errors but providing sources and references in quantity.

Two people read the whole draft and commented on it and to them a special thankyou. Margot Jefferys provided not only pages of detailed criticism, but also constructive comments on the structure as a whole. These have been immensely valuable, despite the fact that I have totally ignored some of that advice. On my head be it! Margot has, over many years, been a tower of strength and guide through the social medical world, historical and contemporary. Jennifer Lorch not only was from day to day continually encouraging and helpful, she also acted as the intelligent lay reader, pointing out where jargon, medical or sociological, had crept in. If I have succeeded in being technical without being unintelligible, it will be due a great deal to her literary skills. My thanks to all those who read parts or the whole for reducing the more obvious bêtises. Of course, what follows is my responsibility alone.

My thanks also to Fiona Stone for typing the first draft throughout and to

Judy Morris for helping to check and collate the final draft; to the Warwick department secretaries who over the years have been unerringly helpful; to Pat Hills for helping to keep my books, pamphlets and photocopies under control. Thanks also to the Warwick University librarians, particularly those in science, social science, history and inter-library loans, and to the librarians of the Royal Society of Medicine for their skilful help.

I would like to make the following acknowledgements. Figure 2.1 on page 29 is reproduced by permission of the University of California Press. It first appeared in A. Kleinman, *Patients and Healers in the Context of Culture* © 1980 The Regents of the University of California. Table 5.1 on page 65 is reproduced by permission of the British Sociological Association. Figure 13.1 on page 186 is reproduced by permission of the Office of Health Economics. Figure 9.1 on pages 134–35, is reproduced by permission of Baywood Publishing Company. It first appeared in Radical Statistics Health Group 'A critique of *Priorities for Health and Personal Social Services in England*', *International Journal of Health Services*, 8, 2, pp, 367–400, © 1978 Baywood Publishing Company Inc. Figure 9.2 on page 138, Figure 13.2 on page 188, and Figure 17.1 on page 232 are reproduced with the permission of the Controller of Her Majesty's Stationery Office.

Without the wisdom and generosity of the Warwick University Sabbatical Leave Committee this book could not have been written, albeit that it was never quite finished in the leave allocated. My thanks to them and to the university.

Finally many thanks to Bill Williams, who first asked me to write the book, and to Gordon Smith of Unwin Hyman for their forbearance and encouragement.

Leamington Spa, 1987

THE SOCIOLOGY
OF HEALTH AND HEALING

1 Introduction: Some Theoretical and Methodological Thoughts

This book sets out to look at the arrangements that are and have been made at different times and places for restoring and maintaining health and for ameliorating suffering, paying particular attention to biomedicine in advanced industrial societies and most specifically in Britain. The intention is to treat these phenomena, including the associated medical knowledge, as socially created. The book is written not only for those who are teaching or taking specialist courses in the sociology of medicine or the sociology of health and illness but for sociologists and social scientists more generally. The ways in which a society copes with the major events of birth, illness and death are central to the beliefs and practices of that society and also bear a close relationship to its other major social, economic and cultural institutions. In particular, the treatment of those who are temporarily or permanently dependent on others is a revealing indicator of the social values lying behind the allocation of material and non-material resources. This being so, understanding the beliefs and practices associated with health and healing and the social processes involved contributes to a deeper understanding of the society in which they are found.

It is also the case, as I shall argue later, that the nature of health work presents particular problems for sociological analysis. Work in this area therefore has important implications for sociological theory beyond the theory required for the analysis of the substantive area itself. There are by now a number of texts for doctors, nurses, health administrators and others associated with health care (for example, Armstrong, 1980 and 1983a; Dingwall and McIntosh, 1978; Maclean, 1974; Patrick and Scambler, 1982; Tuckett, 1976). There are fewer British volumes which discuss health and healing specifically sociologically (Cox and Mead, 1975; Doyal with Pennell, 1979; see also, from the USA, Coe, 1970; Jaco, 1979; Maykovich, 1980; Mechanic, 1978). This work seeks to add a further contribution to the latter. At the same time it is hoped that this book may also be of interest to health-care practitioners and administrators who already have some interest in understanding more about the social aspects of their work. While inevitably the book will contain technical arguments and will therefore necessarily use language in a technical sense, the aim is to write in a way which is accessible to specialists in other disciplines and to an interested lay readership.

THE THEORETICAL APPROACH

Three assumptions underly the theoretical position adopted here. The first, already mentioned, relates to the social construction of all healing knowledge; the second, associated with this, is that health knowledge and practice cannot be seen simply as cultural phenomena but are related to the social and economic structure of the society in which they are found; the third assumes a common, but variable, biological base of which account must be taken. The assumption that health knowledge is socially constructed applies equally to sophisticated knowledge developed and learned in medical schools and to unwritten folklore and practice passed from generation to generation. No assumptions are made about any ultimate or absolute knowledge. The book, therefore, rests upon the assumption that, while quite different from our own, the beliefs and practices of non-industrial peoples are in their own terms logical and rational, as were those of our own people at an earlier period; also, that the beliefs and practices of lay members of our own society, although sometimes at odds with the understanding and advice of medical experts, also have their own logic and rationality. All these various notions are as much to be respected as the understandings of highly trained medical personnel. Associated with this it is also assumed that there can be no simple judgement of what is 'efficacious' in healing practice. Supplementary questions have to be asked such as: 'Efficacious in whose terms? For what purpose? To what end?'

HEALTH IN THE SOCIAL AND ECONOMIC STRUCTURE

The second theoretical assumption is that health knowledge and health practice cannot be understood in cultural terms alone, although it is clearly the case that the relationship of health knowledge to other facets of the culture is important and must be explored. Reference has also to be made to the more material aspects of the societies in question and to structured social relations, particularly relations of mating, procreation and child rearing, economic relations and those associated with the political order. That is to say, it is assumed that the knowledge and practices of members of any society about how to promote, maintain and restore health will be related to and vary with these three major and fundamental sets of relationships: those to do with the reproduction of the society; with the mode of production and distribution of goods and services; and with the maintenance of internal order and external defence. For advanced industrial societies this means that three facets will be crucial: the familial or kinship structure and the associated gender order; the mode of production and the associated social and economic class system; and the various structures of the state.

This relationship, between health knowledge and practice on the one hand and the society in which they are found on the other, is not assumed to be simply one way. It is true that the division of labour in health care can in some sense be said to mirror that of the society as a whole. But it does more than that. The way health work is undertaken plays a part, sometimes a major part, in the creation and re-creation of the society itself. Clearly the beliefs and feelings about such matters as birth, mating, death and suffering which are constantly purveyed by the health carers are critical to the way the society goes about other tasks that are performed.

THE BIOLOGICAL BASE

As much as it is important to stress the social, cultural and economic concomitants of health practice and health knowledge, so it is also important to acknowledge the biological base. The assumption made here is that this base is common to all human beings. Birth, mating, ageing and death are biological phenomena; health knowledge and practices develop in response to them and to the suffering which appears to go along with living. In an attempt to avoid biological reductionism many sociologists have paid too little attention to these underlying physical phenomena, although this tendency is beginning to be overcome (see, for example, Barrett, 1981, pp. 338–9; Strong, 1982; Timpanaro, 1980; U 205 Open University Course Team, 1985a).

What this book seeks to bring out is that the same biological phenomena can be interpreted differently in different times and places for social, economic, or cultural reasons. Such interpretations and the beliefs and actions to which they lead are what I have referred to as social construction. The particular social construction of this kind with which readers will probably be most familiar is the dominant mode of the twentieth century, namely, biomedicine. I use the term 'biomedicine', following Kleinman (1978), to describe what is sometimes referred to as 'modern medicine' (a meaningless phrase because what is modern today is ancient tomorrow) or as 'Western' or 'scientific' medicine. Biomedicine indicates the predominant emphasis of that form of knowledge which is above all focused on the body as a biochemical organism.

In addition to the varied interpretations of the biological base, there is also variation in the biological base itself above and beyond the commonly shared humanity. Empirically the risks to which humans are exposed vary considerably over time and space. In some societies today – as was true in our own in times past – the expectation of life is about 25 years, and to live to 45 is to be old and therefore also to be judged wise. For example, Lewis (1975, p. 67) quotes demographic data which show that in the Sepik society of which the Gnau are a part (see Chapter 2) the population histogram forms a broad-based pyramid, 'a form which reflects the high mortality of infants, and the greater risk there of dying in early or middle life compared to the risks in a country like England'. When they were born, men could expect to live slightly less than 45 years; at 5 years of age their expectation was nearly 48 years. Unlike England today the expectation of life of women at both ages was slightly less than that of the men, although there were slightly more women than men in the oldest age groups. In such societies there are many more children than adults, in contrast to advanced industrial societies with their increasingly large populations of the old and very old and small numbers of children and young people. Societies where epidemic diseases are rife, where flood and famine take a toll, have different survival problems from industrial societies where people are faced with heart disease and cancer. These factors, along with the inevitability of ageing and death following birth in whatever society one lives in, have to be taken into account. They form a major part of the material base upon which ideas and arrangements for health maintenance and restoration are constructed.

To make such assumptions, as is done here, is quite different from espousing a socio-biologism which implies that social life is determined biologically. Such a determinism is rejected here. The notion that the biological organism is separate from its environment is one which has developed since the Enlightenment; it is associated with endless and unrewarding arguments about 'nature' versus 'nurture'. Steven Rose and his colleagues (1984) have argued from biological evidence against the correctness of this division, suggesting that organism and environment are one unitary phenomenon, each being unable to exist without the other. This argument thus surpasses those which suggest organism and environment interact and moves far beyond any notion of biological determinism.

The focus of this book, however, is the social. From this stance the rich variety of human life suggests a series of social variations upon the biological base which make biological determinism improbable. Saying that, however, is not to deny that the kinds of society we invent and particularly the way we handle issues of life, health, suffering and death arise from the way, in different societies, we perceive this essential part of our humanness. And how we perceive it, how we behave in relation to the biological base, also affects our destiny as social beings, for there is no doubt about the social creation of illness and suffering as well as the social construction of the knowledge about it.

WHAT IS HEALTH WORK?

Thinking about these theoretical assumptions makes it plain that the question 'What is health work?' does not have a straightforward answer; it is problematic. It is problematic partly because concepts of 'health' or 'well-being' are also problematic. In our own society health tends to be defined as the absence of organic disease, but we also have other notions of 'being well' and are aware of difficult problems where 'illness' and perhaps especially mental illness are not associated with organic disease processes. As we shall see in Chapter 2, in many societies the definition of health is wider; suffering of the body is not clearly distinguished from suffering of the mind, nor is the suffering of a group – as, for example, from flood or drought – always seen as different from individual suffering as we see it. Misfortunes of all kinds are seen in different societies in different relationships to each other. Furthermore, as Chapters 10, 11 and 12 show, in our own society health and illness are conceptualized somewhat differently in different sections of the population, and not only between the trained and the untrained.

For the purposes of analysis in this book, health work will be defined as all those activities which are involved in:

(1)   the production and maintenance of health;
(2)   the restoration of health;
(3)   the care and control of birth, mating and death;
(4)   the amelioration of irreparable conditions and care of the dependent.

Health is here being thought of in terms of general physical and mental well-being, remembering that the specification of what this is will vary over time and space, as has just been indicated.

WHO ARE THE HEALTH WORKERS?

Looking at health work in these basic sociological terms shows at once that it is a continuous activity. It also becomes clear that everyone is involved in some aspect of health work. In consequence, when thinking about the division of labour in health care we are thinking about how health-care activities are divided among the total membership of the society. In some societies it is a question as to whether there are any health specialists at all (see Chapter 2). In other societies, such as advanced industrial societies and in the ancient civilizations such as India and China, there is a highly elaborated division of labour. But we must beware that in consequence of this we do not exclude some important health workers simply because they have not had an elaborate training. Specialists may well be involved, but so are many others.

Many studies in the past have concentrated upon those who are paid for their work in a narrowly defined health-care sector. This book takes a different approach. Whether the society is simple or complex, all those who are involved in health care are taken into account. Ignoring this precept has had the consequence in analyses of advanced industrial societies of distracting analytical attention from the unwaged workers – most often mothers, wives and daughters – although, as we shall see (Chapters 7 and 16), official policy has often relied heavily upon them.

Health production activities begin with the birth of children and maintenance activities with their rearing. Our own care of our bodies and of our life-style is part of health maintenance work. Most important for health production are the activities of the food getters and the food preparers. In highly differentiated societies the former has become a major industry and the latter rests heavily on the activities in the home of those who care for the household, predominantly unwaged women in most societies. Others of their activities, such as cleansing and caring for household members, are also crucial for health maintenance.

As will emerge in the discussions of the historical development of healing knowledge and the organization of practice, a division has been made between curative and preventive services in the health conceptions of those societies where biomedicine dominates. The preventive services are really simply a negative way of looking at production and maintenance of health and one which has originated from the disease-oriented approach to medical knowledge which is at the heart of biomedicine. Using the definition of health work adopted here, it is clear that the entire membership of the society is involved; in market economics this means the unwaged workers in addition to the paid specialists and their waged supporters. In the analysis of the restorative or curative services in such societies all the unpaid workers who help the patient through illness or accident have to be included in the division of labour along with the highly trained salary or fee earners and the waged workers who provide support services. This is also true with regard to the care of the chronic sick and disabled. There are those who are more frequently involved in unwaged health care than others. These are most often women (see also Stacey, 1984).

HEALTH WORK IS 'PEOPLE WORK'

A large part of health work, particularly the restorative and ameliorative aspects, but also some of the maintenance activities, involves one person or groups of people doing things to or for others (Hughes, 1971). It is 'people work' or 'human service'. It is from this that concepts like the division between professional and client, between doctor or nurse and patient, have become current in societies with highly developed divisions of labour. As biomedicine has developed on a mass scale, health care has come to be looked upon as an industry with the paid workers as 'producers' and the patients as 'consumers'.

Consistent with earlier work (Stacey, 1976), in the analyses which follow I shall consider all those ideas as historically and socially specific to particular societies at particular times. The underlying phenomenon is that the patient is an actor in the health-care enterprise rather than a passive recipient of care.

PATIENT AS HEALTH WORKER

Not only is the patient a social actor but s/he is a health worker in the division of health work. This has already become clear as far as the work of health production and health maintenance is concerned. It is also so as far as restorative and ameliorative health work goes. Everett Hughes recognized this as long ago as 1956 (Hughes, 1971). A 'patient can be said to be a producer as much as a consumer of that elusive and abstract good health' (Stacey, 1976, p. 194).

Everett Hughes's proposal that the patient should be included in the division of health labour flowed from his observations of interactions in health care. Working in the symbolic interactionist tradition, Hughes was not trammelled by preconceptions as to the structure of the social relations he was observing, nor was he seduced by the values of the professional workers involved. He reported what he and his associates saw and he saw that patients were workers. He did not however to my knowledge expand at any length upon the theoretical implications of his observation that the patient is a worker in the division of labour. Nor have others taken up and developed his point. Even so, his pupils have continued to work in the spirit of that observation wherein the patient is a central actor in the analysis and one whose actions and values are crucial to those of the trained health-care workers (for example, Fagerhaugh and Strauss, 1977; Roth, 1963).

An altogether different approach is to think of health work as analogous to industrial production. This model I reject, although it is true that such large-scale organizations as hospitals have to be organized in a way which may be said to be analogous to the organization of a factory or a bureaucracy. The production of the 'illusive good health' is quite unlike the production of material goods; health cannot be compared to a can of peas or to the factory-made pins of which Adam Smith wrote. The trained workers, the relatives and friends, the patient her/himself are working together (more or less co-operatively and with more or less mutual misunderstanding) on the mind or body of the patient. This is a qualitatively different activity from the production of peas or pins. It is also qualitatively different from the human-service activities which managers undertake when, for example, they move personnel about a plant. In human service or people work which is undertaken in health care the outcome is crucially important to one of the workers, the patient. It is crucial to her/him in a way different from its importance to any of the other workers involved. It is interesting that when Stevenson carried the industrial model, the division into producers and consumers, to its logical conclusion he recognized that in human-service industries 'production and consumption occur simultaneously' (1976, p. 82).

In line therefore with this ineluctable conclusion derived from observation and argument, the analysis in this book includes the patient in the division of health labour. Further, in line with my earlier conclusions (Stacey, 1976), I shall continue to call the suffering person a 'patient', which derives from the Latin *pati*, meaning to suffer (*OED*). Issues of whether and when patients should be looked upon as 'clients' or 'consumers', and 'service objects' or 'work objects', are then open for analysis and discussion in relation to the health-care arrangements under review and to the theoretical problem being analysed.

Ruzek (1978, p. 7) has pointed out that some hold it as visionary to see the patient as a producer. This is to confuse analytical rigour with social philosophy. Given the status accorded to the patient in many arenas in biomedicine it may require a feat of sociological imagination to recognize that analytically the patient *is* a health producer. Whether the patient as worker can ever be an equal partner in the health-care enterprise in advanced industrial societies or under what conditions that might emerge is another question which should be kept separate from the observation that the patient *is* a health worker in her/his own case. Questions of exploitation associated with the profit motive within capitalism and the control and autonomy problems associated with service industries have to be taken into account in specific instances. Attention certainly has to be paid to them before the particular nature and characteristics of any people work, doctor–patient, professional health worker–patient relationships can be analysed. The patient remains a health worker notwithstanding. Comparative analyses are possible within this understanding.

These then are the underlying concepts in this book. First, that all members of a society are actively involved in health production and maintenance work; second, that everyone is potentially involved in health work as a patient and that the patient is a health worker; third, that more people than the socially recognized healers are health workers; fourth, that the characteristics of 'human service' or 'people work' involved in health work result in that activity having characteristics which distinguish it from most other social activities. These concepts will be used in the analysis which follows.

When the discussion turns to industrial societies the analysis will use familiar concepts relating to church, state, industry and market-place. In such societies notions of class and status will be central to the analysis and are referred to later in this chapter. There is one further set of concepts which underlie the whole way in which this analysis of health and healing has developed. These are the concepts of the gender order and of the division, found in many societies, into public and private, or domestic, domains. Age grading, the concept of the generational order, is also fundamental to some aspects of the social organization.

THE GENDER ORDER

All societies, so far as we know, allocate roles and responsibilities differentially between the sexes, although the ways in which this is done are very variable (see, for example, Oakley, 1972). The notion of the gender order includes more than simple differential allocation of tasks; it implies that there are authority relations and arrogance–deference relations in the sex roles which are the norm in any one society – the relationships between the sexes are systematically ordered. The order is one of gender, not of sex as such, for it is socially constructed and may be constructed in a variety of ways. By far the greater number of societies which we know about have a male-dominated gender order; that is, the men are accorded a superior position. Feminists have tended to call such societies patriarchal, but this term is avoided here. It is avoided first because patriarchy has a clear technical meaning in anthropology which is well established and the term should for analytical purposes be restricted to that usage. It is avoided also because, as Barrett (1980), McKee and O'Brien (1982) and Rowbotham (1979) point out, the feminist usage of 'patriarchy' is confused, including male authority in the family, as fathers and husbands, and male authority in the society more generally; 'patriarchy', as it has come to be used, includes the domination of women by men and the domination of children by men. When referring to societies in which men have superordinate power or authority I shall therefore use the term 'male-dominated gender order', reserving 'patriarchy' for the specific kinship form of male domination.

THE GENERATIONAL ORDER

The generational order also has to be distinguished. Adults have some kind of authority over children in most societies. Women as well as men have authority over children, although each may have a different kind of authority. In some societies the old are venerated, although that tends to occur most commonly in societies with relatively short life expectancies. In industrial societies, whether capitalist or state socialist, the old, no longer producers, tend to be looked down on. Both the nature of the generational order and its relationship to the gender order are critical for an analysis of the health and healing arrangements in any society.

THE PUBLIC AND DOMESTIC DOMAINS

The analysis of the gender order in any complex society requires the use of the concept that the society is divided into public and domestic domains (Nelson, 1974; Rosaldo, 1980; Rosaldo and Lamphere, 1974; Smith, 1974a; Stacey and Price, 1981). 'Domestic' is used here rather than 'private' because the crucial reference is to the domain of the home, the arena of reproduction. How private that is and in what sense it is private has varied over time and from place to place. The distinction between public and domestic applies to all those societies where social institutions have developed outside the household. The public domain is perhaps most often distinguished where religious, military and political institutions are concerned. For Europe, a distinct phase was marked by the development of the centralized state, beginning after the Carolingian period (McNamara and Wemple, 1974); a second important phase was the removal of productive industry from the home with the rise of capitalism (cf. Smith, 1974a, p. 6). The public domain as used here is essentially a political concept, being the arena in which power and authority over the collectivity are exercised.

The domestic and public domains as empirically existing arrangements are not fixed and immutable (Rosaldo, 1980; Stacey, 1981; Stacey and Price, 1981). The social relations within each domain change, and their relationships with each other change. The boundary of each is never clearly defined, and the distinction between the domains is blurred. A great deal of health work nowadays inhabits an uneasy position between the two domains, but one dominated by men and by public domain values. The understanding of the relationship between the domains is therefore critical for an analysis of health and healing. Furthermore, sociologists have hitherto been poorly equipped to analyse these issues because of a lacuna in sociological theory, which has not developed concepts or theories to articulate the domains to each other.

THE PROBLEM OF THE TWO ADAMS

This situation has come about because of the historical and structural specificity of sociological and anthropological theory (Reiter, 1975; Rosaldo, 1980; Smith, 1974b). Elsewhere I have noted that around 1950 there still existed two quite unrelated theories about the division of labour:

> one that it all began with Adam Smith and the other that it all began with Adam and Eve. The first has to do with production and the social control of the workers and the second with reproduction and the social control of women. The problem is that the two accounts, both men's accounts, have never been reconciled. Indeed it is only as a result of the urgent insistence of feminists that the problematic nature of the social order related to reproduction has been recognised.
>
> (Stacey, 1981, p. 172)

I argued that the sociological analysis of the division of labour in health care was impeded by limitations in all the general sociological theories of the division of labour, be they Durkheimian, Marxian, or Weberian in origin. All these theories (which, following O'Brien, 1981, I now call 'malestream,' since patently they are not all mainstream) are historically specific. They began to be developed in the nineteenth century by men to deal with problems of social order in the public domain of industry, church, state and market-place. The domestic domain, an important part of which was the woman's domain, was recorded and analysed only through men's eyes, men who mediated between the public and domestic domains (cf. Smith, 1974a, p. 6). Only men were permitted into the public domain at the time sociology was founded. They did not see the sexual division of labour as sociologically problematic – it was 'natural' – and this assumption was still made by most around 1950, as my analysis (Stacey, 1981) showed. This lacuna, I argued, not only meant that sociology was playing an active part in continuing the invisibility of women and their world to theory, but also more generally was feeding the ideologies which supported the continued oppression of women.

One ideology which it fed was the division into public and domestic domains. It is important to recognize that while the division into public and domestic domains has empirical reality at one level, at another it is an ideological distinction, which began to take its present form during the Industrial Revolution. Its clearest statement is perhaps to be found in the cult of domesticity (Davidoff, l'Esperance and Newby, 1976; Lown, 1983 and 1984). This ideology, expressed as a distinction between private and public rather than domestic and public, was accepted almost unquestioningly by most sociologists until relatively recently. Thus we not only have to note changes in the empirical relations between public and domestic domains, we also have to distinguish ideology from reality.

My second point, and the one which is critical for the present work, is that, because sociological theory fell into this ideological trap, the consequent lacuna, whereby the relations between the domestic and public domains were not analysed, left sociologists with problems when dealing with substantive areas in the division of labour such as health, where many of the tasks to be performed straddle the domestic and public domains and involve ideologies associated with both. Nursing, for example, is work done unwaged in the home or for a fee, salary, or wage in the public domain. It is because sociological theory was developed by men in the public domain that sociologists have tended to include in the health division of labour only those who are paid by contract for their work. Thus the unwaged workers and their patients were excluded (see also Stacey, 1984).

A QUESTION OF THE SOCIAL STRUCTURE

In one sense the existence of the public and domestic domains can be said to be a matter of perception; women and men perceive the world differently because of their different locations in the social structure. The central focus of men's work is outside the home, and even today, when there have been so many changes since the nineteenth century, much women's work is still centrally located in the household. Furthermore, the rewards and sanctions of the domestic domain are quite different from those of the public domain. The rewards and sanctions of the public domain are those of the market-place and of bureaucracy; they include wages, salaries, fees and profits and are contract based. In the domestic domain relationships are based on status, not contract, are ascribed rather than achieved; rewards are mostly non-material or take the form of 'gifts' (cf. Bell and Newby, 1976). They take a form which is more akin to the feudal than to the capitalist or the bureaucratic.

SOCIAL STRUCTURAL CHANGES IN AND BETWEEN THE DOMAINS

Since the founding fathers (yes, all men) wrote, there have been many changes within and between the public and domestic domains. Capitalism has developed from small-scale enterprise to monopoly capitalism and the associated development of international oligopolies. Contemporarily, consumer capitalism involves market control of demand, and the machinations of finance capitalists appear to render the governments of nominally sovereign states powerless to control their own affairs. The nature of the domestic domain has changed; no longer is there an arena in which women have undisputed authority. The so-called 'democratic egalitarian family' has ensured that. Increasingly men consider themselves authorities equal with women in the kitchen and child rearing. Men by no means (except for a rare few) do half the housework or half the child rearing, but they 'help' when it suits them and they also 'interfere' (Stacey and Price, 1981, ch. 6). Women have lost that limited area of authority in the domestic domain which they commanded in more highly sex-segregated societies. At the same time women have not gained equality of status or of power in the public domain, whether in paid employment or in politics.

It is not only in the interpersonal relationships between the mates that change has occurred. The domestic domain has also been 'invaded' by the state. While it is the case that social control is exercised by family and kin, the control functions of the state have also to be considered. The programme to ensure the surveillance of all children's health has, from the beginning of the twentieth century, taken employees of the state into the homes of ordinary people to instruct them how to rear their children. It may still be 'natural' that the mother should also be the child rearer. It is no longer believed that she 'naturally' knows how to do the job properly. The way in which paid women health workers have been used to instruct unpaid women health workers (the mothers) is part of the history of the development of medicine which we shall investigate (Chapters 7 and 16).

The entire history of the development of biomedicine itself constitutes a chapter in the changing relationship between the public and domestic domains leading to the creation of a contemporary and very uneasy territory between. The development of the hospital to the situation in which most Western countries now have a 'hospital centred health care system' (Davies, 1979, pp. 53–72) has created a territory in the public domain which nevertheless is based upon a division of labour derived from the gender order established in the domestic domain and with the same male-dominated gender order. The rise of the professions and the debates about altruism versus self-serving professional activity are at least in part also located in the domestic–public domain shifts. These analyses form a major part of the discussion of the development of modern biomedicine in Chapter 6 and recur in Chapter 13.

THE CRITICAL IMPORTANCE OF ECONOMIC AND SOCIAL CLASS

I have developed at some length these arguments about gender and the public and domestic domains because they are still not well understood in malestream sociology. However, the analysis which follows is based as much on the importance of class in the social structure and in the development of health and healing practices in contemporary industrial societies and their contemporary functioning as it is upon gender. Both these major structural divisions are crucial to any satisfactory analysis. By social and economic class I am referring to those major divisions in contemporary society which derive from the structure of capitalism and of the state. From the point of view of individuals this means that their position in the class structure derives from their relationship to the mode of production and within the authority structure of the state. Chapter 5 will show how modern medical knowledge could not have developed as it has except within a hospital-based system to which the nineteenth-century working class had recourse. It will also emerge (Chapter 6) that the development of the medical profession in its present form was similarly reliant upon the development of the class system within industrial capitalism.

The class analysis and the gender analysis are essentially complementary. The many debates about the nature of the professions – what their relationship, if any, to the class structure might be – is better understood when class and gender are considered together (Chapter 6). No analysis of male domination taken on its own can fully explain the authority relations that have emerged within women's occupations, in the development of line management in nursing, for example. If men exploit women it is also true that men exploit other men and women other women. ('Exploit' is used here in a lay not a technical Marxian sense.) It is also the case that the manner of women's exploitation of each other is crucially related to the generic exploitation of women by men. Gender and class then are the crucial dimensions in the analysis of the division of labour in health care in capitalist industrial societies. These are applied to a division of labour which includes public and domestic domain workers, and the patients as well as the professional and the waged workers. It remains to indicate the methods which are to be used.

The book is divided into two parts. The first is comparative and historical. The second is constituted of an analysis of contemporary health concepts and practices.

AVOIDING ETHNOCENTRICITY

In order both to get as detached a view as possible upon our own health-care arrangements and to understand the nature of health and healing in a general way, it is essential to avoid ethnocentricity. This can partly be done by the way in which the conceptual framework is established. This I have tried to do by using terms and concepts which are not tied specifically to the organizations, institutions, or ideologies of a particular time and place. The methodological approach can also help to loosen our involvement in the faiths and the conflicts of our own time and place. Thus one assumption was that the beliefs and practices of all peoples, formally trained or not, scientific or not, were of equal value and should be judged in the first instance by their own internal logic. Within such a framework an examination of the beliefs and practices about healing in other times and places can help to liberate our thinking. Members of a group are liable to imagine that the way things are done with them is 'natural' and 'right' and perhaps even the 'best'. This is probably necessarily so, otherwise none of us would have the confidence to act in everyday situations. When, however, we come to study our institutions and those of others systematically, we have to suspend this belief, for otherwise we would work with an 'absolutism' (Dingwall, 1976, p. viii) which is inimical to proper scholarship. For these reasons the book proceeds in Chapter 2 with a study of the beliefs and practices of a range of peoples who go about similar problems in quite different ways from each other.

In addition to helping to reduce our ethnocentricity, an understanding of such a variety of beliefs and practices can help us to see in what way the creation of healing knowledge is related to other facets of society; this comparative method can help us identify differences and similarities and possibly spot generalizations across time and space if these exist. This can help to illuminate the nature of our own medical system and the beliefs about illness, health and healing which are held among the lay population.

HISTORICAL DEVELOPMENT

An examination of the historical development of biomedical knowledge and of the health-care systems of industrial societies can also serve the same purpose. But it can do more than that. As Chapters 3–8 seek to show, it can help us see the way in which present-day understandings have been created over the centuries and are rooted in times past; how the historically specific nature of the knowledge that developed was vitally linked to the culture and structure of critical periods from the early modern period.

Specifically the historical analysis is informed by the class and gender structures and ideologies of the period in which biomedicine as we know it developed. The changes in responsibility for healing between the domestic and the public domains, between women and men, emerge as critical to a proper understanding of biomedical knowledge and practice.

The historical method is also applied in these chapters to the development of the interests of the state in health care. Here we see the debate between the curative and preventive modes in their nineteenth-century form and how these emerged by the mid-twentieth century in the domination of the clinical model and the curative mode. The role of the state in regulating relationships between the domestic and public domains is particularly important and is returned to again in Part Two.

Having established the importance of the historical and comparative methodologies, the analysis in Part Two then uses a different approach, taking facets of contemporary health knowledge and practice and analysing each systematically. While concepts are referred to throughout, they are seen to be of such importance for contemporary society that three chapters (10–12) are devoted to them: the way in which concepts relate to values in the macro-society, to its social structure and to the division of labour in health care. It will also be noticed how concepts may change when health-care arrangements change.

Chapter 13 looks at the social organization of health-care delivery and its relationship with the division of health labour, while Chapters 14 and 15 consider the unpaid labourers, that is, the patients and the carers in the domestic domain.

The way in which the domination of the clinical, hospital-based conceptualization of health care emerges in practice is examined in Chapter 13, while the implications for practice of the conflicting ideologies of welfare and profit and the organization of the capitalist pharmaceutical and hospital supplies industries are analysed in Chapter 16. In this chapter Marxist and neo-Marxist analyses of profit-making industries in the exploitation of health problems are discussed. In Chapters 13–15 substantive data relating to the nature of people work in human service are examined: the power and authority relations which are involved and the conflicts which ensue. Particular attention is paid to the implications for professions and occupations of activities which straddle the domestic domain of the home and the public domain of market-place and state.

The final chapter, Chapter 17, addresses the substantive issue of the control of human reproduction. It seeks to analyse the implications of the medical take-over of fertility control and childbirth and the implications of the new reproductive technologies including the possibility of genetic manipulation. These are crucial issues for the reproduction of our society, not only at the biological level but at the social level also. It is proposed that once again medicine and science are actively involved in recreating the power and authority structures of the society, but that those who are doing the re-creation are inadequately informed of the possible unintended consequences of their apparently humane actions.

In studying our own society, so far from being in danger of 'going native' we are already native. We believe in our knowledge systems, in the findings of modern medicine and in the dominant hierarchical values of our societies. Or if we are sceptical about the first and in opposition to the second, our scepticism and our opposition are still creations of those dominant values and developed in the light of them. Furthermore, we have stakes in the system as it is. Social scientists as much as practitioners can easily slip into treating some actors as 'objects'. I find it morally imperative to attempt to use theories and methodologies which help to avoid that danger. I hope that the application in practice of the theoretical decision to include all the actors in the division of labour in health care, be they trained or untrained, paid or unpaid, will have the merit of ensuring that the method of analysis cuts across all the occupational, administrative, professional and institutional boundaries of contemporary and other societies. While perhaps the study may consequently appear of less immediate relevance to one working within a particular framework (such as that of a health-care administrator or consultant surgeon), the end result of the analysis should be a deeper understanding of those institutions and may perhaps suggest ways in which the contemporary division of labour in health care could be modified for the better well-being of the population.

Part One

2 Health and Healing in Other Societies

CHANGES IN THE MODE OF STUDY

In Chapter 1, I pointed out that the approach of this book is to examine the health knowledge and healing practices of each society in their own terms, to look for their own internal logic and see how they fit with the rest of the knowledge and practices of that society. Further, I wish to try to relate healing systems to their social and economic arrangements more generally, particularly to the economic relations and the form of government.

To take the first point: it has by no means always been the case that scholars have sought to understand a society in its own terms, in the meanings that beliefs and practices have for its members. Many of the accounts we have of the healing arrangements of other countries are consequently unsatisfactory. The earliest were simply travellers' tales; many of the more systematic accounts were made by people who did not question the wisdom or morality of imperial rule and were certain of the superiority of biomedicine. Early anthropologists and sociologists assumed a linear theory of social development. being convinced that their own society was the most advanced and 'highest' and therefore best. Later the Americans took over this position and added Europe to the areas of the world in need of development. We have to be aware therefore of what we are reading and how it was written.

Recent developments in medical anthropology have to a large extent broken away from this tradition, although not altogether. As Paul Unschuld (1978, pp. 75–7) has put it: 'The study of health care systems of different cultures has proceeded to a point where most authors are aware of "category fallacies" that result from imposing our own notions on a culture alien to us.' Gilbert Lewis (1975, 1976, 1980 and 1986) has in his work made a particular point of trying to avoid imposing his meanings upon those of the Gnau, the people of South-East Asia he studied. He shows how he was making false assumptions based upon his own preconceptions. A striking example is his discovery that some of the Gnau do not believe that birds die. He points out that he had presumed that something that was so obvious to him – that birds do die – would also be obvious to the Gnau, and he was wrong; he would in any case have assumed that all would agree upon the answer to a question like that, and they did not. The discovery led him to understand that the Gnau have two senses of life: consciousness, movement, action, on the one hand; and life in contrast to death, as a passage of time, as a span with a beginning and an end, on the other. Lewis had been among the Gnau for two years before by chance he came upon these discoveries (1980, pp. 136–7).

Paradoxically, starting from different societies' own conceptions aids comparative study. Such an approach helps us to see the fundamental assumptions that we make about our society, to recognize that, just as much as some people leave indeterminate things we are clear about, so we leave indeterminate some things which are clearly explained in other cosmologies. Biomedicine does not explain why particular individuals should be smitten with illness or bear a handicapped child when others do not suffer the same fate; nor does biomedicine seek to explain those incredible spells of bad luck from which all of us from time to time suffer.

Among the more recent developments in medical anthropology there has also been a considerable effort made to develop theories whereby it is possible to relate knowledge of one society to that of another. Some of these have been essentially in cultural terms, as in the work of Horatio Fabrega (1973)) and Arthur Kleinman (1980), for example. Others such as Allen Young (1976a, 1976b, 1978 and 1986b) and Ronald Frankenberg (1980 and 1981) have specifically been concerned with the beliefs and practices of a society as well as with their relationship to the mode of production.

Whatever we believe, if we are to study health and illness in our own society or in others we have for the time being to suspend belief in biomedicine and also in the notion that healers are necessarily either always altruistic or always simply concerned to gain power and prestige.

The best of the earlier writers were able to learn from their studies of other peoples notwithstanding their own great faith in their own medicine. Some of these works are really worthwhile – for example, Carstairs (1955), Cassel (1955), Marriott (1955). At the same time we have to remember the circumstances in which biomedicine was spread throughout the world, initially by European traders seeking for profit. Biomedicine was established in foreign parts to sustain the health of the European military and governmental establishments, of the traders and, later, the settlers. Along with these activities the Western invaders upset the social and economic arrangements, altered the food supply, disrupted the home life of much of the indigenous population and introduced infectious diseases such as measles to which those peoples had no resistance. Saying this is not to promulgate some myth of a golden age. The social existence that European conquerors disturbed was by no means always a peaceful or an idyllic one. The point is that conquest by trade or by arms, or by both, disturbed all preceding arrangements, affecting the whole society, including its healthiness in physiological and psychological senses.

Until about the mid-1970s the data that were available were largely of three kinds:

(1) Studies which sought to answer the question why biomedicine was not accepted among non-European peoples: these studies were embedded in the assumption that such people would be much better off if they accepted biomedical treatment, and how could we convince them of that?
(2) Studies which asked why people who had a choice of healing systems chose this or that one, and for what they chose it: the best of these assume people's choice is rational in their own terms.

(3)   Accounts which attempt to describe health and illness practices: many are ethnographies which lack an explanatory component.

Since the mid-1970s there has been much more variation on these themes. The status of indigenous healings systems has been raised. This partly derives from the increasing self-confidence and independence of post-colonial societies and their rejection of matters associated with their imperial oppressors. It partly derives from a recognition on the part of the World Health Organization that neither is there enough money for hospital-centred health care nor is it (and the associated high technologies) what is most importantly needed by poor and largely rural populations in many parts of the world. There has therefore been an increasing stress upon the importance of indigenous culture and of indigenous medicine as part of that. Biomedicine remains of high status in many parts of the world, nevertheless. As Frankenberg (1980, p. 198) has put it, support for traditional medicine is often only skin deep. Furthermore, there is nowhere in the world where an indigenous culture survives unalloyed. Many, of course, had experienced invasions before those from Europe – as, for example, the Amhara in Ethiopia, whom Young (1976a) describes.

The question 'How can we persuade them our method is best?' has been replaced by 'What methods would be most appropriate?' In medical anthropology and sociology therefore attention has been turned towards facets of this question. These have included increasingly sophisticated attempts to understand the cultural relationships between various healing systems and also, most important in my view, attempts to understand the issues in structural terms including the part played by imperial conquest, international manufacturing and finance capital; not only the relationships between biomedicine and indigenous healing practices, but also between those and other elaborated health-care systems, such as the Chinese and the Ayurvedic and Unani of the Indian subcontinent.

From the earlier studies we can learn a number of things which I will shortly illustrate:

(1)   Not all peoples necessarily distinguish physical illness from other kinds of misfortune, either in the body of knowledge which seeks to explain it, or in the methods of amelioration.
(2)   The problems and their solutions are seen in group terms rather than in individual terms.
(3)   In some societies matters of illness and treatment are matters for negotiation; in others they are matters of authoritative pronouncement.
(4)   Biomedical doctors were astonished to find that their ideas were not readily accepted as superior to the 'primitive' ways of the conquered peoples.

In subsequent studies greater attempts are made to ground the observations theoretically, to categorize healing systems in relation to their social organization, the systematization of their knowledge and its mode of transmission. These works recognize that there have been many mixtures of healing systems for many years before biomedicine came on the scene. It is not the mixture which is surprising, but the twentieth-century domination of biomedicine, a matter hitherto taken for granted by many. Yet even where biomedicine dominates there remain many other systems of healing, as we shall see. The question of how and why choices are made between cosmologies and practitioners remains important even when one ceases to ask it for the simple and ethnocentric reason of 'Why don't they come to my clinic, and how can I make them?'

In approaching all of this we shall, as I indicated in Chapter 1, be assuming the universality of the human and biological base, reminding ourselves that the material, physiological and mental problems with which peoples have to deal nevertheless vary over time and space; their longevity, sex ratios, food supply, social mode and success of production, and reproduction vary. The variations which are imposed upon the common human theme by the social and economic arrangements and to some extent the ecology are enormous.

HEALING AMONG THE GNAU

Let us first look at the Gnau of New Guinea, whose health practices and beliefs have been recorded by Gilbert Lewis (1975, 1976, 1980 and 1986). Lewis is a biomedical doctor as well as a social anthropologist and he does make certain assumptions about the relative superiority and correctness of biomedicine. At the same time he has given us a vivid and sympathetic description of the health practices of the Gnau. The Gnau are particularly interesting both because their way of understanding illness and misfortune is quite different from ours and copes with some problems that our cosmology leaves untouched and because of the division of labour in the caring and healing processes.

Lewis reports that for the Gnau disorders of the body as we understand them are things which are undesired: *wola*. As well as meaning 'ill', *wola* means 'bad', 'evil', 'wretched', 'harmful', and 'forbidden', 'potentially dangerous'. In the form *biwola* it is also used for 'aged' or 'old'. The Gnau therefore have no word to distinguish illness in general from other generalized misfortune in the way which 'sickness' or 'illness' does in English. At the same time the Gnau are capable of making this distinction, which has been imported into their society. Thus Lewis tells us that they use the pidgin English 'sik' and use it only for bodily misfortunes. In addition to *wola* there is an intransitive verb, *neyigeg*, which roughly translates as 'to be sick', which seems to mean that someone is suffering in her/his person as a whole and applies to illnesses which we would call internal. *Wola* on the other hand may affect part or all of the person. Thus a limb or an organ may be *wola*, but the person as a whole may be well or the person may be affected in her/himself. In the case of what we understand as insidious diseases or disabilities (cf. chronic illness and handicap) the Gnau would say 'ruined' or 'wretched' and use *biwola* as for old, aged.

To be sick, or *neyigeg*, is only one aspect of *wola* and contains the risk of death. *Neyigeg* is caused by evil beings, probably ancestors, or by destructive magic and sorcery. Conventionally, when a Gnau is sick s/he withdraws into a passive and wretched state, shuns company and conversation, speaks in an altered tone of voice, lies apart miserable in dirt or in a dark hut with the door shut. The patient (and that no doubt is the right term since 'patient' originally means sufferer) shuns certain food, eats alone, begrimes her/himself with dust and ashes. This behaviour constitutes an appeal for help and it obliges others, especially close relatives, to find out and treat the illness. The patients do not themselves report the illness to anyone; illness is displayed and not described. Nor does anyone examine the patient.

While many societies have counterparts to our pharmacists and medical doctors in herbalists, diviners and healers of various kinds, this is not the case among the Gnau. They have no clearly distinguished specialist or expert healers. Having defined themselves as ill, the Gnau are passive in their treatment. Almost any adult will do to help the sick, although usually it is a senior man who comes to the aid of the sufferer. The patient's withdrawal into the passive and wretched state is to deceive the spirits who have caused the illness into believing they have succeeded in their intention to destroy the sufferer. The task of the helpers is to assist in mitigating or defeating the evil which has caused the patient *neyigeg*. It is important to be clear about the division of labour: no specialists, and it is the patient who decides that s/he is ill and also who decides that s/he is recovered; passivity in treatment and generalized help from others during the period of distress. Malingering is not a relevant concept. As Lewis says, who would wish to continue to lie wretched in the dirt for longer than was necessary for safety? It has to be said also that the social division of labour is not highly advanced among the Gnau; their methods of treating the sick, which assume competence upon the part of all adults, are not unusual in terms of the rest of their social organization, in which most skills are generalized (Lewis, 1976).

There is, however, a clear division of labour between the sexes. 'The distribution of most job activities is segregated according to sex' (Lewis, 1975, p. 340). This, along with the rules and customs connected with marriage and reproduction, constitutes what I would refer to as a clear gender order. I shall return to this later (see page 30).

There is the question of the domain wherein treatment takes place. It is generally undertaken by people of the village and most often by near kin. In that sense it is a domestic matter, for there is not an elaborated distinction between public and domestic domains as there is in advanced industrial societies. Sometimes Gnau attend clinics or hospital elsewhere, but this is relatively rare. They knew that Lewis was a biomedical doctor and they did call him to cases of illness – he treated them, although he could not practise in their village as he would have at home in England. Gnau are aware of a world outside their village. They recognize 'the Administration', an outside authority which imposes upon the village the few differentiated tasks that there are, designating villagers for various governmental and administrative offices.

THE DOMAINS IN KISHAN GARLHI

This difference between the family, the village and the outside world becomes clear in McKim Marriott's (1955) early account of North-West India, where he found biomedicine had a marginal position. Stung by the failure of his clinic, he sought to explain his experience in structural terms, suggesting that the people of Kishan Garlhi recognize three great social realms: those of kinship and family; village and caste; and the outside world. The first was controlled by limitless demands and mutual trust; the second in part by particular obligations and formal respect; and the last which included government, the market-place and Western medicine, was controlled by money and power. Frankenberg (1980 and

1981) is particularly concerned with this last domain and its impact on the first two.

In Kishan Garlhi, indigenous medicine was practised within the family, and the presence of the family was essential for healing consultations. Western notions of privacy and individual responsibility were not relevant, for the group was responsible for illness treatment. The power to treat was diffused among many people, but not among all people, as with the Gnau. Among the people of Kishan Garlhi there were many with the power to heal and many possible treatments. The Western doctor coming from that third outside world was accorded high status, but his behaviour was not appropriate. His attempt to talk person to person to the villagers caused suspicion; furthermore, because his consultations were confidential to the sufferer, it was not possible for the family to negotiate about the illness and the treatment as they were used to doing. In addition, the fact that the doctor made inquiries suggested that he did not know what was the matter; therefore he lacked authority. Finally the issuing of a prescription suggested that his power was limited, because others made up and administered the medicine. McKim Marriott's own commitment to biomedical theory is revealed when he says that the social framework of the treatment could be altered to make it more acceptable to the local people without altering its scientific value. This implies that the method of delivery of health care may be varied independently of the content of the health knowledge – an interesting but questionable notion.

ILLNESS CAUSATION AMONG THE ZULU

John Cassel's (1955) work among the Zulu in 1940 was also written from a basis of the presumed superiority of biomedicine and the help that the system could bring to a people who were, in biomedical terms, suffering severely from malnutrition and tuberculosis. Based on a health centre at Polela, his work, and that of his colleagues, took the indigenous belief system seriously. Cassel and his colleagues did not presume that the local Zulu failed to co-operate with the health clinic because they were 'ignorant' or 'superstitious' or 'stupid'. Their presumption was that the Zulu way of explaining illness and misfortune differed from theirs and needed to be understood if the Zulu were to be persuaded to 'better' ways. For this reason the report of the work is instructive.

The aim of the Polela health centre was not to impose new health concepts and practices on the community, but to integrate them into the culture through popular participation. It was notable for those days that all the health educators employed by the Polela health centre were African, and all discussions were held in Zulu. Moreover, it is now forty years later that the World Health Organization is promulgating vigorously the use of indigenous people in health improvement schemes and taking the policy further to include the integration of indigenous healing practices. Cassel reports that by working through the local beliefs partial success was achieved in improving dietary practices to relieve the severe malnutrition. There was a great deal less success in encouraging the Zulu to accept treatment for pulmonary TB and in checking its rapid spread. The Zulu were not prepared to accept the biomedical germ theory, for they were convinced that the illness was caused by the machinations of an ill-wisher who had introduced poison which remained in the stomach and for which an emetic had to be administered by a specially skilled witch-doctor. The hospital, furthermore, was heartily disliked because it was an alien place 100 miles away perceived as somewhere people went only to die.

An interesting illustration is given of the incompatibility between the two kinds of healing and explanatory systems. Four years previously the daughter of a family had left home to marry and contracted TB in her marital home. The TB was diagnosed at the health centre, but treatment was refused. The daughter, ill as she was, returned to her parental home. Over the subsequent four years eight members of that household became infected with tuberculosis; four died, four were seriously ill. Because of this the family head, who was a Bantu witch-doctor, agreed to talk to the health centre staff and he agreed to let the ill people go to hospital.

The doctor then took this opportunity to teach about the biomedical theory of the spread of infectious illness. He described the course of the disease through the household from the initial infection the daughter had brought back from her marital home. At this the father became angry and withdrew his consent to hospitalization. The doctor had thus lost his prime goal of hospitalization to cure the illness in these cases. Furthermore, he did not at first understand why. After a long discussion it emerged that his explanation of the spread of the disease from the daughter amounted in the terms of the Bantu cosmology to accusing the daughter of having the power to spread disease. This power only sorcerers and witch-doctors have. To accuse the daughter was to ascribe to her powers she did not and should not have, a disruptive and dangerous suggestion. The biomedical doctor achieved his goal only when he had withdrawn this accusation, after which hospital was again agreed to. Did the daughter recover? And what of the others? We are not told. That was not the point of the account.

Cassel (1955) saw the problems of biomedical doctors largely in cultural terms, as a question of conflicting belief systems; for Marriot (1955) there was that, but also a question of social structure and the relationship between the imperial domain and the domains of the kin and the village. Others have seen the defeat of particular attempts at establishing Western health care in more overtly conflictful terms involving both culture and structure.

DISPUTES AMONG THE HEALERS

Oscar Lewis (1955), for example, discussing why a clinic failed in Tepoztlan, Mexico, saw the outcome as the result of a power struggle between the indigenous healers, specifically the *curanderos*, and the biomedical doctors at the clinic. The researchers had gone to Tepoztlan to study the culture and the people. In exchange for their co-operation in the research the villagers asked for practical support. The Mexican government supplied a doctor for six months, and the village helped to establish a Western-style medical co-operative. This had an initial success, and then suddenly the villagers abandoned it. Apart from the clinic there were three types of healer in Tepoztlan: *curanderos*, *mágicos* and 'el doctor'. The *curanderos*, mostly women, treated with herbs and charged a fee of about 25–50 centavos. The two *mágicos* used spiritualism, magic and the women's herbal remedies and charged 1–10 pesos. These two groups of healers were Tepoztecans. 'El doctor' was an outsider but he was not qualified. He charged 100 pesos for his treatments. The clinic charged 1 peso for theirs.

Lewis (1955) puts forward a number of reasons for the failure of the clinic. There was the readiness on the part of the people to distrust innovations and a generalized lack of interest in changing the local ways of doing things; the fee was too high for many; and there was a lack of rapport between doctor and patient derived from their different cultural backgrounds and understandings.

More positively, there was continued faith in the practices of the *curanderos*. In addition Lewis stresses the readiness of local interest groups, headed by the leading *curandero*, Don Rosa, to see the medical co-operative as a threat. He killed the clinic by discrediting it. The researchers were administering a Rorschach test to all the schoolchildren. Don Rosa persuaded the parents that this was an immoral activity by distributing pornographic pictures which he had acquired in a neighbouring town, saying that these were the tests which were being given to the children. It was not only the *curanderos* who felt threatened. So also did the mayor, because the research team was doing something to improve the lot of the Tepoztecans and he, the mayor, was doing nothing. In addition the researchers had championed the poor farmers, the faction which was out of power. The schoolmaster also opposed the innovations represented by the clinic because he was in a marginal position in the village and was therefore currying favour with the education committee. It was safer for him to abuse the clinic to them than to support it. The local synarchist (fascist) was also involved. The upshot of all these actions and alliances was that the clinic was roundly defeated, and the previously installed healers were once again left with the field to themselves.

The struggle for clients, the struggle to maintain power and prestige, is something to which Una MacLean refers with regard to Nigeria (1971 and 1976). Reporting the elaborate indigenous division of labour in health care, she also indicates that this is further complicated by the presence of biomedicine, which presents a real challenge to the indigenous healers. MacLean notes that in face of this competition Yoruba healers are codifying their knowledge in books and forming organizations to resist the threat it represents. In the case of India the long-established and codified healing systems are demanding from government the same sort of privileges which have been accorded to biomedicine (Frankenberg, 1981; Jeffery, 1977). When looking, therefore, at those studies which discuss to which healers ordinary people resort, it is important to recall that as well as offering their healing skills practitioners of all cosmologies have certain vested interests to defend.

A HIERARCHY OF RESORT?

In analysing the hierarchy of resort to plural healing systems among the Manus in the Admiralty Islands in the South Pacific, Schwartz (1969) makes clear the long historical sequence of the imposition of biomedicine in various guises. The Manus have been colonized for a hundred years by, in turn, Germany, Australia, Japan, the USA and again Australia. During this time the Manus experienced increases in suffering by reason of dysentery, influenza and tuberculosis and nearly all of them had malaria. Beginning with the 'doctor boy' or 'aid post orderly' the Manus had long had available to them, and indeed imposed upon them, some version of biomedicine. They have never fully accepted this system however, and Schwartz found that after the Second World

War their acceptance of biomedicine declined. They accepted it but only as a lowly part of their cosmology, simply as a lower-level description, empirical, with no explanatory value. They explain illness and misfortune in terms of ghost ancestor supremacy or powers from the living through magic or sorcery. Biomedicine therefore does not have a causative explanation which fits into the bio-social-moral frame within which their explanations are cast. It is thus not useful for serious illness. The Manus categorize illnesses rather than cures and, indeed, they categorize illness into native and European. The sudden illness of a child, for example, may be due to ill feeling between her parents, and it is that ill feeling which should be treated. The impersonal and amoral biomedicine is not applicable in such a case.

In addition to the aid post orderly and other healers trained in biomedicine, the Manus have a variety of healers available to them. The village leader may be the person who makes a diagnosis. In the case of ill feeling between parents, for example, this was so, and he organized a ceremony to reconcile the parents; but the child was not better, so the village all joined in hymn singing and prayers. The child developed bad convulsions, which were thought to be caused by a ghost ancestor, the spirit of one who had died in violence. This called for a specialist, an exorcist, who used a charm. None of these attempts were of any avail, and the child died. Schwartz (1969, p. 204) uses this account to illustrate what she calls 'acculturative' practices, where a variety of healing practices are used. In addition the example illustrates the division of labour among the healers, who also include herbalists, not mentioned in this particular account.

There is a question as to whether it is correct to think in terms of a hierarchy of resort, implying as this does that the alternatives are given a rank order in the minds of people to whom they are available. Indeed, in Schwartz's account while it is clear the biomedicine takes a lowly place in the Manus' cosmology, it is not clear what the overall ranking might be. It is perhaps rather more satisfactory to think in terms of available resources from among which people chose. This seems to be the approach taken by Judith Lasker (1981), who surveyed the choices made by people on the Ivory Coast. She shows that when they suffer people mostly go to the healer who is available because they do not have much choice. The person locally available may be a biomedic or an indigenous healer. Nevertheless, people are selective about some things; for example, the indigenous bone setter who sets broken bones without the heavy plaster cast used by biomedics is preferred, and in this case the nearest healer may well not be chosen, despite the extra costs involved. It appears to be a mistake to imagine that people necessarily hold alternatives ready ranked in their heads (a mistake as much in the West as anywhere else). It seems much more likely that people store a variety of information which they use as seems appropriate to them and when feasible.

EXTERNALIZING AND INTERNALIZING SYSTEMS

Allan Young (1976a) has distinguished between ways of thinking about misfortune which emphasize casual or aetiological explanations compared with those which emphasize processual or physiological explanations. The first have the form of narratives in which at least some important events take place outside the sick person's body; and the second work by means of images and analogies which make it possible for people to order events within the sick person's body from the onset of the symptoms to the conclusion of the sickness episode. Young further distinguishes polar types of belief systems: internalizing and externalizing. Externalizing systems concentrate on making aetiological (i.e. causal) explanations for serious sickness; diagnostic interest focuses on discovering what could have brought the sick person to the attention of the pathogenic agent, e.g. grudges, witchcraft, or external events. Gnau healing and belief systems fall clearly in this category. Although in the course of healing Gnau do collect and apply herbs, they do not have a great herbal knowledge. The focus of their treatment is to pacify or cheat the offended forces. Young argues that peoples who have externalizing systems make only gross symptomatic distinctions, since internal physiological events are either ignored or not elaborated. Lewis, it will be remembered, when he was called to Gnau patients was not expected to examine them.

By contrast physiological explanations are essential to all the internalizing systems. These include not only biomedicine, where we expect explanations about what is going on inside our bodies, but also the great formalized healing systems of the Indian subcontinent, Ayurvedic and Unani. These healing systems all conceptualize in terms of the course of the illness inside the body; but as we shall see later (Chapters 10–12), they do also include notions of invasions from outside.

For the moment it may be helpful to look at the Amhara of Ethiopia, whom Young (1976a) has studied and who, he argues, have an incomplete internalizing system. This incompleteness is associated with the form of the division of labour; healing is only partially professionalized, and both physiological and aetiological explanations are found. There is no one theory of health, illness and treatment; literate and oral traditions exist side by side and have done so for two millennia. The Amhara identify most of the body's internal organs as we would and emphasize the heart and stomach for explaining sickness. Divine providence ensures that the body's organs work together in a state of harmonious well-being, but this may be upset by any of five categories of agents. These agents include excess of commonplace activities, corrosive substances which can be ingested or breathed into the body, poisons administered by an enemy and various magical practices. The Amhara do not link the agents to the illnesses in any very specific way. Overstimulation of the heart is essential to the way the agents most often work.

There is considerable division of labour in Amhara health care, and healers are distinguished by their healing activities. There are activities which return body parts to their appropriate position (e.g. setting bones); which excise (e.g. removing tonsils, teeth); which return body parts to normal motility (e.g. reducing a fever); which remove the causal agent from contact with the afflicted person (e.g. purges, emetics); spirits who lift their agents from the sufferer in return for supplications. In any treatment a number of these may be combined. Twenty names are used for healers, the most general distinguishing the *habesha hakiym*, or Abyssinian healer, from those who cure by the techniques of biomedicine. The *habesha hakiym* fall into four categories: chirurgeons, who do things such as setting bones, taking out teeth and excising tonsils; the herbalists, who reduce fevers and remove causal agents by emetics, purges and the like;

spirit healers, who also remove causal agents by, for example, emetics but who invoke spirits as well; and a final miscellaneous category of cuppers, tattooists and midwives. It may be Young's concentration on the public domain which leads him to put midwives in a miscellaneous category with cuppers and tattooists. Would a woman's account have differed?

There is therefore a division of labour and a specialization of skills which we did not find among, for example, the Gnau. Young (1976a) reports, however, that the secular healers are indistinguishable from other Amhara except for their curing and they are known for their specific ability which is often limited to competence in regard to three or four specific illnesses. In contrast, the power of the spirit healers appears to be generic, and they are distinguished by their spirit helpers. The herbalists are stratified according to the power of their medicines and the method of administration. There are also household remedies which are a matter of common knowledge; these may be used by suffering Amhara in combination with professional remedies.

This division of labour and these skills are associated with a variety of ways of explaining illness and suffering. The beliefs of the Amhara do not form one systematic whole. In some societies one can distinguish a series of folk beliefs which can be contrasted with a 'great tradition'. This is not the case with the Amhara. They are not interested in the abstract, and it is only at the abstract level that the inconsistency of their beliefs emerges. They are interested in the contingent and the practical, in what are the most effective ways to manipulate people in order to reach socially desirable goals in everyday life. Their ideas about healing, both the externalizing and the internalizing facets, reflect these ideas about the organization of social life in general.

Young argues that the Amhara beliefs and practices about health and healing are no less rational because they are not linked by one coherent theory. Lewis also noted that not all Gnau made the same interpretations. Each of us also knows this to be true of our own culture. The important feature is that the Amhara beliefs and practices bring order into their life and provide a framework in which Amhara can work to overcome misfortunes, including physical illnesses. The essential commonality between the attempts of all people to make sense of the world around them is argued by Robin Horton (1970).

MAKING SENSE OF LIVING

Horton shows that there are not the great differences between Western scientific thought and African thinking that many of us who consider ourselves Western scientists have liked to believe. He argues that the quest for unity underlying apparent diversity, for simplicity underlying apparent disorder, for regularity underlying anomaly, is universal. All peoples at all times try to make sense of the world around them, of experiences and events which otherwise would appear as simply confusing.

Scientific theory replaces common sense; just so, Horton argues, does mystical thinking replace common sense. Processes of abstraction, analysis, reintegration are present in both. The differences between mystical and scientific thinking lie in what Horton calls the closed and the open predicaments. Mystical thinking is closed; it cannot imagine any alternative, and its proponents do not permit thinking about alternatives. Failures of prediction are not taken as evidence of the incorrectness of the theory, but are used, as the Amhara use them, as occasions for producing more evidence so that the prediction may be improved. Western thought, on the other hand, Horton argues, is open; it is part of the scientific process of Western thought that disconfirming evidence should be constantly sought and admitted when found, so that fundamental propositions are open to alteration and disproof.

The existence of a theory, whether scientific or mystical, has implications for the division of labour. Where there is a highly elaborated system of thought, whether mystical or scientific, there are specialists who have the particular knowledge and the responsibility for purveying it. These specialists tend to claim esoteric knowledge, i.e. knowledge which is not available to the population at large. Young (1976a) explains that lay Amhara would not seek to question too deeply any apparent contradictions in the beliefs of that cosmology. It would be indiscreet; they might be thought to be seeking powers which would be dangerous and not appropriate for them to possess. As soon as theories develop which are specialized in this way, there is a gap between the specialist and the lay person. Furthermore, a power relation develops between them. The notions of power and powers are something to which we shall find ourselves constantly returning as the arguments of this book develop.

Horton makes too little (as Dingwall, 1976, has argued briefly) of the various ways in which Western scientific thought is less than open in practice. While Horton is correct to argue that the structure of Western science is by definition open, he underplays its closedness in relation to the bulk of the lay population. He recognizes that there is a difference in the Western world between scientists and lay people who have not been trained in scientific method and have not seen scientific proof. In the Middle Ages in Europe many Christian relics were sold. Among them were pieces which were said to have come from the cross upon which Jesus was nailed. It is now widely said that many of these relics were fakes, that there were many more pieces sold than could have come from the one cross. Yet the people believed, or so we think. In this context I have, since the first Moon landing, annually asked my students, 'What proof have you got that people have really landed on the Moon, one of the greatest scientific achievements of our age?' They have to admit that they cannot really prove that the whole space age programme is not a gigantic spoof set up in some television studio somewhere. Nor can they justify their belief that the Moon rock distributed to many laboratories really is Moon rock, or that TV transmissions come by satellite. They have no more scientific proof to hand than had those who believed in the veracity of the pieces of the cross. They do have circumstantial evidence, of course, but no real proof. In the end they trust the scientists. It becomes a matter of faith.

Horton's (1970) point about the style of theorizing is, however, well taken, and particularly his careful arguments about the nature of mystical theorizing. There is the difference that because of the openness of the scientific system a scientist if asked would feel that s/he had some responsibility to try to explain her/his procedures and to explain the methods of proof used. This, as we have seen, would not be the case with the Amhara. In their case power is felt to inhere in the knowledge itself. In the case of Western science, the power is not in the knowledge but in the manipulations which can flow from that knowledge. And in any case contemporary twentieth-century science requires large teams of people and apparatus, so that no one person could exercise the power. (This is a different point from what one person can do in activating the equipment once it has all been set up.)

Most people in the West nevertheless are in much the same position in relation to scientific knowledge as are the Amhara and other adherents of mystical systems. It is true that Western peoples want to know 'what is the matter', as do peoples elsewhere, in the sense of knowing how to put it right. Many lay Westerners are prepared 'to leave it to them that know' (see Williams, 1981a, 1981b and 1983) and have difficulty in understanding complex scientific explanations. Many also assume, as do believers in mystical systems, that to have knowledge is to have power, believing that 'if "they" only knew what was the matter, if "they" only knew what caused it', they, the professional healers, would then have the power to heal. Within the cosmology of Western science this does not follow. The differences between lay Westerners and lay Amhara in relation to healing knowledge and the related cosmology are also reduced when one considers presumptions that medicine is an 'art' which is based on esoteric knowledge learned as much from experience as from books, esoteric knowlege not generally available to the populace at large. These claims are added to the complexities and mysteries of modern science. Sections of the Western population ask questions in the scientists' terms and know how to ask them. Many do not. The questions many ask require empirical answers of a different order: the eyewitness account, the lesson from experience, an empiricism different from scientific proof.

There is a further point which Horton develops insufficiently; it is the conservatism which enters into the formal arrangements for the control and creation of scientific knowledge, the production of new scientists and the allocation of resources. There can be vested interests in the old ways which block the emergence of new ways of thinking, vested interests in the maintenance of existing ways of practice.

Such conservatism can of course occur only where, as well as a highly developed division of labour, there is also support for the status quo from other organized groups in the society. It is interesting and important to note how this division occurs and in what ways it relates to other aspects of the society. In many societies healing begins in the domestic domain, and much, possibly all, of it is confined to that domain. Depending on the healing arrangements of the society it may fan out from there to the public domain.

HEALING AND THE GENDER ORDER AMONG THE YORUBA

Una Maclean (1971 and 1976) has described for Nigeria how in the case of illness a Yoruba man may (1) request one of his wives to prepare herbs, (2) attend for consultation with a professional herbalist, or (3) consult a *babalawo* or diviner who will uncover why the patient is suffering in this way, focusing on the client's personal relationships and the details of his life. Both the herbalists and the diviners, who are usually men, have been carefully trained in their skills; they are specialists. The Yoruba skills relate not only to empirical knowledge of herbs but to a careful understanding of the elaborate Yoruba cosmology. It is an essential feature of Yoruba medical philosophy that witchcraft, the anger of the ancestors and the whims of capricious gods are the prime causes of personal disease and disaster.

Maclean is one of the few writers who has directly addressed the issue of the gender order with regard to the question of the sex of the sufferer and the healer (1969, 1971 and 1976). She points out that among the Yoruba the women have a fair measure of independence, are engaged in trading and are responsible for the maintenance of the children while they are young. In the division of labour in curative healing, however, the practice of medicine is traditionally a male concern, while the sale of materials for herbal or magical remedies is the responsibility of the market women. The society is male dominated, and even women's reproductive role is in some sense second-hand. Men desire to maintain the lineage, and sons are essential to carry on the spirit of the ancestors. Women are not full social beings in that they do not have ancestors but they are nevertheless keen to have children. Children will ensure the regard of their husbands and of others in society and also ensure a more enduring bond between husband and wife. Given a high infant death rate women are constantly worried about their reproductive capacity; no wife wishes to leave her husband's descent line to rival wives in a polygamous household. The advice she gets, however, will mostly be from men, whether she goes to the hospital (sometimes in defiance of the senior man of her people, who would previously have prescribed) or to the indigenous healers. Those healers will however rely upon the largely female herbalists for the preparation of potions and infusions.

Maclean's survey found no class of midwives among the Yoruba. We know that in many places childbirth is firmly in the domestic domain of the women. This is of course not to say that male members of the tribe are not involved and do not have some control of the proceedings even where birth itself is attended by women exclusively and where knowledge about pregnancy, parturition and child rearing is held by women and passed down the female line. In such societies men may wait outside the place of the women's labour to receive the news, and later the child, into their society.

In societies where there is a division between the domestic and public domains there are two issues involved; one is the location of healing, whether in the public or domestic domain; the second is the nature of the gender order, whether and in what way each domain is controlled by women or by men. In many societies healing takes place in the domestic domain, where it may be controlled by women, or by men who instruct the women, or it may be shared. Some studies which distinguish the location of healing do not report on the gender order.

KLEINMAN'S THREE ARENAS OF HEALING

Arthur Kleinman (1978, 1980 and 1986), for example, in presenting a theoretical model of medical systems as cultural systems which he hopes could be used cross-culturally, refers to what he calls three *sectors* or *arenas* in which healing takes place. These he calls the popular, the folk and the professional. He presents the relationship between these diagrammatically as shown in Figure 2.1.

The *popular arena* is the nearest to what I have referred to as the domestic domain; the 'popular arena comprises principally the family context of sickness and care, but also includes social network and community activities' (Kleinman,

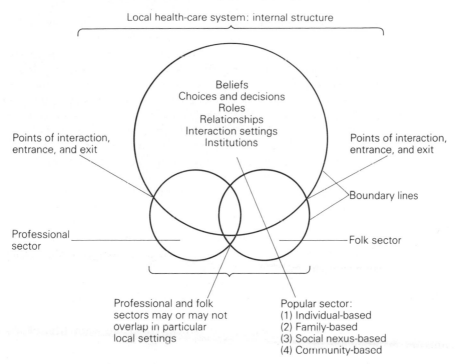

Local health-care system: internal structure

Beliefs
Choices and decisions
Roles
Relationships
Interaction settings
Institutions

Points of interaction,
entrance, and exit

Points of interaction,
entrance, and exit

Boundary lines

Professional
sector

Folk sector

Professional and folk
sectors may or may not
overlap in particular
local settings

Popular sector:
(1) Individual-based
(2) Family-based
(3) Social nexus-based
(4) Community-based

Source: Kleinman, 1980, p. 50.

Figure 2.1 *Health-care systems.*

1986, p. 33). In this domain, Kleinman argues, between 70 and 90 per cent of sickness is managed. By the *folk arena* Kleinman (1978 and 1986, p. 33) means the 'non-professional healing specialists'. In his view medical anthropologists have until recently underemphasized the popular arena at the expense of the folk arena. The first point is consistent with my complaint (see Chapter 1) that sociologists have underrated the importance of the role of the unpaid worker in industrialized market economies. The *professional arena* 'consists of professional scientific ("Western" or "cosmopolitan") medicine [biomedicine, in the terms used here] and professionalized indigenous healing traditions (e.g. Chinese, Ayurvedic, Yunani, and chiropractic)' (1978, pp. 86–7; 1986, pp. 32–3).

What Kleinman develops from this division is an attempt at a theoretical explanation of the relationships between these domains. His model presents difficulties. Although he argues that 'an autonomous anthropology of suffering and human services would offer distinct advantages not to be gained from a medical anthropology dominated by biomedical paradigms' (1978, p. 89; 1986, p. 40), there seems to me to be no doubt that Kleinman is really concerned only with the way in which knowledge so developed could increase the power of biomedical practice. Indeed, the summary of the values of his model (1978, p. 85; 1986, p. 30) makes this plain.

Ronald Frankenberg (Thomas, 1978, p. 95) in commenting on this paper argued, correctly to my mind, that any analysis of cultural systems must be located within a system of political economy. He argued that health systems can be understood only by characterizing the social formations in which they are embedded and that to do this the relations of production have to be analyzed. These relations, he argued, 'do not only include the production of goods and services, but they also include the production of health and disease and above all the production of knowledge' (p. 95). Elsewhere (1980) he argues that pluralism in healing practices occurs only in class-divided societies. Lewis points out that the Gnau do not have a stratified society; it is also the case that they do not have a division of labour in which there is any specialized medical service. One may see a connection here with the mode of production. Yet Lewis argues that he cannot find a causal connection clearly running from the form of their society to the form of their religion (1975, p. 350) and by implication to their religious beliefs, although he considers some of the detail of their mode of production.

While Frankenberg's points have value, Kleinman (1980) and Marriott (1955) are correct to draw attention to the domain issue. In many healing systems, it is not only family and friends but the whole village which is involved in the healing process. What Kleinman and Marriott miss, and what Frankenberg does not point out in his critique of Kleinman, is that the relations of *reproduction* are as important as the relations of production, and crucially important in health matters.

Kleinman stresses how the majority of work associated with health production, maintenance and restoration takes place in the domestic domain. In his study (1980) of illness and healing in that domain in Taiwan, he and his associate interviewed the women, that is, the mother and the grandmother of the household. As have so many before him when studying illness in the family, he took accounts about the whole family from the women (cf. Brown and Harris, 1978). However, no attention is paid to sex in any of the tables that follow. Nor does Kleinman ever discuss the implications of the sex of the healers. The assumption seems to be that healers are men. Careful inspection confirms this. We learn that Chinese-style doctors are mostly middle-aged men (p. 209) about half of whom have family members (both men and women) who are training, or have trained, as Western-style doctors. Ch'ien interpreters, who practise divination, are (p. 246) middle-aged or elderly men (although we learn that two-thirds of their patients are women). Some mention is made of 'special ritual practitioners' for children, who are 'usually old women in the neighbourhood' (p. 193). In the overview of the elaborate division of labour in health care which he describes in chapter 2, Kleinman does not refer to sex or gender at all. Nowhere is there any reference to what it may mean that most practitioners are male, while nine-tenths of healing takes place by his own reckoning in the domestic domain, where, as he says, male members do not know the range of healing activities in which the women (more culturally traditional) are involved (pp. 196–7).

THE GNAU GENDER ORDER

While, as was indicated earlier (page 19), Gilbert Lewis does not use the concept of the gender order in his analysis of the Gnau (1975 and 1980), he makes the division of the society into a male world and a female world abundantly clear. It also seems to me that some of his stresses reveal the socially inevitable bias of his informants and the information and interpretations he received to the male world and its members. Undifferentiated though the Gnau society was in many ways, Lewis (1980, p. 166) was able to identify some sort of public domain commanded by men, some collective areas over which men have authority, perhaps political. 'The men hold the public eye. They lead, the women follow' (1975, p. 346).

The women are the subject of bride-wealth. A woman leaves her natal home for the home of her husband; then part of the bride-wealth is paid by her husband to men of her family. But the marriage is not for real until the women have produced, and especially sons. Then more of the bride-wealth is paid over (1975, pp. 29–31). Lewis's view of the Gnau is of a geographically stable society in which people are and remain located in a particular village – except for some of the women. A woman's account would have been unlikely to give the impression of such stable location as Lewis recounts (cf. Sharma, 1980). But his ethnography is good, and we are given enough data to begin to grasp such differences. It becomes clear that the worth of women depends on their reproductive success, the production of boys being deemed more successful than that of girls, while the worth of men depends upon their hunting prowess and fighting achievements. Important though the reproductive abilities are, it is also made clear to the reader that the male achievements rank higher (1980, p. 158). The question of the kind of biological base to which people are relating also becomes clear in this analysis. Kalimao, for example, had given birth to two living children; she had had three others who had died in early infancy or just after birth: such are the personal meanings of a high infant mortality rate.

Gnau society is therefore less undifferentiated than one might at first assume and certainly more differentiated than a reading of Lewis (1976) without benefit of Lewis (1975) might lead one to expect. The Gnau are highly differentiated by gender, and the society is patrilocal and patriarchal. Theirs is a male-dominated gender order. The social order is closely associated with the biological differences between men and women but is socially elaborated in ways which by no stretch of the imagination could be said to be determined by those differences. It cannot, for example, determine why early in the morning the women and girls 'go to fetch water and walk with a smouldering lump of wood held close to their chest to warm them', while the men sit by the fire as they wait to eat (1975, p. 62). Nor does it explain certain differentiations in the illnesses which women and men experience.

Generally speaking women and men are liable to suffer from similar types and similar amounts of ailments, but women and children, especially female children, are liable to share illnesses caused by a different set of hazards from men and males in general. Women were particularly at risk from the spirits of their husbands' clan or lineage. Men were more ready to take what Lewis categorized as trivial illness more seriously than women, and he suspected that younger women made demonstrations of illness at times when their domestic duties were particularly heavy. He notes also that the condition *beng beng* is nowadays experienced only by women. Sufferers from *beng beng* exhibit frantic uneven breathing, while rapid cries seem to be jerked out of them. *Beng beng* is not itself an illness in Lewis's view. The condition has developed only since the 1950s, was apparently imported with the millenarian cargo cults (see Worsley,

1970, on cargo cults) and is said to be due to spirit possession. Occasionally after experiencing *beng beng* women would behave as if ill in the conventional withdrawn manner. They would be treated for illness, but *beng beng* itself was not thought of as an illness. Lewis does not explore in detail why this should be a particularly female behaviour, although he notes that at one time both men and women were involved in the cargo cult. Then men also exhibited the behaviour, and some men, but not women, were jailed for it by the Administration, which wished to eradicate the cargo cult. This hints at an underlying relationship whereby the male-dominated gender order of the Administration recognized the male-dominated gender order of the Gnau and acted accordingly. Did the prison experience 'cure' the men as a social category, leaving the women victims of *beng beng*? A more complex analysis of domains and the gender order would be needed to answer such a question.

Lewis provides the ethnographic data but not the conceptual framework within which we might begin to analyse these problems. Kleinman appears to be blind to the sex and gender implications of his otherwise perceptive domain analysis. Kleinman is not alone in this blindness. A special issue of *Social Science and Medicine* devoted to sex, culture and illness (1978) is entirely concerned with the way sex and gender affect the patient, and not at all with the way they affect the division of labour among the healers. This is a serious omission in an area where the public and domestic domains, the relations of production and reproduction, are both involved. These two are interconnected but semi-autonomous areas, both of which, and the relations between them, have to be understood if health beliefs and practices are to be satisfactorily analysed and explained. The importance of this and of the relations between the sexes delineated in the changing gender order as capitalist society develops will become abundantly clear as we trace the development of biomedicine in European history.

3 The Plurality of Healing Systems in Tudor and Stuart England

Steven Feierman (1979) has pointed out the similarities between Tudor and Stuart Britain and many parts of the twentieth-century Third World in terms of the variety of healers and healing knowledge available. This variety he refers to as a 'plural healing system', although to what extent these multifaceted arrangements amount to one 'system' is somewhat doubtful. He then presents the problem of how it should have come about that in less than three centuries from the end of that period biomedicine in Britain came to dominate over all other types of thought and practice about illness and healing. Biomedicine did not become the only healing system; many alternatives continued to exist (see Chapter 11); but biomedicine undoubtedly gained the most prestige, authority and economic power.

How this came about will be the subject of the rest of Part One of this book, for some historical understanding is necessary for a competent analysis of the late twentieth century. This historical approach should provide at the minimum a sense of perspective, but should also reveal some of the antecedents of contemporary beliefs and practices, alliances and conflicts. This chapter and those that follow do not pretend to be a full history; for that readers should turn to the works of medical and social historians, some of whom are cited in the chapters that follow. Rather, the aim is to illustrate the developments which have taken place.

THE SIZE AND STRUCTURE OF THE POPULATION

The scale of the Tudor and Stuart period was Lilliputian in comparison with the dense populations and large-scale organizations of the twentieth century. 'Few persons in the old world ever found themselves in groups larger than family groups, and there were few families of more than a dozen members' (Laslett, 1971, p. 7). Furthermore great assemblies were small by our standards. 'The largest crowd recorded for seventeenth century England, that is the Parliamentary Army which fought at Marston Moor [1644], would have gone three, four or even five times into the sporting stadium of today' (1971, p. 10).

Most common people passed most of their life in what I have called the domestic domain; that was where production and reproduction both took place. But there was already a public domain which was the domain of the men. The Christian church had long existed as a large-scale organization and, apart from the great and powerful abbeys (Clark, 1968), was run by men. The central state – that is, parliament, the judiciary, the military – was a crucial part of that male public domain, which also contained the schools and the two ancient universities. In the cities already by the sixteenth century municipal government was well developed and was controlled by local powerful men. The market-place was different; women went there to trade produce as well as to purchase. Otherwise in any large public congresses if women were present at all it was as spectators.

The domestic domain was organized around the patriarchal family, using that word in its technical sense to mean a domestic group in which the husband-father had power and authority. The family was not only patriarchal, it was also patrilineal; name and property passed down the male line. 'In general, families in early modern England were rather more nuclear than extended; large numbers of children were unusual; and marriage after the age of twenty was the rule, even among the aristocracy, and took place comparatively late in life, given ... the shorter life expectancy' (Pelling, 1985a, p. 78). Some households included relatives other than the children of the couple, as well as paid servants and apprentices. These last stood to the head of the family and his wife in a relationship similar to that of their sons and daughters.

THE GENDER ORDER, THE PUBLIC DOMAIN AND THE CLASS SYSTEM

There was a clear sex segregation of tasks and roles. Women ran the household, prepared meals, made butter, cheese, beer and bread, looked after the cattle and took the fruit to market. The men did the ploughing, hedging, carting and the heavy work of the harvest. These were skilled, if laborious, tasks for both men and women, essential parts of both production and reproduction. Women's position, while not without power and influence (cf. Stacey and Price, 1981), was legally inferior and subservient. In legal terms, they were non-persons; they along with the children and the servants were subsumed into their fathers, husbands, masters.

From this order of generation, gender and status the public domain derived. It was the domination of men in the familial order which led to their commanding position in the wider world, in church and state, positions denied to all others. The majority of people, about 94 per cent in 1500 and 80 per cent in 1700, lived in the rural areas (Pelling, 1987, p. 108). Although many no doubt passed their life in their own parish and the area around it, there were increasing indications of mobility during the Elizabethan period (1558–1603) and thereafter. The numbers of people living in a village were not large, perhaps not more than two hundred and possibly only twenty or thirty (Laslett, 1971, p. 56, discussing late Stuart times). Even cities and towns were small by our standards. London, then the fourth largest city in Europe, had perhaps 200,000 people in 1600 (Pelling and Webster, 1979, p. 188); while Norwich, the second largest city in England, had about 17,000 in 1575 (Pelling and Webster, 1979, p. 226).

The people's life, in contrast to that of the gentry, was one of considerable privation. Only a small part of the population were members of the gentry and aristocracy, perhaps 4 or 5 per cent (Laslett, 1971). These were the only people for whom the nation was a meaningful concept in terms of social interaction. The men from this small section of the population in a sense constituted the national public domain, owning most of the power and the wealth and never doing manual work. Looked at in this way one might say that the common people, like the women of the aristocracy and the gentry, were confined to the domestic domain. But upper-class women might have considerable managerial powers there, especially in the absence of their husbands. In the towns, freemen had established their own governments, and there were numerous self-governing guilds which included women as well as men. People of both sexes were expected to work, and many were engaged in highly skilled occupations. There were numerous signs of change in the class order; rising professional groups, lawyers, clergymen, merchants and officials were beginning to present a challenge to the older orders (Thomas, 1971).

HEALTH, ILL HEALTH AND LONGEVITY

By our standards one might say that life was nasty, brutish and short for the people of Tudor and Stuart England, and in Keith Thomas's view (1971, p. 4) they were exceedingly liable to pain, sickness and premature death. Estimates of the expectation of life vary; one (Thomas, 1980, p. 6) is that in 1650–75 the expectation of life among *noble* boys was only 29.6 years, a third dying before they were 5. Thomas (1980, p. 6) also quotes John Graunt's estimate for 1662 that of every 100 live children born in London 36 died in their first six years and a further 24 in the following ten years; thus only 40 per cent survived beyond the age of 10 (see also Forbes, 1979, p. 10). However, as Margaret Pelling (1985a, p. 78) points out, a person in Shakespeare's England 'surviving to the age of thirty could expect to live another thirty years'. Schofield and Wrigley, whose evidence comes chiefly from rural parishes, have estimated that the expectation of life in Tudor and Stuart England was thirty to forty years – an unusually high level by the general standard of early modern Europe (1981, p. 95). Roger Finlay (1981, tables 5.15, 5.16 and 6.3) has calculated life expectancies of both sexes combined for various parishes in London (a somewhat unique city in terms of its size, growth and health problems) in the period 1580–1653 as ranging from 21 years to 34.6. Ronald Sawyer (1983), having examined the extensive records between 1601 and 1612 of Richard Napier, a licensed doctor and rector of Great Linford in Buckinghamshire, reminds us that not all were destined to live short and unpleasant lives, notwithstanding a good deal of accident, ill health and suffering. Nevertheless the best of the estimates indicate a short life compared with an expectation of more like seventy years nowadays. Compared with the 1980s the 'Elizabethan period was dominated by young people: over half the population was under twenty-five' (Pelling, 1985a, p. 78).

Webster (1982c, p. 115) reminds us that mortality rates do not of themselves tell much about the healthiness of the population. It is possible for the infant death rate to improve while the general health of the population is worsening. While historians have paid attention to the professionals, this has been at the expense of attention to the health of the people. We are still a long way from understanding with any precision the health of the people in Shakespeare's England, but 'the experience of ill-health was an important factor in the situation ... bodies were wracked by pain deriving from stone, hernia, gout and syphilis' (Webster, 1982c, pp. 115–16; see also Pelling, 1986, for an account of the health of the people of London in the Tudor and Stuart period).

Attention to the dramatic events of epidemic diseases such as influenza, typhus and smallpox as well as plague (Thomas, 1971, pp. 8–9), important though these were, has also, according to Pelling (1985a, p. 79), distracted from the endemic or chronic diseases, which affected the way people thought about their daily lives. Epidemic and endemic diseases should, however, not be too sharply distinguished; for the bubonic plague, cause of the Black Death when it first appeared in England in 1348–9, had been endemic for three centuries, finally to die out only after the epidemics of the mid-1660s. (For a comprehensive account of the impact of the plague in Tudor and Stuart times, see Slack, 1985; and for its effects specifically on London, see Slack, 1986.)

Although relatively rare, 'famine was a real cause of death, particularly in the disastrous years 1596–98' and is sporadically recorded in parish registers in the sixteenth century (Pelling, 1985a, p. 78). Undernourishment was more common. These conditions varied from time to time and parish to parish. Blight in the crops and disease among cattle were ever-present hazards. To some extent there may have been connections between such natural disasters and epidemics, but Paul Slack (1979, 1985, pp. 73–6) argues that a variety of influences in living conditions were at work. Of other misfortunes which befell, fire in the town was perhaps the most disastrous (Thomas, 1971, pp. 17–20).

A 'Census of the Poor', which was carried out by the municipal authorities in Norwich in 1570, provides a unique opportunity to gain a better idea of the health of the period and has been analysed by Pelling (1985b, pp. 119–20). About a quarter of the native-born population was described as poor. 'About nine per cent of the adult poor (that is, over the age of sixteen) were described at that time as being in some way sick or disabled, although many did some work nonetheless. A further 1½ percent ... all ... aged, were described as past work.' The sick poor were 'sick, sickly, or very sick ... weak, diseased, bedridden, lame, crooked, or suffering from stone, gout, dumbness, deafness, broken legs, diseases of the mouth, broken ribs, thigfola (?fistula [a type of ulcer]), or were one-legged or one-handed.' The pox, lunacy and blindness were also reported (p. 120).

THE WORLD OF SUPERNATURAL POWER

Overlapping with the ordinary physical world was a sphere inhabited by strange, evil creatures, half-animal, half-demon. A world full of 'power', both good and evil. This cannot be dismissed as a delusion or fantasy of a minority; it appears to have been fully credible to all the villagers and to the presiding magistrates [at the witch trials of 1566 and 1579], who included the Queen's Attorney, Sir John Fortescue (later Chancellor of the Exchequer) and Thomas Cole, Archdeacon of Essex.

(Macfarlane, 1970, p. 96)

The familiar of the witch Agnes Waterhouse was said, at one of the Essex witch trials from which this evidence comes, to have appeared to a girl while she was churning butter. This apparition had a face like an ape, a chain and silver whistle about his neck and a pair of horns on his head and was carrying the key of the milkhouse door in his mouth.

Nor was this a matter only of pagan belief. The church also recognized 'powers'. Indeed, the medieval church was involved in healing which one can describe only as magical in so far as saints, shrines and images were thought themselves to have healing properties (Thomas, 1971, ch. 2). The church recognized, although it did not approve of, the powers which some women and men had for good or ill. The church saw this world and the next in terms of a struggle between the forces of God and the Devil, between good and evil.

. The church was bitterly opposed to those who exercised 'powers' other than those it had itself bestowed. Witch-hunts were mounted throughout this period. But it seems that most blessers, witches, wise women and men applied their nostrums or their incantations invoking God – as, for example, those who healed by touch: 'God bless; I touch; God heals' (Thomas, 1971, p. 238). In many cases healers advocated, as did Margaret Hunt in the 1520s, that their patients should recite Paternosters, Ave Marias and Creeds each in ritually defined numbers and repetitiously (Thomas, 1971, p. 211).

The belief in supernatural powers was shared by the highest and the lowest in the land; it took a variety of forms. As we have seen for other non-industrial societies there was a contradictory array of beliefs. The 'powers' could cause material and spiritual disaster as well as ill health and death. As among other peoples we have looked at, there was not a sharp distinction between the causes and cures for physical illness and those for more general disasters.

THEORIES AND BELIEFS ABOUT HEALTH AND ILL HEALTH

According to Pelling (1982, p. 485; 1985a, p. 79) the high incidence of serious disease did not mean that people were worried only about the life-threatening conditions. The evidence is that they were constantly concerned with their health, watching small signs for possible future degeneration, fearing threats to their senses, suffering disability deriving from childbirth and seeking to relieve pain in backache, headache and toothache. Particular attention was paid to the excretions and to the appearance of the skin, not only the consequences of disfiguring diseases but also boils and pimples. Mental suffering was also a major preoccupation. As Pelling says (1985a, p. 80), these circumstances must have created a high demand for medical attention.

The causes of illness and disaster and the methods of healing and restoration of order ranged widely. The ordinary folk believed in empirical causes and cures and had considerable knowledge of herbs; some had skills in bone setting and other specialisations, and experimented with new ideas or treatments, as well as believing in powers for evil or for good, which could make ill or cure. The physicians, whose education was highly abstract, also had a range of explanatory theories. The theories of the Greek physician Galen were currently undergoing a great revival, especially in the Italian universities as one aspect of the recovery by humanists of ancient texts in the original. Galenic medicine was based on a theory of 'humours' which involved notions of balance, especially between hot and cold and wet and dry. The moods and temperaments of the patient were involved with the humours and the balance which had to be achieved and sustained.

Alchemical medicine continued to be strong and important. It had a considerable grip in the sixteenth century. Roger Bacon was the major authority, and alchemy was an entrenched interest in court circles. As Charles Webster comments (1979, p. 309), the extent of the general diffusion of ideas about magic and alchemy can be gauged by the number of sixteenth- and seventeenth-century plays on the subject, such as Marlowe's *Dr Faustus*, Greene's *Friar Bacon and Friar Bungay*, Lyly's *Gallathea* and Jonson's *Alchemist*.

Alchemy, which was associated with the mythological tradition of ancient Greece and Arabia (Sheppard, 1972; Webster, 1979), received an impetus in the sixteenth century that continued until the end of the seventeenth. Alchemy fitted well with ideas rife at the time of the Reformation; it played a unifying role, its various branches drew upon the skills of linguists, scholars, mathematicians and natural philosophers. The College of Physicians of London, entrenched in the Galenic tradition, was threatened by these alchemical ideas and therefore attacked their protagonists (Webster, 1979, pp. 313–14).

Official medicine had been challenged on the Continent in the sixteenth century by Paracelsus (the Latin name for Dr Theophratus Bombastus ab Hohenheim), who substituted a functional conception of physiology, the living organism, for the ancient anatomy of 'humours' and 'qualities' (Guthrie, 1960, p. 156–61). Paracelsus was an outcast of the medical school. Many legends grew up around him, and a following developed throughout Europe in the later sixteenth and seventeenth centuries. Paracelsus believed in the light of nature which was God-given and stressed experience and experiment in the practitioner's method. He developed the idea of the 'ens' (which in his view was linked with the stars); from this the entity theory of diseases later developed. In the theory of ens the label rather than the patient becomes the object of treatment, because the disease rather than its origin becomes an independent entity. The importance of the transformation of notions about disease will become apparent in Chapter 4.

Paracelsus also made contributions which were important in the development of pharmacology. He learned a great deal from indigenous traditions and cunning folk about the properties of herbal medicine, and he replaced the traditional pharmacopoeia with what he had learned.

The lively English tradition of alchemy provided fertile ground for Paracelsianism and for the development of chemical therapy (Webster, 1979, pp. 313–16). From 1640 Paracelsus became a dominant influence in English medicine. His ideas had been largely assimilated by 1600 although in 1560, nearly twenty years after his death, they had been unknown in England (Webster, 1979, p. 323 and 1982b). His work had a particular appeal to the lower ranks of the medical profession for it refined and revitalized their own ideas and practices (Weber, 1979, p. 327). It furthermore fitted well with the notions of the Protestant Reformation and became entrenched in all European Protestant countries. Allen Debus (1972) has drawn attention to the compromise which began to develop between the Galenists and the Paracelsians as evidenced in the Pharmacopoeia of 1618 issued by the College of Physicians, albeit to try to retain some grip upon the apothecaries (Pelling and Webster, 1979).

However, strange it may seem to us, many of the tools of rational science were developed in association with ideas which we would call mystical. The importance of alchemy to the development of chemotherapy has already been mentioned. The association of the advance of mathematics with astrology or what we might think of as fortune-telling is equally striking in its apparent (to our eyes) contradiction (Keller, 1972).

This glimpse at the links between what we would see as magical or mystical

ideas and the development of empirically based science may help us to
understand how it was that the systems of knowledge of the common people and
of the *cognoscenti* were not mutually exclusive as we might expect them to be if
we made a judgement simply from our own position of knowledge (Pelling and
Webster, 1979). The ideas which were put together in theory were also tried out
together in practice.

THE DIVISION OF LABOUR IN HEALTH CARE

Given the plurality of healing systems, the wide range of beliefs and practices and
the high demand for health care, how did people choose, and who chose what?

The choice available was wider in the towns than in the countryside. There
people had to rely more upon folk healers, although there were barber-surgeons
in a number of villages. There was more choice in the towns, especially for those
who could pay more although according to Pelling (1987, pp. 106–9) this was
not the only governing factor, since fees varied, payment in kind was possible,
some practitioners treated some cases free, and even the less well off were
prepared to pay if they thought it worthwhile. While the élite physicians could
be afforded only by the upper class, it seems to have been the case that they, as
well as the common people, consulted the cunning folk and various other healers
as well as consulting physicians.

The Importance of Domestic-Domain Healing and of Women Healers
There is no doubt that the greatest amount of health maintenance and health
restoration went on in the home. Alice Clark (1968, pp. 254–8) has drawn
together records from great houses, books of advice and memoirs which make
this clear. The women learned from their mothers, as had their mothers before
them. As she points out, humbler housewives had much similar knowledge and
skills, although it is true that upper-class housewives took it as part of their
responsibilities to minister to their poorer neighbours as well as to their own
household.

It seems likely that, in addition to using their empirical knowledge, ritual
healing in which prayers, charms, or spells accompanied the medicine was also
sometimes administered in the patient's family (Pelling, 1987, p. 109; Thomas,
1971, p. 210). Nor would this have necessarily been confined to the common
people.

Folk Medicine in the Health Division of Labour
When the skills of the household were exhausted there were a variety of healers
to whom recourse might be had, diviners, wise women and cunning folk, who
continued to be important for the majority who lived in the country. These wise
people would also help in time of misfortune. As among the Amhara, upon
whom Young reports (see Chapter 2), folk healers were generally indistinguishable from other people. They were housewives, weavers, carpenters, ordinary
folk. They had knowledge or powers which they used when they were applied
to for help, but there was some specialization.

During the sixteenth and seventeenth centuries these popular magicians went
under a variety of names – 'cunning men', 'wise women', 'charmers',

'blessers', 'conjurors', 'sorcerers', 'witches' – they offered a variety of services, which ranged from healing the sick and finding lost goods to fortune telling and divination of all kinds.

(Thomas, 1971, p. 210)

The terms Thomas points to are the same as those used to describe the three 'Wise Men' or Magi from the East. These people purveyed the traditional folk medicine upon which the majority of Tudor and Stuart people depended. It was a mixture of accumulated experience based on nursing and midwifery combined with inherited lore about the healing properties of plants and minerals, but including ritual healing.

The Gender Order among the Folk Healers

Was there any clear gender order among the folk healers? The evidence is scanty because too few people have paid attention to this aspect. It is to overstate the case to imagine, as Barbara Ehrenreich and Deidre English (1974b and 1979) do, that all witches were healers who were women (cf. Versluysen, 1980). It is even more inaccurate to refer to all folk healers as 'cunning men' as Thomas tends to do in his study of magical healing. Having used the generic male term, he then frequently illustrates his point from examples of wise women.

It is not clear whether there was a gender distinction between diviners (who found out the matter) and healers (who attempted to put it right). No such distinction appears to be reported. In Tudor and Stuart England both women and men are reported as empirics, using herbs and potions. When some healers were brought to trial they defended themselves by saying that they had not used 'powers' at all, they had simply used their empirical knowledge of healing, applying herbs and the like (Thomas, 1971, pp. 226–7).

There were certainly good reports of some of the women healers. Clark quotes authorities which suggest that within the knowledge of the period the healing these women undertook was competent. When Adam Martindale was very ill he failed to get help from various learned men who were consulted:

> in this great straite God sent us in much mercie a poore woman, who by a salve made of nothing but Celandine and a little of the Mosse of an ashe root, shred and boyled in May-butter, tooke it clear away in a short time, and though after a space there was some new breakings out, yet these being annointed with the same salve … were absolutely cleared away.
> (Life of Adam Martindale, 1632, p. 21, quoted in Clarke, 1968, pp. 257–8)

The Array of Practitioners of Medicine

'Medicine' is here used, following Pelling and Webster (1979), to relate to the healing skills exercised by a wide array of practitioners. The line between a folk healer and other medical practitioners was probably not as clear as we in the twentieth century might expect, since knowledge from various sources was combined in practice.

At one time historians made a rather clear distinction between qualified and unqualified practitioners, the latter being referred to as 'quacks'. It was also assumed that the qualified healers were divided into the three categories: physicians, apothecaries and barber-surgeons. The extent to which that three-fold continental division really applied to Britain has now been called into question. R. S. Roberts (1962 and 1964) has noted that the 'greater part of general medical practice lay in the hands of wise country people who were sound empirical practitioners protected by the Act of 1542', sometimes inaccurately referred to as 'the Quacks' Charter' (1962, pp. 363 and 377). He has also shown that the official records, such as Raach (1962) drew together in his *Directory of English Country Physicians*, may have concealed more than they revealed. Not only were some of the university-qualified physicians listed merely retired to the country and not in practice there, but those who were in practice, although they may have been licensed as physicians or surgeons, did not practise in that manner. There was already, Roberts argues, a category of general medical practitioner, who may or may not have had formal training and who practised in part or all of the three activities of apothecary, surgeon and physician – albeit 'general practitioner' may not have become a formal title until the nineteenth century (Peterson, 1978). In the country, physicians and surgeons were licensed by the bishops. In London, Henry VIII incorporated the physicians into the College of Physicians and the barber-surgeons and surgeons into a company, for the health problems of London were recognized as special (Roberts, 1964, p. 217). However, here too apart from during a short period the exclusive appellation of physician, surgeon, or apothecary bore little relationship to the reality of practice.

Later writers have taken these arguments further. In order not to be misled by the appearance of titles and licences, when Pelling and Webster studied medical practitioners of the sixteenth century they included, entirely correctly to my mind, 'any individual whose occupation is basically concerned with the care of the sick' (1979, p. 166). They anticipated criticism for including the empiric (a person who treated symptoms without formal qualifications or theoretical justification) along with the 'professional'. They correctly justify themselves by saying that previous studies have excluded the most numerous practitioners. This variety is also attested to by Lucinda Beier (1981). The host of healers of all kinds is made plain by Margaret Pelling's study of Norwich (1978a; Pelling and Webster, 1979). She looked at medical practice between 1550 and 1640 and chose Norwich because it was likely to give the most substantial picture of provincial practice, it being a major urban centre of the period, with a population maximum during that time of 17,000 and experiencing massive fluctuations because of migration and the plague.

Pelling (1978a, p. 30) tells us that

the provisional total of Norwich practitioners 1550–1640 is 174, comprising: 22 doctors of medicine, medical licentiates, or practitioners of physic; 46 members of the Norwich Barber Surgeons' Company; 34 other surgeons and barber surgeons, some of them also members of the Company; 36 apothecaries; 13 women practitioners including midwives; 14 stranger practitioners (of all types); 5 itinerants; one 'astrologer, glover and empiric'; and 3 bone setters all of whom were employed by the city authorities.

In a later work (Pelling, 1982), she indicates two groups of practitioners excluding midwives: Group A, active in Norwich between 1550 and 1640 who bore some part in the formalities and responsibilities of the city and the barber-surgeons' company; and Group B, of practitioners in many ways similar but not so involved. Group A, of about 150 practitioners, included physicians, surgeons, barber-surgeons, lithotomists (i.e. those who cut to extract stones), bonesetters 'and many to whom it would be difficult to give a single occupational designation' (p. 507). Group B, approximately 120 practitioners, differed from Group A principally in that it included two important minorities 'regularly missed from formal records used for occupational analyses, women and strangers' (p. 508). In addition to these two groups there were the apothecaries, about forty in number.

'Sixteenth-century Norwich was ruled by an independent and durable oligarchic structure in which craft and trade organisations had constant reference to the mayor and alderman' (Pelling and Webster, 1979, p. 208). This group constituted the public domain in my terms. One could argue that Group A practitioners were in, or closely associated with, this public domain of political power, while Group B were not. They may have practised in an essentially similar way; they included some of the better-known physicians; some of the 120 might later qualify for office perhaps, but it is unlikely that at that time the women would.

How the Practitioners Were Used

Pelling (1982; see also Pelling and Webster, 1979) calculates a ratio of about 1:200 practitioners to the Norwich population. Who went to them and how were they employed? There were two principal modes: consultation by private individuals on behalf of themselves or others and employment by the city authorities on behalf of the sick poor.

So far as the private consultations are concerned, the high level of concern about their health demonstrated by the first Elizabethans has already been remarked (page 37). Pelling (1985a) tells us further that 'all the evidence suggests that the "patient" in the early modern period was extremely "active", being critical, sceptical and well-informed'. These well-informed lay people, when sick,

> chose freely among the range of practitioners according to their own and their friends' judgment of the nature and seriousness of their condition ... It is also possible to argue that the relations between doctor and patient were more evenly balanced than is the case today. Patients bargained with practitioners as in a commercial transaction and settled on an agreed product or 'cure'.
>
> (Pelling, 1985a, p. 80)

Among the variety, the most numerous single category was the barbers and barber-surgeons, who were organized into the only isolable medical institution, the Norwich Barber-Surgeons' Company (Pelling and Webster, 1979). They offered their medical services through their barber shops, which were associated with their dwellings and where they offered other goods and services besides barbering and medicine. Many other trades were commonly connected with

barbering; Pelling (1982, pp. 504–5) records that those most commonly associated were wax and tallow chandling, music, malting, brewing and the retailing of
drink. In her account of the barber-surgeons of London in Tudor and Stuart
times, Pelling (1986) plots the distribution of freeman barber-surgeons and
shows their connection with areas of fashion, entertainment and ill repute
(p. 85); their shops were outlets of news, printed and verbal (p. 86). Their work
was closely connected with ameliorating or disguising the effects of disease and
deformity; clothing, cosmetics and wigs were all deployed, the last two by the
barber-surgeons who also treated the pox (syphilis – a major disfigurer) with
mercury.

Medical consultations took place openly and possibly by proxy in the barber's
shop. In this sense it was a public affair; there was nothing confidential in the
consultation. Pelling (1982, p. 506) argues that 'the insistence of later medical
men, especially physicians, on the decorum and exclusiveness of the doctor–
patient relation can be seen as a means of dissociation from the older craft
origins'. The friends who were present at these transactions were later found as
parties to legal proceedings when patients were alleging that a contract had failed
(Pelling, 1982, p. 506). These consultations, taking place among friends and
family, are reminiscent of the more public consultations reported in many of the
anthropological studies discussed in Chapter 2 and are analogous to those of
Marriot's (1955) third realm of village and caste. The contrast with present-day
consultations is similar to that between traditional Chinese and Western-style
doctors in Northern Taiwan (Ahern, 1987).

HEALTH CARE FOR THE POOR

The well-organized city authorities in Norwich recognized the social importance of illness and made arrangements not only for prevention but also for the
care of the sick (Pelling, 1985b). Norwich had introduced a compulsory poor
rate as early as 1549, but its provisions for medical care were independent of this
and lasted into the eighteenth century (p. 117). The numbers of sick poor have
already been referred to (page 36). From the 1570s, when the census had been
taken, the city provided that the proctors or keepers of the city's lazar-houses
(from Lazarus, the leper) should receive the diseased, including the leprous, and
that poor women should take them into their homes. Also from this time the city
employed healers for the poor. At least an eighth of the Norwich practitioners
discussed above were employed in this way, the city choosing representatives of
the full range of practitioners available and roughly in the proportions that they
existed in the city. Over a third were women, including a surgeon and other
healers; the men, the remaining two-thirds, included barber-surgeons, surgeons,
bone setters, some apothecaries and physician-surgeons 'and recruits to medicine from other trades' (pp. 121–2).

Payment was by contract, as it was for individual treatments. Conditional
contracts were the most usual whereby the practitioner was paid something on
account and the remainder when the contract was fulfilled. This encouraged
practitioners not to take on cases they could not cure and also to attend to their
failures. Cases against practitioners taken to law fitted more readily 'into the
framework of breakdown of agreed contracts than into the modern category of
malpractice suits' (Pelling, 1985b, pp. 122–3). Lazar-house keepers also accepted

as part of the bargain they struck with the city a responsibility for the future maintenance of a poor person if they could not effect a cure. They took these possibilities into account in striking the bargain (p. 129).

Undoubtedly the Norwich city authorities were concerned with the public good in their provisions: to reduce the costs imposed by the sick poor who by treatment might be returned to work, including attempts to cope with intractable conditions such as blindness; to reduce the dangers of infection, especially the serious consequences of syphilis, the 'French pox', in the late sixteenth and early seventeenth centuries and the great plague epidemics between 1580 and 1625. The city did not employ town physicians or medical officials on the continental model but made *ad hoc* arrangements with 'general medical practitioners' and flexible contracts with lazar-house keepers (Pelling, 1985b, pp. 135–6). There was active municipal involvement nevertheless, which endured through the dissolution years in the second half of the 1530s and on through the civil wars, the Commonwealth and the Restoration.

SURGEONS, BARBER-SURGEONS AND PHYSICIANS

In Norwich as in London and doubtless most other centres, academically qualified physicians were relatively unimportant; many licensed physicians were unqualified, and practice was dominated by the more numerous surgeons and barber-surgeons. In any case the 'licensed had no monopoly of skill or virtue' (Pelling and Webster, 1979, p. 216). By the end of the sixteenth century the élite of the London Barber-Surgeons' Company were 'making a more active and original contribution to medicine than their colleagues in the College of Physicians' (Pelling and Webster, 1979, p. 177). The surgeons were craftsmen who learned by apprenticeship: cutting and manipulation, bone setting, skilled manual labour applied to the human body. Surgeons had been organized into guilds since the Middle Ages. In 1520 they joined with the more numerous barbers to form the Barber-Surgeons' Company of London.

In the sixteenth century academic training was reserved for a small minority. This does not mean that the majority were ignorant. Most learning was through apprenticeships; knowledge was passed by word of mouth, and practice was learned from observation. This applied largely to healers of all sorts in public and domestic domains. Following the communication revolution caused by the invention of the printing press, there were a number of popular books describing the various forms of healing. These seem to have been read not only by the practitioners but also by educated laymen (Pelling, 1985a; Slack, 1979; Webster, 1975).

The élite however received academic education at Oxford or Cambridge or on the Continent. Among medical practitioners this élite group was organized in the College of Physicians, established in 1518. The College's charter gave it a monopoly to practise 'physic' in London and to license physicians to practise in other parts of the country. We may most easily think of 'physic' as internal medicine. Physicians examined, diagnosed and prescribed. Fellows of the College could not dispense drugs. Their prescriptions were made up by apothecaries or druggists. The College was a small body; for the late sixteenth century Pelling and Webster (1979, p. 188) estimate that there were between thirty and fifty members. Furthermore its pretensions to control medicine outweighed its effectiveness. It was unable to control the large numbers of unlicensed practitioners in London. In addition, there were a miscellany of licensing authorities in the country as a whole, including the universities and the ecclesiastical authorities.

THE APOTHECARIES

The apothecaries were among the groups of healers that the College could not restrain from practice. They were tradesmen who from the fourteenth century were in London part of the Grocers' Company or Guild, one of the medieval guilds into which merchants and tradespeople were organized. In 1617 the apothecaries were granted independence from the grocers, and the Society of Apothecaries was incorporated, thus establishing a distinct occupation. They were allowed to manufacture, sell, or apply drugs and medicines, but grocers were not. Among the trades apothecaries ranked above barber-surgeons.

Although it was not the apothecaries' task to diagnose and prescribe, they sometimes took on this role. Physicians treated the upper class; middle- and lower-class patients increasingly came to apothecaries for treatment. During the great plague of 1665–6 when the upper classes fled from the capital to the country the physicians went with them. The apothecaries continued to be available to give medical aid to the populace, which, as Carol Kronus (1976) points out, reinforced the legitimacy of their claim to be giving a public service. From the time of the plague onwards the apothecaries flourished and increasingly offended the physicians by treating patients and growing wealthy on the sale of drugs in addition. At the beginning of the eighteenth century (1703) the (now) Royal College of Physicians eventually lost a lawsuit to restrain the apothecaries from practising, when the House of Lords gave the apothecaries the legal right to practise. They could now all legally do what many had been doing for many years.

In this way the healing occupations began to be more formally sorted out, although never so precisely in practice as the formal organization might lead one to expect. Thus, for example, George Birch of Norwich (died 1632), a man of high civic status, was grocer, apothecary and alderman, treated one particular household but also 'ministered physic and surgery' to the poor as an employee of the city (Pelling and Webster, 1979, p. 221).

CONCLUSION

So far as social class is concerned, in terms of its origins, the College of Physicians of London is the only group one could say was clearly associated with the upper class. The fellows were a very small élite group, rarely more than fifteen before 1575 (Pelling and Webster, 1979, p. 169). Some gentlemen graduates of Oxford lived in the country but not necessarily practising there. Members of the upper class sought treatment from qualified and licensed physicians and might have them, or others, attached to their household to be available as needed. The upper classes might also consult other healers who they learned had a good reputation for dealing with the kind of illness which was assailing them.

In London physicians licensed by the College ranked highest in prestige, but there were others who practised without a licence. In the provinces physicians were not identifiable as an organized group and might be found in the barber-surgeons' company or with the apothecaries. These arrangements were found in London also. The apothecaries had greater prestige and wealth than the barbers and barber-surgeons, who were the most numerous.

The sick among the common people, apart from the poor who had provisions made for them in cities like Norwich, 'shopped around' on the basis of their knowledge of healers and their healing practices – restrained, but not entirely so, by what they could afford. These constraints were tempered by the use of payment in kind, variable fees and the occasional offer of free treatment, such arrangements applying to wise men and women as well as to other practitioners (Thomas, 1971).

So far as the domain of healing is concerned, most took place in the domestic domain: some in the homes of the healers, again including wise women and cunning men as well as apothecaries, barbers and surgeons. Some took place in the shops of tradesmen who practised medicine, a relatively public place but usually attached to the practitioner's domicile. Some healers purveyed their wares from market stalls (some were genuine, some mountebanks). Some patients were admitted for healing to the homes of poor women or to modest institutions such as the Norwich lazar-house represented. Only the market stalls and the lazar-houses could be said to be in the public domain.

All categories of healers included women, except for the London College of Physicians, which had excluded them from the outset. Women seem to have constituted, in Norwich at least, about a third of the healers who were paid for their work and were almost certainly the majority of all those who cared for the sick when one includes housewives. From the Norman conquest women had been licensed to practise. The bishops were particularly concerned to license and control the midwives, because of the importance of controlling new life and admitting members to the church. It is said that in the fourteenth century Cecilia of Oxford was appointed Court Surgeon, and some women apparently were members of surgeon's guilds as, for example, of the Norwich Barber-Surgeons' Company. The same was true of the apothecaries. Women were permitted in trade in the Middle Ages, and this continued – although it is unclear, as Pelling and Webster (1979, p. 222) point out, whether by the sixteenth century women could take out freedoms, run businesses and indenture apprentices in their own right rather than in that of a deceased husband. It does seem also likely that the *feme sole* (i.e. a woman living on her own) had some capabilities in her own right that neither the married woman nor she who was still under the authority of her father had. Until the seventeenth century helping women in childbirth was exclusively women's work. How male surgeons began to invade this territory will be reviewed in Chapter 4. Women, however, were not involved extensively, if at all, in the administration of the municipalities, the guilds and companies, and not at all in the London College of Physicians, which was firmly placed in the male public domain.

Healing it seems in the sixteenth and seventeenth centuries was still primarily a domestic-domain activity; even healing as a trade was not far from the domestic domain. At the same time public authorities – municipalities like Norwich and the civic authorities in London – were concerned about and involved with health matters, preventive and curative. The great Elizabeth and the short-reigning Mary apart, members of those authorities were all public-domain men.

4 Eighteenth-Century Foundations for the Development of Biomedicine

In Chapter 3 we saw how many different healing systems there were in sixteenth- and seventeenth-century England. Within the ancient and sometimes magical or metaphysical ideas the beginnings of great changes could be discerned, although it was to be nearly a century before biomedicine began to develop towards its present form and another century and a half before it came to have powerful tools at its command (Macfarlane, 1970; McKeown, 1971). This chapter will try to describe and analyse some of the changes which took place in the eighteenth century, which laid the bases from which biomedicine developed, led to its domination over all alternative healing systems and established a division of health labour which its practitioners also dominated.

Two aspects of these changes which particularly concerned the delivery of health care were the increasing wealth of the nation and the development of the market. The mode whereby these were used had much to do with the ideas of the Enlightenment prevalent in the century. The threat which rulers felt from the increasing numbers of urban workers was also important. Nor can the biological base be ignored, for the threat of epidemic disease continued to give cause for concern. Ideas, actions and institutional changes were intermingled in ways whose connections we cannot always be sure about or even begin to see.

ENVIRONMENTAL HEALTH

Enlightenment thought applied to health matters led to a great interest through-out Europe in environmental medicine. Ludmilla Jordanova (1981) argues that concern with the needs of the whole population was an essentially Enlighten-ment concern, although municipalities in England had already taken action as we saw in Chapter 3.

Claudine Herzlich (1973, p. 19) has pointed out that the distinction between Hygeia, the goddess of health, and Aesculapius, the god of healing, between the importance of prevention and the importance of cure, has a long history. This distinction is associated with that between environmental causes of ill health and internal causes, and is also associated with the externalizing and internalizing systems of healing knowledge to which, as we saw in chapter 2, Young (1976a) has drawn attention.

In eighteenth-century Germany and France great stress was laid on the belief that diseases had external removable causes, which led to a search for new forms of practice and the development of 'medical police'. As expressed in France, for example, this involved various aspects such as health administration for the whole country, the control of medical practice and practitioners, legal aspects of medicine and the science of hygiene (Jordanova, 1981, p. 13).

The English brand of Enlightenment individualism did not take kindly to the implications of 'medical police', but the notion of environmentally controllable health hazards was present nevertheless. As noted in Chapter 3, municipalities like Norwich were already taking action in the sixteenth century. Furthermore, given the sectarian divisions in Britain, there was no single medical establishment and no one set of medical ideas. 'The locus of the English medical Enlightenment lay with the private, the individual, the local, the personal, the voluntary' (Porter, 1979, p. 32). Roy Porter points to three important changes in England at this time. First, secularization: in the seventeenth century deviants had been stigmatized in religious terms, called, for example, witches or possessed; in the eighteenth century they were defined in medical terms as masturbators, mad, or epileptics. In Porter's view, although not all would agree, 'eighteenth century doctors and patients alike lost that sense of spiritual meaning of suffering, and of the curative efficacy of faith and prayers' (1979, p. 32). They had lost the faith in 'powers', a loss which, Thomas (1970, p. 71) pointed out, preceded by a century the beginnings of the development of an efficacious medicine. Second, philanthropy went along with the Enlightenment, leading to an increase in the provision by the rich for the poor. Enlightenment values not only increased the provision but altered its direction away from religion to medicine. Third, in Enlightenment thought pain ceased to have a positive value: the *philosophes* (many of whom were also physicians) hoped scientific medicine would defeat pain. From this, Porter argues, ultimately came the shift of the medical goal from care to cure.

Late twentieth-century readers will be familiar with a sharp distinction, now commonly drawn, between cure and care; this had not yet been made in the eighteenth century. Nor was there a clear distinction between curative and preventive medicine. The same practitioners might well be involved in curative medicine in a hospital setting, as well as in what later came to be called public health. Medical men, furthermore, had wide-ranging interests in science, philosophy and many facets of the commonweal. Jordanova (1979) discusses the relationship between the earth sciences (geology, geography, meteorology) and biomedical sciences (physiology, biology, hygiene), and she shows how much stress, within the then contemporary notions of 'naturalness', was laid upon the environment. Those who espoused these ideas included influential people who were concerned with criminals and the poor as well as with medical education, insanity and hospital organization (Jordanova, 1979, p. 123). They saw a prospect of controlling and thus improving the social order as well as the health of the people by regulating the environment and the personal behaviour of individuals. Many of the hospitals and the asylums for the insane founded in the late eighteenth and early nineteenth centuries were inspired by environmentalist considerations. 'The total institution [see Goffman, 1961] was a perfectly controlled environment which would cure the inmates both morally and physically' (Jordanova, 1979, p. 134).

REPEATED EPIDEMICS AND CONSTANT AILMENTS CONTINUE

The control of infectious diseases had long concerned both medical and public men charged with responsibility to keep order, as we have seen (Chapter 3). Although Fraser Brockington (1965) refers to the first quarantine regulations being promulgated in 1743, there was by the eighteenth century already a tradition of attempts at control. There were quarantine regulations, but they were irregularly applied, being the responsibility of the municipalities (Slack, 1976).

In the case of epidemic diseases personal suffering became of public interest. In the eighteenth century, as there had been in Tudor and Stuart times, there was also much pain which had to be suffered alone, or with the help of others in the domestic domain or of a practitioner personally consulted. The diary of Richard Kay, a Lancashire doctor in the first half of the eighteenth century, is instructive. It is similar to documents which could be quoted from the earlier period. Kay, untouched by the questionings of some of his contemporaries, was extremely devout and religious. In addition to describing graphically the sufferings of his patients he also describes his own. He frequently records how 'this day' he has had to spend time in his closet. On 24 November 1738 it was 'Tumour in my Goom [gum] which is this Afternoon burst'. From 13 February 1739 he reports bad toothache. On 15 February he records: 'This Day I've spent some time in my Closet. O my Tooth, my Tooth, no remedy takes Effect, I've had continual pain of it all Day.' It appeared to ease by the 16th, 'but my Head worse' (quoted in Brockbank and Kenworthy, 1968, pp. 25–6). Among the ailments Kay records in addition are: 'Scorbutic [scurvy-like] pains in my Back Belly and other Places' (p. 61) for which he took some 'physick' (7 May 1743), recorded again on 20 August of the same year (p. 69). In January 1745 his teeth are bad again for three days, and he complains of cold. In April he is taking 'physick' for an unnamed illness; in May has a bad inflammation of his right eye; in July has uneasiness of his left groin, back and hips. In January 1749 he again complains of scurvy. He died at the age of 35 in 1751 apparently in an epidemic of fever. Throughout, in a manner continuous with earlier centuries, he takes his suffering to be a visitation from God and prays that God will take it from him. Dr Kay's diary illustrates some of the sufferings of the period and the concern for health which is continuous with that described by Pelling for Shakespeare's England, referred to in Chapter 2 (page 35). Bear in mind that Kay's standard of life and general well-being are likely to have been better than those of the general run of the population.

Kay was in a position to dose himself with whatever was available or to consult his father, also a doctor. Lay people experiencing pain or suffering still had a wide variety of persons to whom they could have recourse. Indeed, during the eighteenth century they were increasingly being plied with alternatives.

Concern continued for the care of the sick poor. For example, Joan Lane has extracted all references to 'surgeons, their practices, patients, fees, contracts, practice areas and recorded treatments to the poor' for 89 out of Warwickshire's 215 parishes for the period 1750–1800 (Lane, 1981, p. 10). She concludes that the 'overseers' tried to 'provide medical attention for the regular and occasional poor from the locally raised poor-rate at their disposal, that was not appreciably worse than other villagers enjoyed' (p. 13). She noted a particular interest in smallpox on the part of the surgeons, who had practices in towns and villages throughout Warwickshire, and of the overseers, an interest not unconnected she believes with the costs of the several severe outbreaks they experienced during her period.

PHYSICIANS, SURGEONS, APOTHECARIES AND OTHERS

So in the eighteenth century who was available to treat the population of all classes? In formal legal terms there were three categories of recognized healers or practitioners, derived from the three, officially recognized organizations of medical practitioners: the Royal College of Physicians of London, initially established, as was noted in Chapter 3, as the College of Physicians of London in 1518; the Company of Barber-Surgeons, which resulted from the merger of the Barbers' Company with the small élite of surgeons in 1540; and the Worshipful Society of Apothecaries, which had split off from the Grocers' Company in 1617. It was in the mid-eighteenth century (1745) that the surgeons broke away from the barber-surgeons to form a separate company of surgeons; at the end of that century, in 1800, the Company was reformed as the Royal College of Surgeons of London (Pelling, 1987; Waddington, 1984).

In accounts of the rise of the professions this tripartite division is taken to be of central importance, as for example in the discussion by Larson (1977, around p. 87) and by Waddington (1984, ch. 1), although the latter is careful to indicate that practice, in the eighteenth century as well as the early nineteenth, did not follow the legal situation with any precision. There are two problems with this focus on the tripartite division which have been pointed out strongly by Pelling (1987). The first is that, as these organizations were London based and concerned principally with the practitioners of health care in London, concentrating on them thus ignores practitioners' organizations in the provinces; secondly, looking only at these three formal groups and at other institutions, such as hospitals, we ignore a great deal of health care and healing which was undertaken, whether for love, cash, or kind, by others than licentiates of formal companies. In practice, it seems, there were more practitioners than those organized in the three major categories. Furthermore, the lines between physicians, surgeons and apothecaries were not so clearly drawn in practice as the legal position and the official histories would lead one to suppose.

CREATING THE QUACKS TO CREATE THE PROFESSION

One of the critical changes associated with the development of capitalism was the emergence of the labour market, not only for manual workers but also for healers. Magali Larson (1977), Roy Porter (1983) and Ivan Waddington (1984) stress the importance of the market in the development of medicine as a powerful occupation. The medical market expanded. Improved communications, both the written word and transport, made it increasingly possible for healers of all kinds to sell their skills and their cures to an ever-larger clientele. It was in this context that the 'anti-quack literature' developed. Orthodox practitioners were conscious of competition from the unlicensed. Indeed, anti-quack rhetoric was already in existence in the sixteenth and seventeenth centuries as one set of healers attempted to discredit others (Beier, 1981). Licensed physicians and other orthodox practitioners attempted to distinguish themselves from the medical fringe, the quacks, charlatans and mountebanks, who were untrained and who, they said, exploited the ignorance and suffering of gullible people. Orthodox practitioners described themselves as 'professionals' who could be trusted because they were well trained and also behaved properly (Beier, 1981; Porter, 1983). With their 'anti-quack literature' they sought to smear the unlicensed and dissuade people from consulting them (Beier, 1981, p. 30).

The licensed did not succeed in their attempts in the eighteenth century, perhaps because there was nothing they had to hand to demonstrate their superiority; also because, as Waddington (1984) points out, it was not until the nineteenth century that there was a body of centrally organized practitioners in any position to control medical practice.

Quacks may have been characterized by their knavishness, their gift of the gab, but Porter (1983, p. 13) is convinced that it would be a forlorn task to try to draw hard-and-fast lines between 'proper' practitioners and quacks using criteria such as integrity, scientific method, or therapeutic efficiency. Some quacks were well trained and successful. The competence and success rates of licensed physicians also varied. Furthermore 'orthodox' medical men and quacks overlapped and mingled. Porter's argument is that what quacks and also licensed doctors were involved in was the creation of a medical market and one that would become national. Both had to make a living.

The plurality of healers which was noted in Chapter 3 with regard to the seventeenth century carried over into the eighteenth. Healers of all sorts did not spend all of their time in medical practice; they were involved in many other kinds of trade and occupation. It was not a distinction between being a professional or being a tradesman which was the mark of an acceptable or unacceptable practitioner. The distinction between trade and profession was one created, like the creation of the quacks, in the interests of particular groups within the array of practitioners. As Porter (1983) argues convincingly, it was still true in the eighteenth century that practitioners, including licensed practitioners, were involved also in trade.

Waddington (1984, pp. 34–5) notes that, in the first half of the nineteenth century at least, many practitioners were involved in a second occupation, sometimes turning to writing but quite often also making up and trading in potions and running shops. Jeanne Peterson (1978) also stresses the varied tasks many practitioners undertook until well into the nineteenth century. Pelling (1982 and 1987) argues, however, that what was happening was not so much a question of medical practitioners in some sense of professionals having a second and less professional occupation, but of people combining work of different kinds, skills or trades, as a matter of course. Medical practice by the licensed as well as the unlicensed was combined in this way, just as a variety of other activities were. Porter (1983, p. 19) suggests that 'orthodox' or 'proper' medical men tended to leave many of the more tiresome ailments to the 'advertising professors', as Oliver Goldsmith called the more aggressive entrepreneurs among the quacks. Furthermore fringe practitioners in the seventeenth and eighteenth centuries were not practising radical alternatives to orthodoxy; there was no one medical orthodoxy. Their offerings were as scientific (although some might say scientistic) in the Enlightenment mode as those of the licensed. The quacks did not exist as such – there was simply a wide range of practitioners. The existence of quacks was created by those wishing to claim orthodoxy. As Lucinda Beier has it, the 'history of the creation of the medical fringe is the history of the birth of the medical profession' (1981, p. 80; see also Loudon, 1986).

MEDICINE AND THE GENDER ORDER

As well as vilifying the quacks, some medical men were also vilifying the midwives; indeed, women as such were often included in the unacceptable outgroup of practitioners. Already by 'the seventeenth century the barrier which excluded men from midwifery had broken down' (Clark, 1968, p. 265). Until the arrival of the *accoucheurs* (to use the French term) or 'men-midwives' (to use the less euphemistic but perhaps more honest Anglo-Saxon) early in the seventeenth century, attending women in childbirth had been an exclusively female occupation. The knowledge and training which midwives received came from their own experience of having babies, by example and from working with and listening to older midwives (Eccles, 1982; Oakley, 1976).

The dispute which developed in the seventeenth century and continued into the eighteenth was partly an aspect of the decline in ecclesiastical administration; it was a dispute both between two modes of medical knowledge and between the material interests of two sets of practitioners. It was also more than that: a challenge to the gender order. The ultimate outcome was one in which formal training took precedence over experiential knowledge. Depending how readers assess the value of each, so will their judgement vary.

Clark (1968) sees the disadvantages from which the midwives suffered as resulting from their exclusion from public-domain education. In this Jean Donnison (1977) and Audrey Eccles (1982) would agree. Clark's account is one of the way in which women were systematically denied access to knowledge, training and practice. Adrienne Rich's (1977) account, on the other hand, stresses the knowledge from experience, the empathy which was available to the women midwives, their knowledge of female anatomy which eighteenth-century men lacked.

In previous times women had had a legally inferior but not unpowerful position in a highly sex-segregated gender order. Theirs may have been a minor place in the male world order, but they did have a place of their own which they commanded and from which they could exert influence. It was focused on the domestic domain, was centralized in the kitchen and included midwifery, labour in childbirth being essentially women's work. From the seventeenth century and gaining a great deal of impetus in the eighteenth century this position was challenged; the apparent security of the women's domain was threatened. The men began to be interested in the problems of childbirth deriving from the new scientific approaches being applied to medicine. Given the exclusion of women from the universities and from the reconstructed companies of physicians and surgeons, the new medical knowledge which had been released first as a result of the Renaissance, and later more imperatively in the Enlightenment, was denied to women. The use of the forceps to aid difficult deliveries was also a factor in the unequal struggle. Originally in the exclusive control of the Chamberlen family, women, not being in the reformed Company of Surgeons, were not permitted to use the instrument (Donnison, 1977; Oakley, 1976; Rich, 1977). It is not surprising that within a patriarchal gender order highly placed women should in all these circumstances turn to male medical advisers over against their historically conventional female helpers. Furthermore, the new *accoucheurs* would have come from a higher social status if not class than most of the midwives by this time. Thus it came about that first in France and later in

England the highly born and highly placed, probably the wives themselves, began to call in the *accoucheurs* or the 'men-midwives' to attend women in childbirth.

There is no doubt that those who accepted male attendants were, and saw themselves as, very daring, for they were flying in the face of many taboos which sustained the former gender order. It would not have occurred to them that this radical departure, which they saw as very up to the moment and the best available, was involving them in supporting the beginnings of a new form of subordination for women. The tragic history of Mary Wollstonecraft, the late eighteenth-century feminist, in this regard is well known. Mary stood out against the fashionable trend, apparently 'because she thought it indecorous to have a male doctor in attendance' (Tomalin, 1985, p. 272). It is particularly ironic that she should have died in childbirth. When the placenta did not come away, her midwife, who was midwife in charge of the Westminster lying-in hospital, sent for a medical man, the chief obstetrician of that hospital, whose efforts to remove the placenta appear to have introduced an infection, from which Mary died ten days later (Tomalin, 1985, pp. 272–80).

Those medical men who wished to gain a foothold in midwifery were faced with two problems. On the one hand they had to convince pregnant women and their husbands that they had more to offer than traditional midwives; second, they had to convince their male colleagues that this was really 'fit work for men'. (See Loudon, 1986, pp. 92–4, for the various aspects of their problem on the latter point.) The very title 'man-midwife' cannot have offered immediate help on either score. The campaign of vilification against midwives which these medical men entered into has made it difficult to get a clear view of the sort of women who were midwives and how competent they were. Eccles's (1982) account, for example, being drawn (however carefully) from literary accounts reveals throughout a bias towards the strongly stated position of the articulate men.

The campaign against the midwives has to be seen, like the campaign against the quacks, as the activity of a group of people who were trying to make space for themselves. Utterances associated with the campaign make it hard to be clear what the situation really was. Indeed, David Harley (1981) has accused Jean Donnison (1977) of being caught in a trap, along with Hilda Smith (1976) and Jane Donegan (1978), in that she accepts the accuracy of the stereotype that the 'midwife was an elderly widow or spinster, economically marginal and largely unlettered' (p. 6). He notes the resemblance of the stereotype, as do Rich and Donnison, to the victims of witchcraft prosecutions. Harley's examination of diocesan licensing records (midwives had been required to be licensed with the church authorities since 1512: Donnison, 1977, p. 5) finds many literate and respectable midwives. In Lancashire and Cheshire they included wives of prosperous merchants and yeomen, although their number declined as the eighteenth century wore on, perhaps because of the developing cult of domesticity among the better-off men, who encouraged their wives to stay home. 'Gentility and household management appear to replace skilled work and social involvement as marks of community leadership' (Harley, 1981, p. 9). Donnison is well aware of the varied social backgrounds of midwives. Her implied confidence in the available new knowledge from which women were excluded perhaps leads her to devalue the old knowledge as much as an opposite confidence leads Rich to value it. What is clear is that the new knowledge was men's knowledge, that it lacked some data which women had and that the men were determined already by the seventeenth century to carve a place for themselves in this hitherto exclusively female world.

However, most women in the eighteenth century continued to be attended by women when they were in labour, whether the midwives were licensed or unlicensed. The fee itself would have prevented poorer women applying for a licence, as Donnison (1977, p. 7) points out. Most healing and caring was still undertaken by women in the household too.

THE DEVELOPMENT OF THE HOSPITAL

What perhaps in the long run was most important for the transformation of medical knowledge, and was certainly the most visible of the eighteenth-century developments in England, was the establishment of the hospitals. There had been hospitals in the medieval period. They were associated with religious foundations and had not initially catered for the sick, or not only for them; they were hospices for those needing shelter and care. Indeed, when new hospitals were opened after the Reformation they were frequently referred to as 'infirmaries' to distinguish them from 'hospitals', which cared for the elderly rather than treating the sick.

On the Continent there was a more continuous tradition of these ancient religious foundations, many of which were transformed to accommodate more of the sick and also to be a locus for developing medical skills. In some places the Catholic foundations were continuous, in others Protestant organizations took them over. In England however there was an abrupt break because the dissolution of the monasteries left the country with few places outside the home where the sick could be treated. In the few hospitals that survived there was no doubt less discontinuity. Carole Rawcliffe suggests that, for those which were refounded, the break was not abrupt because the secular authorities had long exercised influence (1983, p. 26). Henry VIII had promised that the sick would not suffer, and the result of petitions was that by the end of the sixteenth century five royal or chartered hospitals had been established.

Paul Slack's (1980) view is rather different, however. 'The five London hospitals', he argues, 'can be compared only with poor-relief institutions in major cities on the continent ... they were unique in England' (p. 108). Their architects had seized upon the opportunity created by the dissolution to establish in London institutions on the lines of the continental welfare schemes (p. 110). The motives behind them were a mixture of the fear of disorder, disease and decay; a quest for civil harmony and civic decency; and the triumph of Christian charity (p. 114).

However one may interpret the history, the hospitals were very different from twentieth-century hospitals. Of the five, the Bridewell was a prison or reformatory; Christ's Hospital was for corrupt, fatherless and helpless children; St Mary's Bethlehem was a lunatic asylum. Two of the ancient hospitals continued to care for the sick poor and thereby to remove the dangers they presented from the streets: St Thomas's and St Bartholomew's. These had been refounded twelve and fourteen years respectively after the dissolution of 1539 (Woodward, 1974, pp. 2, 147). It was not until 1720 that the Westminster

Hospital was founded, the first of the new hospital development. St George's, the London and the Middlesex followed within the next quarter-century. Before the end of the century some twenty-eight or thirty were also founded in the provinces (Abel-Smith, 1964; Webster, 1978, p. 214; Woodward, 1974, p. 147).

Initiatives for the new hospitals (infirmaries) came from local dignitaries, clergy, Nonconformists and royalty. Doctors themselves were associated with these developments from the outset (Woodward, 1974), but Abel-Smith (1964) is probably right to suggest that in the eighteenth century the major initiative was lay. The hospitals were founded on the philanthropic principle, which had acquired a new importance associated with the ideas of the Enlightenment, as we have noted. 'Infirmaries were one of the most characteristic expressions of Christian philanthropy of the eighteenth century' (Webster, 1978, p. 214). The increasing wealth made the new initiatives feasible. Governors and subscribers came from a social élite and from among those who were aspiring to improve their social position. In addition to the hope of a better place in the next world there were 'temporal inducements' for an upwardly mobile subscriber to have his name associated with those of high status (Woodward, 1974, pp. 17–22). The subscription also gave power, for, except in case of accident or emergency, the only way to get treatment in a voluntary hospital was by recommendation of a subscriber. The whole was part of that patronage system which was 'the other face of property' (Perkin, 1969, p. 51).

Webster (1978) shows that the infirmary movement related to the needs of the agricultural labourer rather than the industrial worker, in terms of the rules of admission and the conditions treated; most were built in small county towns, few in expanding industrial towns. The numbers of infirmaries established declined from the 1740s, rather than increasing as one might expect if the philanthropy was designed to ameliorate the consequences of the Industrial Revolution. Based on an examination of infirmaries established in expanding northern towns, Webster shows the crises of finance and space which developed for infirmaries in places like Manchester and Newcastle. He points also to the unmet needs. Rules 'inherited from the Reformation forbad the admission of children, pregnant women, the consumptive, the dying, the epileptic and those suffering from venereal or infectious disease' (p. 215).

In Manchester a struggle between a conservative faction and a small group of laymen and doctors associated with the Literary and Philosophical Society resulted in radical change. 'They believed it was essential for the evolution of a well-ordered industrial society for "the useful classes" to be restored to health, as it was for machinery to be repaired, or factories planned for maximum efficiency' (Webster, 1978, p. 217). They amended the rules so that those who could not be admitted and who could not attend as out-patients should be visited in their homes by the medical staff of the infirmary. Visiting the homes of the sick poor increased these medical men's conviction of the importance of public health and the limits of the contribution which infirmary care could make. The active group won in a confrontation such that home visiting was extended, and fever wards and more surgical wards were built. In the 1790s cases of fever contracted in the hospital were being treated there, and a 'house of recovery' for those who contracted fever outside the infirmary was opened; a dispensary was also opened to make medical care more widely available.

In Manchester the 'expansionists' were 'predominantly radical and Unitarian ... their critics ... tory and anglican' (Webster, 1978, p. 219). Each had strong and differing partisan loyalties associated with the French Revoloution. In Newcastle the story was different. Here the conservative faction had greater power, and expansion was ultimately possible only in consequence of the intervention of the Bishop of Durham, who was devoted to bettering the conditions of the poor. In both Manchester and Newcastle plans for a Board of Health which would be responsible for public health, for preventive measures in the towns, had to be sacrificed. This was something which 'the philanthropic spirit of their age proved unwilling to countenance' (p. 223), just as in many places the infirmaries did not respond to the escalation of ill health and the changing pattern of disease which accompanied the Industrial Revolution. Separate fever hospitals and dispensaries were a response to that rigidity.

In the eighteenth-century voluntary hospitals, physicians and surgeons had honorary appointments, giving their services free, although this might involve only a weekly ward round, much of their work being done by their pupils or by apothecaries. The latter were the only salaried members of the staff, the only ones in full-time attendance, and were worked hard. In giving their services free the physicians and surgeons enhanced their reputation with their private patients, who were also donors, thus building up their practices among well-to-do fee-paying patients upon whom they waited in their own homes. But this was not all; the hospitals began to be centres for teaching and research; and the pupils also paid fees (Abel-Smith, 1964; Woodward, 1974).

HOSPITALS FOR WOMEN

The infirmaries were opposed to admitting women and to lying in wards. In Manchester, Charles White, a leading British obstetrician, opposed an extension of the infirmary charity to include the delivery of parturient women in their own homes and instead founded his own lying-in charity under his own control (Webster, 1978, p. 218). It is rare to find mention of the lying-in hospitals, although, as Margaret Versluysen (1977) points out, there were two lying-in wards and four separate lying-in hospitals established in London between 1739 and 1765. They accounted for only a fraction of London births in the period, but they are of considerable importance to the manner and control of childbirth. In trying to answer the question 'why was secular maternal hospital provision created in this period, by whom and for what reasons?' Versluysen (p. 34) argues as follows. In the seventeenth century, medical men who took up midwifery were in a difficulty because they were seen as intervening in what had previously been an exclusively female domain, and consequent professional antagonism developed. Nevertheless, by the 1730s the numbers of male mid-wives had expanded dramatically. However it was the women, the midwives, who had the practical clinical experience; the men's knowledge was theoretical, as we have already noted. In this situation, Versluysen argues, the lying-in hospital resolved the tension in favour of the medical men, for in that context the matron-midwife 'was unambiguously defined as a less skilled, inferior type of midwifery practitioner' (p. 35).

Outside the context of the lying-in hospital medical men had to be restrained in their approach to parturient women, attending cases only where midwives called them because 'abnormalities' had developed. They sometimes crept into the chamber of the labouring woman in such a way that she was unaware of their presence. They could avoid all that in a hospital where only the poor went. Foucault (1973, p. 85) notes that only unmarried women were admitted to the maternity hospital in Copenhagen, a practice recommended in Paris in the 1790s. Such women could be investigated with impunity and used for research and teaching.

We can only speculate how different the story might have been if Mrs Cellier's attempts to establish a College for Midwives in 1687 had succeeded (Versluysen, 1981, pp. 33–4). Given the control of the public domain already excercised by men we can see with hindsight that her attempts would inevitably have been frustrated.

THE BIRTH OF CLINICAL MEDICINE

In the context of the hospital, modern clinical medicine was born. Throughout Europe developments were taking place which were to change the mode and locale of healing and also of childbirth by the mid-twentieth century.

At the outset of this chapter we discussed the ways in which the Enlightenment influenced public health provisions. It had other profound influences. The rationality which accompanied the Enlightenment facilitated major changes in medical knowledge, which have been extensively explored by Foucault (1967 and 1973). When reading Foucault's analyses it is important to remember differences in French and British history, in terms of both revolutionary and political history and the development of hospitals (see Jamous and Peloille, 1970, and Waddington 1973a, on French hospitals; and Jordanova, 1981, on the French public health movement).

The new clinical medicine which began to develop at the end of the eighteenth century required knowledge of the human body hitherto denied. It required the breaking of centuries-old taboos about the violation of the human body and challenged religious authority. It was to have importance for the place medicine would take in society beyond the lessons it taught medical students and researchers about human anatomy. It also related to fundamental underlying changes in society. The breach of these taboos occurred differently in various European countries. In Britain bodies were snatched illegally from graves; in many parts of the Continent the bodies of the poor were available earlier, although not always without difficulty.

Whatever mechanisms were employed to effect the change, it is clear that the conscience and the susceptibilities of the people at large were being modified more or less against their will. However, as Waddington (1973a, p. 221) has pointed out, it was the early availability of corpses which put French medicine in the forefront of the new clinical developments.

THE NEW GAZE

Michel Foucault (1973, pp. 124–5) argues that corpses had been dissected a lot earlier than regular medical histories have hitherto allowed, occurring in the middle of the eighteenth century. The knowledge was not fully exploited until the century's end. The opening up of corpses, Foucault argues, and particularly of newly dead corpses, led to the new understanding of life, death and disease.

He quotes Bichat, who wrote that all had been confusion in twenty years' bedside observations but 'Open up a few corpses: you will dissipate at once the darkness that observation alone could not dissipate' (1973, p. 146). Formerly death and disease came as external invaders. Old paintings and poems depict death hovering over a house or entering a window. Disease was an entity as Paracelsus had suggested. Now, Foucault argues, death came to be understood not as one indivisible but as a myriad of deaths of parts of the organism at different times. Disease now took on the 'internal, constant, mobile dimensions of the relation between life and death. It is not because he falls ill that man dies; fundamentally, it is because he may die that man may fall ill' (1973, p. 155). Disease, previously indivisible, could now be spacialized and individualized. This understanding followed the new way of looking at human bodies which involved observation, feeling and listening – or in Foucault's terms the 'new gaze' with its trinity of sight, touch and hearing.

The nub of Foucault's argument is that the understanding of the body and of disease was transformed by this new clinical 'gaze'. In Armstrong's terms, a 'new concept of the body' emerged (1983b, p. xi). Doctors began to look below the surface signs and symptoms to what happens underneath. The questions that they asked the patients changed. 'Where does it hurt?' replaced the more general question 'What is the matter with you?' The new question relates to something which can be identified in the body. Thus we find physicians using ear-trumpets to listen to the heart beat and they feel and observe the body. In the new clinical medicine observation gave way to examination (Waddington, 1973a, p. 214). A new nosology, or classification of disease, resulted. It was one, however, with a masculinist vision, as Ludmilla Jordanova (1985) has graphically shown in her analysis of the way William Hunter presented images of pregnant women in his obstetrical atlas of 1774.

The new clinic, Foucault argues, was more than the old empiricism; in the new clinic the first application of analysis took place. Signs and symptoms were distinguished. The symptom is the form in which the disease is presented, it allows the disease to show through. The sign announces what has been, what is, what will be. With the new medical gaze the symptom becomes a sign, and the sign says what the symptom is. The analysis reveals an ordering which is the natural order itself. In the eighteenth century the notion of the natural order had, among some members of the intelligentsia, come to supersede the beliefs in deities and powers which held so much sway in the sixteenth and seventeenth centuries. Thinkers were attracted by theories which avoided supernatural explanations and stayed firmly within the realm of observable nature (Jordanova, 1979, p. 135). This was important for environmental medicine but also for clinical medicine.

In his stress on the important changes taking place in the eighteenth century and making such sharp contrasts between the 'old clinic' and the 'new clinic', Foucault apparently undervalues the many changes that had been taking place previously. Britain, and especially England, may have been behind the Continent in the development of medical knowledge in the sixteenth, seventeenth and eighteenth centuries; nevertheless we should note that in the seventeenth century Sydenham had already sought to overcome the divorce between the abstract learning of the university trained and the empirical knowledge of the practitioners by insisting on the importance of clinical medicine at the bedside. Earlier that century Harvey had established that blood circulated in the body. In dating the birth of the clinic at the end of the eighteenth century, where, as he says, the medical historians themselves commonly date it, perhaps Foucault has himself accepted too readily biomedicine's own account of its history.

As I hinted, the historical specificity of the development of ideas and institutions in France may be more important than Foucault and his disciples allow. Roy Porter (1979) has drawn attention to this in discussing the relationship of medicine and the Enlightenment, as did Jordanova (1981) in discussing medical police. Porter contrasts twentieth-century scholars whose interpretation he calls 'naïve optimistic', who see the Enlightenment as a panacea in medical terms (and cast medical history in terms of an upward progress thereafter), and those he calls 'conspiratorial pessimistic', who have a decidedly more jaundiced view, among whom he includes Foucault. Porter argues that the special conditions of life in eighteenth-century England rule out both these interpretations.

On the one hand, the absence of a militant, exclusive medical profession is suggestive of the lack of the genuinely efficacious scientific medicine which the 'Naïve Optimistic' school expect to find. But equally the absence of a bureaucratic medical profession means that the conspiracy for the medicalization of life through the state, presumed by the pessimists, is a mirage.

(Porter, 1979, p. 38)

From the point of view of the argument of this book, however, Foucault's work is important for a number of reasons. First, because he shows how the new ideas arose in particular socioeconomic circumstances and in their turn led to further changes; how the unity of hospital and teaching was needed for the development of the new clinical medicine which was linked to the locale in which healing took place. The hospital provided the necessary conditions which the home did not; and although this is not Foucault's language, he shows how the development of biomedicine could have come about only in a class-divided and sex-segregated society in which the poor and the fallen provided good clinical material for research and teaching.

By 1900 the scene was laid in the arenas of public health and curative medicine, in both home and hospital, for the development and triumph of biomedicine in the nineteenth century as a male-dominated and class-based profession. Confidence was increasing in the power of medical men. By that time, nevertheless, the curative powers of medicine had not greatly improved on the performance recorded at the start of the century. The consequences of the Industrial Revolution and the associated urbanization would soon present statesmen and practitioners with new problems.

5 Hospitals and Public Health: Control, Exploitation and the Development of Medical Knowledge

The English hospital system developed in a fragmented way. This chapter will trace how, by the end of the nineteenth century, a complex array of hospital provision had developed. The voluntary hospital movement continued, gaining greater momentum after 1850. Voluntary hospitals treated the deserving poor, Poor Law hospitals the paupers (i.e. the undeserving poor); asylums separated the insane and isolation hospitals the infectious.

During the century also concern with epidemics was associated with movements for sanitary reform which later developed into the public health movement. Originally a matter for laymen, by the end of the century medicine had firmly taken over the provisions. The causes of epidemic diseases and the manner of controlling them were hotly disputed for the first three-quarters of the century. Ultimately a generally agreed biomedical model gained acceptance, making the claim to a unified medical profession much more plausible. The disputes were associated with inter- and intra-occupational differences and with a dispute about women's status in which most medical men sided with the dominant male opinion.

THE BACKGROUND OF RAPID ECONOMIC AND SOCIAL CHANGE

The increasing size of the urban industrial population posed problems of health and social control. Population increases were remarkable, as was the rapid growth of industrial towns. At the same time the increasing wealth of the nation and the optimism and general belief in progress were conducive to social and medical transformations.

> During the course of the nineteenth century the British economy grew prodigiously. Exports rose sevenfold ... imports still faster ... Production in the leading industries advanced in step with trade: coal output rose more than twentyfold ... pig-iron more than thirtyfold ... raw cotton consumed more than thirtyfold ... paper more than fortyfold. Older industries ... grew less fast, but newer ones ... still faster ... population more than trebled, while per capita industrial production and real income quadrupled.
>
> (Perkin, 1969, pp. 3–4)

It was in this context that the new medicine and the new medical men flourished.

THE VOLUNTARY HOSPITALS

The second phase of hospital development was inspired not so much by laymen as by the doctors themselves, although they continued to rely entirely on philanthropic lay people for the necessary subscriptions and donations. The doctors were anxious to increase the 'material' they had available for teaching and research and to achieve positions for themselves (Abel-Smith, 1964, pp. 16–18). At the end of the eighteenth century only three London hospitals took medical students, most instruction taking place in private, profit-making, schools; medical education was a combination of theoretical instruction, such as the 'physic' taught at Oxford and Cambridge, and rather casual apprenticeships. The fusion of which Foucault spoke had not taken place (see pages 57–8). But by the 1820s and 1830s medical education was transferred to hospitals and institutionalized there. By the 1850s the hospital medical school had co-opted or destroyed private medical education (Peterson, 1978, pp. 63–5). Hospital staffs therefore came to be known as those with the most advanced knowledge, and for the doctors 'charitable work became the key to fame and fortune' (Abel-Smith, 1964, p. 19).

Initially the hospitals founded were general hospitals. By the mid-nineteenth century there was, however, little room at the top for ambitious medical men as their numbers increased. Nor was there space in the general hospitals for younger men to develop their more specialized interests (Abel-Smith, 1964, pp. 20–2). Consequently the general hospitals were succeeded by the foundation of numbers of specialist hospitals: for example, for eyes from the early years of the nineteenth century, for children from 1851. These specialist hospitals were partly the result of the refusal of the general hospitals to treat certain types of case; for example, they would not take children, nor would they treat eye problems (Abel-Smith, 1964, pp. 22–31).

The voluntary hospitals had a preference for cases which would respond to available treatment. These provided the most interesting teaching material and were the best advertisements for the skill of the physicians and surgeons. Such cases either recovered, or if long-standing, were 'relieved' as living testimonials to the doctors who treated them. Those who died were removed from the scene. 'Boring' cases of any sort were not acceptable. Nor would the voluntary hospitals take infectious diseases, nor VD, nor TB (although Woodward, 1974, has demonstrated variation in these limitations). Furthermore beds were available only to those whom the subscribers favoured, for theirs was the right of admission.

The living conditions in the voluntary hospitals were rigorous by any modern standards, and there is some dispute about how dangerous they were. Woodward (1974, ch. 10) is inclined to think that they were not the death-traps that so many have made them out to be. In particular he considers that the remarkably high death rates reported by Florence Nightingale in her third edition of *Notes on Hospitals* derive from a serious mistake in the denominator on which they were based. He is inclined to conclude, contrary to the views of McKeown and Brown (1955–6) and notwithstanding all the difficulties in the statistics, that the voluntary hospitals may well have helped patients and certainly did not do tremendous harm to any large number of them. Woodward's concern is to some extent misplaced. The dispute about the accuracy of the statistics Nightingale presented using Farr's methods 'can best be understood if this skirmish is seen as a reflection of a larger conflict within the medical world of London' (Eyler, 1979, p. 183). J. M. Eyler is arguing, as Porter (1979, p. 34) did for the eighteenth century, that it is the shift in medical conceptualization and of the focus of medical treatment which is critical rather than the impact of medicine on the health and longevity of the people of the period. It remains the case however that the presence of 'hospital diseases' was a worry, of which puerperal fever in the lying-in wards and hospitals was a most dramatic example.

THE WORKHOUSES AND WORKHOUSE INFIRMARIES

Because the voluntary hospitals were restrictive in the patients they would admit, other hospital provisions developed. Sick paupers and those with diseases that the voluntary hospitals turned away had to be provided for by the Poor Law. In 1861 there were 11,000 patients in voluntary hospitals, a great increase from the 1,600 of 1789, but there were 50,000 sick paupers (Abel-Smith, 1964, p. 46). The flood of people to the towns in the eighteenth century, which increased in the nineteenth, dislocated the networks of healers based upon the domestic domain upon which the great majority of the people had relied. Notwithstanding the serious hazards of eighteenth- and nineteenth-century hospitals the common people therefore turned to them for succour in times of illness. Those sufferers who were not 'good clinical material' or not well connected could not gain admittance to the voluntary hospitals. They had no alternative but to turn to, or were forcibly removed by, the Poor Law, which had to accommodate sick children, mental cases, those with TB and VD and the chronic sick (Abel-Smith, 1964, p. 49). There thus developed two classes of institutionalized patients: the deserving and the undeserving poor. The former had the privilege of admission to voluntary hospitals; the latter suffered the workhouse.

Initially, after the introduction of the new Poor Law of 1834, the intention had been to treat the sick at home and to institutionalize only the able-bodied poor. There was however inadequate medical relief to do this, and medical officers therefore admitted the sick if they did not recover quickly at home. But the workhouse had been established on the principle of 'less eligibility' and was hardly suitable to be run as a house for the treatment of the sick (Abel-Smith, 1964, pp. 46–9). The treatment of the sick was confused with the discouragement of pauperism (Crowther, 1981, p. 156). It was not until 1867 that the president of the Poor Law Board publicly recognized this (Crowther, 1981, p. 168), but notions about malingerers and the need for deterrence remained for many years.

The workhouse hospitals where the majority of cases were treated were not connected with the medical schools at all. Until the latter part of the nineteenth century all medical officers were under lay control. The sick poor were nursed either in the workhouse itself or in a workhouse infirmary controlled by the Poor Law guardians through the workhouse master. There were no separate fever hospitals, so in times of epidemic the workhouse infirmary became overcrowded (Crowther, 1981, p. 160)

Whatever may have been the rigours and hazards of the voluntary hospitals the workhouses were deplorable by comparison. Anxiety about them had mounted such that in 1866 two inquiries were held: one by the *Lancet* and the other by special inspectors of the Poor Law Board. These exposed dreadful conditions. There was inadequate ventilation; the sick were mixed with other inhabitants. There was 'a special air of bescrubbedness, rather a powerful odour of soap and water, about the wards of the workhouse infirmaries' (*Lancet*, quoted in Abel-Smith, 1964, p. 52), but this was only a veneer of hygiene; there was a shortage of toilets and baths. In Kensington and Paddington the inspector found patients washing in their chamber-pots and was told they liked it that way. He later found out that they did it 'against their will and their former habits at home'. Only a few guardians provided toilet-paper on the grounds that the poor were not in the habit of using it, but 'there were ... "numberless instances" of closets being blocked with "old towels, dusters and dish cloths" – and leaves of Holy Scripture' (Abel-Smith, 1964, p. 52).

Concerns such as these led to the Metropolitan Poor Act of 1867, which provided for infirmaries with an administration separate from the workhouse (Crowther, 1981, p. 162). Under this the Metropolitan Asylums Board was set up to administer hospitals for lunatics, fever and smallpox cases. From 1871 the Local Government Board became responsible for the Poor Law.

Dispensaries were a way of providing for the sick without having to admit them. As early as 1769 a dispensary for sick children had been set up in Red Lion Square in London; children were rarely admitted to hospital in the eighteenth and early nineteenth centuries (Abel-Smith, 1964, p. 13). After the revelations of the mid-1860s various further developments were planned by the Poor Law Board, which now had increased powers. An increased emphasis on dispensaries was part of this movement to provide more adequate infirmaries. Dispensaries were to be sited not more than a mile from any patient's dwelling – and preferably nearer. As well as helping the patient this would reduce the number of home calls the medical officer had to make (Abel-Smith, 1964, pp. 83–5).

Not only were the workhouse hospitals in no way connected with medical education; for much of the century the bulk of nursing was done by paupers. Nursing reform, discussed in Chapter 6, was a matter for the voluntary hospitals. The medical officers, furthermore, had no security of tenure and ordinarily took workhouse positions part-time while hoping to develop a private practice (Abel-Smith, 1964, p. 58).

There was a good deal of variation in the Poor Law hospitals as well as in the voluntary hospitals, since both Poor Law guardians and subscribers were locally based (Abel-Smith, 1964; Woodward, 1974). This was a muddle in Abel-Smith's eyes, but 'the poor had gained the right to institutional care when they were sick' (1964, p. 65). Some today may feel this was perhaps a dubiously valuable right. Josephine Butler, an upper-class woman, was among contemporaries who opposed the development of large-scale institutional care (Butler, 1954, p. 60).

SOCIAL CLASS AND THE HOSPITALS

Throughout this period the well-to-do and the aristocracy continued to be treated at home. Subscribers did not become patients in their hospitals. They paid for physicians and surgeons to attend them in their own homes; when they were not tended by women of their own household, they engaged women as nurses to care for them there. The slow capitulation of the aristocracy to the notion of hospital treatment can be highlighted by the royal behaviour. It is only in the last quarter of the twentieth century that the British royal family has conceded the superiority of the hospital as a locale for treatment. Until recently surgeons as well as physicians waited upon royalty for all consultations. When operations were carried out at Buckingham Palace or babies were delivered there, a room, not necessarily the same room, was specially prepared. Royal babies up to Princess Anne's first child were all delivered at home. When in her 80s Elizabeth the Queen Mother went to hospital for the removal of a fish bone from her throat, it was the first time in a long life that she had been hospitalized for treatment. So far as humbler mortals are concerned, it was not until late in the nineteenth century that middle-class people began to go into hospitals.

This class division in the locale of health-care delivery was critical for the development of modern medicine, as the works of Abel-Smith (1964), Jewson (1974 and 1976), Peterson (1976) and Waddington (1973a, 1979 and 1984) all make plain. In two frequently quoted papers Jewson discusses the way in which doctor/patient relations, the development of biomedicine and the form of medical knowledge are closely interconnected. He argues that Galenic notions served well a physician faced with treating an eighteenth-century aristocrat. Jewson understands the relationship between such a patient and his physician as one of patronage. A powerful patient could determine the conditions on which the service was rendered. A medical theory which took account of the patient's moods, as Galenic medicine does, fitted well a social relationship of that kind. Jewson then takes his argument further and shows how treatment in hospital changes a person into a case, and then, later again, the case becomes a laboratory specimen. This progression follows the move of the 'gaze' in Foucault's terms (see page 58) into the interior workings of the body and later to the details of the cells.

Jewson's diagrammatic summary of this process is reproduced in Figure 5.1. Jewson (1976) argues that to be able to treat patients as cases, and parts of them as laboratory specimens, was crucial for the development of clinical biomedicine. In so far as effective medicine resulted in the nineteenth century, the rich private patients benefited from the experiments carried out on the poor.

Margaret Pelling (1987), however, has raised objections to this line of argument, which, she correctly points out, is a development from S. W. F. Holloway's (1964 and 1966) work. She argues that private transactions may not have been a major part of medicine in the early modern period; further, that Holloway has asserted rather than demonstrated the domination of a patronage relationship in the eighteenth century. The arguments she complains, have not been precisely articulated in historical terms. She would agree that practitioners were not infrequently attached to aristocratic households, to be available to give advice and treatment as needed. Her objection is to the assumption that such relationships were characteristic of medicine before 1800. The argument, she claims, relates only to minorities. There is, she believes, more continuity between the periods before and after 1800 than the Holloway–Jewson arguments would suggest. There was also extensive provision for the sick poor before 1800, as we saw in Chapter 3.

	Patron	Occupational role of medical investigator	Source of patronage	Perception of sick-man	Occupational task of medical investigator	Conceptualization of illness
Bedside medicine	Patient	Practitioner	Private fees	Person	Prognosis and therapy	Total psycho-somatic disturbance
Hospital medicine	State; hospital	Clinician	Professional career structure	Case	Diagnosis and classification	Organic lesion
Laboratory medicine	State; academy	Scientist	Scientific career structure	Cell complex	Analysis and explanation	Biochemical process

Source: Jewson, 1976, p. 228.

Figure 5.1 *Three modes of production of medical knowledge.*

REGULATION OF THE WORKING CLASS

Mitchell Dean and Gail Bolton (1980) have argued that this is not all; the hospitals and the workhouses where the sick poor were nursed acted to regulate and control the labouring population and those who could not work, thus reinforcing distinctions between the rich and the poor. They see the development of the hospital system as part of the resolution of certain critical disputes about administration in the nineteenth century. Policy-makers at that time, they argue, had to resolve a problem between the *laissez-faire* dictum against interfering with the 'natural' existence of the poor – without whom there could be no wealth – on the one hand, and the wish for security, happiness and order, on the other. While poverty was inevitable they believed nevertheless it produced a moral and a political danger for the social order. The resolution lay along moral lines. Dean and Bolton quote Robert Southey, who wrote in 1829 that government should see 'the moral improvement of the people as its first duty' (Dean and Bolton, 1980, p. 81). Those who wished for intervention spoke of 'care', the means whereby socially dangerous features could be kept under control. The management of the poor would lead to the well-being and the orderliness of the population. The poor were the 'other' to polite civilized society. I shall discuss the implications for the division of labour in Chapter 6. Here we should note that the discipline, the religious observance, the hierarchy of the hospital and the workhouse constituted them as two of the places where this moral control was exercised.

Foucault (1967, 1973, 1979 and 1980) also sees the removal to hospital in power terms, but power conceived rather differently. We have noted how the new clinical 'gaze' altered the spatial understanding of the body; there were other spatial changes in social relations. Bentham's Panopticon was a prison built in such a way that every inmate was separate but constantly observed. Although possibly only one was ever built, Foucault takes it to symbolize a major politico-social shift represented in the nineteenth-century development of large-scale institutions, hospitals, mental asylums and prisons. He sees a crucial change in the way social relations were constituted and understood and the power which inheres in them was exercised and experienced. Instead of residing in a visible person, e.g. a sovereign, power was diffused and evaded designation.

EPIDEMIC DISEASES

The recurrent epidemics to which nineteenth-century English people, just as much as their eighteenth-century forebears, were subject were a feature of the biological base of the society as a whole, although not all sections suffered equally. These epidemics were seen to be especially associated with the poorer quarters of towns. Disease and social disorder were also associated in the nineteenth-century mind. Some epidemic diseases were thought of by those who suffered them as foreign' others were 'English' diseases (Morris, 1976). The latter were endemic in the population, i.e. they recurred from time to time and followed an understood course, were taken for granted and were in no way so frightening as the epidemics of 'foreign' diseases which were not understood and seemed to take a dreadful toll. Our lay understanding of nineteenth-century epidemic diseases is much coloured by these 'foreign' invaders like cholera and the attempts to combat them. We hear less of the endemic killers such as typhoid. This perspective has arisen, in part at least, because those social and public administrators who were seeking means to control all epidemic diseases and their associated civil disturbances, and whose attention was forcefully drawn to the new epidemic diseases, capitalized on the panic created by 'foreign' invaders (Pelling, 1978b).

In the late eighteenth and early nineteenth centuries, associated with observations of the geographic scatter of epidemics, there was a powerful 'geography' of disease, which Foucault describes for France. A disease was said to arise from Marseilles, Bicetre, Rouen, Paris or Nîmes (1973, p. 23). These were 'natural' loci, unlike the unnatural locus of hospital diseases. The notion of 'natural' diseases was strongly associated with the concept of environmental causes of disease and miasmatic ideas.

RURAL AND URBAN EPIDEMICS

Many generalizations have been made about the health conditions of the common people in the nineteenth century and their relationship to industrial capital. Probably it is not true as an overall generalization to say either that the life circumstances of ordinary people were worse in the towns than they had been in their villages of origin, or the other way round. It must have depended where they came from and where they went to (Smith, 1979; Thompson, 1963). For one who had moved into the 'booming suburb' of Croydon, where there were 13,000 people in 1848, no sewerage facilities at all and only rudimentary drainage, almost any rural conditions might have been better; however, for one who was living in the woollen township of Hepptonstall, with the sewer passing under the flagstones of the cottage floor, the water supply already polluted higher up on the moor and a devastating typhus epidemic raging, no large town would have been worse (Smith, 1979, p. 197; Thompson, 1963, p. 320). What people faced depended upon who were the local authorities, what their relations with central government were and, furthermore, whether they were blocked or helped by old landed gentry or rising industrial bourgeoisie.

Whatever rural conditions may have been, it is undoubtedly the case that conditions in the towns were far from healthy (although there was contemporary dispute as to why they were unhealthy). Lack of appropriate means of disposing of human excrement, lack of clean water supplies, the contamination of food and drink and the crowding of people into small areas without adequate drainage or ventilation are not seen as conducive to health whether a person believes in miasmatic theory, contagion, bacteriology, or latter-day immunology. Frederick Engels's (1971, pp. 108–24) graphic account for 1844 is well known and worth rereading. He uses miasmatic theory to explain the health consequences of the conditions he describes.

Mrs Layton (Llewellyn Davies 1977) records her late Victorian childhood in Bethnal Green. There were about forty cows kept in sheds at the back of their house and let out into the adjoining yard by day, causing a multitude of flies in summer.

> The smell was at times intolerable ... Sanitation was never considered. The water-butt was placed outside the closet, which had no flush of water and smelt abominably. The ashes and the house refuse were put in one corner of the yard only a few yards from the water-butt. This applied to all the other houses in the neighbourhood.
>
> (Llewelyn Davies, 1977, p. 3)

Mrs Layton believed this was the cause of the various kinds of fever and smallpox which continually broke out and of the cholera which once killed hundreds.

Leonora Davidoff and Catherine Hall (1987, p. 382) describe the absence of clean water and hygienic sewerage disposal in Birmingham in the early years of the nineteenth century. 'Moving to the leafy purlieus of Edgbaston did not necessarily solve the problem'; even here in the 1840s there was a lack of proper drainage, and cesspools overflowed into local wells.

Buying (doubtful) drinking water in 1848, indeed water for all purposes, at *8d* for a weekly load and *1s 3d* on washing days and sending children out to crap in the local lane (Smith, 1979, pp. 197–8 and 216) are conditions which twentieth-century British residents find it hard to imagine. Gradually piped water was extended, its quality improved, and soap came into use, but it was not until the 1890s that domestic piped water supply became safe, uninterrupted and more generally if not universally available (Smith, 1979, p. 228).

SPATIAL SEPARATION OF SOCIAL CLASSES

While in some circumstances rising bourgeoisie and labouring poor might both lack sanitation, it is also the case that from the late eighteenth century the residential areas of the better-off were increasingly separated from those of the workers. A new status system was developing and a class system being articulated (Davidoff and Hall, 1987; Perkin, 1969; Thompson, 1963). In these circumstances it became necessary for the living conditions of one part of the population to be explained and described to the other and above all to those responsible for government and the maintenance of law and order. This in Perkin's view was the great contribution of Edwin Chadwick.

> His great *Report on the Sanitary Condition of the Labouring Population of Great Britain*, of 1842, although based on the false 'miasmatic' theory of the causation of disease, for that very reason focused public attention on the foul privies, cess pools, drains, sewers and polluted water supplies of the slums from whence the poisonous miasma arose.
>
> (Perkin, 1969, p. 170).

This report drew attention to the startlingly different life chances of people living in well-to-do as opposed to impoverished areas of the great new cities such as Manchester (see also Smith, 1979, pp. 195ff.).

MIASMA, CONTAGION AND THEIR VARIANTS: CAUSES OF EPIDEMICS

Perkin refers in this quotation to the miasmatic theory, which Edwin Chadwick espoused, as 'false'. Certainly it differed from the theories of contagion of the period. Both differ radically from the 'germ theory' which was developed later and from late twentieth-century notions of immune systems. Chadwick's views, which underlay the early public health legislation, were supported by some medical men, notably Southwood Smith, who worked closely with him (upon whose reports Engels relied heavily), and by Florence Nightingale. Miasmatic theory was based on the notion 'that epidemic disease was caused by *miasma* ['a noxious emanation' – *OED*] from decomposing organic matter. Bad smells were therefore dangerous and everything must be done to improve sanitation and drainage so that air should not be corrupted and cause epidemics' (Poynter and Keele, 1961, p. 92). Marshes were a source of miasma, as were cesspools, dung heaps, rubbish dumps and slums, indeed any areas where accumulations of fetid materials led to bad smells. Disease and disorder could both emanate from the slums.

Empirical observation had long made it plain that some sorts of disease spread rapidly from person to person causing untold suffering in a population. This was believed to be a characteristic of bubonic plague (*the* plague), and efforts to contain it are documented from the time of the Black Death in the fourteenth century – although, as we now know, bubonic plague was not passed from person to person by contact but through the agency of rats and fleas (see Slack, 1985). Attempts were made to regulate entry into the country, thus hoping to control contagion.

The empirical observations about the spread of disease led to a variety of versions of contagion as a cause of epidemics. At its simplest the theory of contagion suggested that epidemic diseases were spread by contact of one person with another or with materials, such as cloth, which passed from one person to another. In some of these theories transmission was not thought of as occurring through the agency of any sort of organism, but as being quite mechanical (cf. Morris, 1976, pp. 170–1). One of the many attempts at understanding and explanation which led to further contemporary confusion was the development of *contagium vivum* theories, i.e. theories which suggested that the transmission by contact was not strictly mechanical, but was perpetrated by a living organism variously thought of as a fungus or as 'animalculae' (Pelling, 1978b, ch. 5). There was not, however, one theory of all epidemic disease. Contingent contagionism, i.e. the notion that a disease is sometimes contagious and sometimes not, became increasingly popular among medical men in the nineteenth century; this view is somewhat hard for the twentieth-century mind to comprehend (Pelling, 1978b; personal communication, 1987).

Cholera, which struck England in 1831, having seemingly advanced across Europe from India, was unknown to all but a few English army doctors who had seen it in India and later in Russia. It came to Britain at a time of extensive change in the social and economic structure of the country, developing trade and empire, and change also in the theory and practice of medicine. At first there was difficulty in diagnosing it in the early stages; those who could make the diagnosis lacked the appropriate social credentials and therefore were easy to disbelieve. For example, the Sunderland Board of Health employed an army surgeon, James Butler Kell, who had experience of cholera but lacked local social status and was a surgeon, not a physician. Neither merchants nor their labourers wanted the economic loss which was associated with quarantine (Morris, 1976, ch. 3). Furthermore the spread of the disease did not seem altogether to indicate that it was contagious – some contacts got it, others did not. The empirical evidence confused those practitioners who were in contact with the disease as to whether a contagionist theory was appropriate; whether it was appropriate to deal with it as plague had previously been dealt with. The high incidence of the disease in the poorer quarters of towns encouraged belief in some version of environmental causation.

In 1948 Akerknecht developed a sociological analysis of medical theories about epidemic disease which stood unchallenged for about thirty years. His thesis was that 'an attitude of thought appropriately called anti-contagionism attracted liberal-minded activists early in the century, just before its final downfall' (Pelling, 1978b, p. 298). Miasmatic theory was one of those 'anti-contagionist' theories. It was closely associated with the practical programme of clean water, sewage disposal, drainage and refuse disposal of the sanitarians. These were the actions and arguments which underlay the Public Health Act of 1848, the culmination of the Utilitarian campaign of Edwin Chadwick and Southwood Smith. The contagion theory on the other hand was associated with the quarantine laws. Any person or ship arriving from a place where an epidemic raged or having had contact with a person suffering from epidemic disease was to be quarantined by regulation. Such regulation necessarily impeded normal social intercourse and, along with that, trade. Merchants found their ships impounded and unable to discharge cargo. Restriction on the free movement of goods thus upset mercantilists and capitalists and also those who, like colliers, casters and keelmen, moved products such as coal in the case of the cholera epidemic in Newcastle in 1832 (Morris, 1976, p. 46).

Ackerknecht's error, in Pelling's eyes, is on the one hand to put all theories of contagion together with *contagium vivum* theories, and thus to ally them to later nineteenth-century germ theory, and on the other hand to see all theories involving miasma or 'filth' as anti-contagionist. (For an alternative view, see Cooter, 1982.) Indeed, the error of this can be illustrated from what Pasteur said to Napoleon III in 1863: 'all my ambition was to arrive at knowledge of putrid and contagious diseases' (Poynter and Keele, 1961, p. 116). Ackerknecht has obscured a struggle between those medical men who supported the public health movement and joined with government in the General Board of Health and with which Chadwick was associated and those who were the élite of orthodox medicine.

> Forty years after John Snow had demonstrated that cholera was conveyed by contaminated water and nine years after Koch had identified the micro-organism which caused it, the RCP still gave no special warnings about care in handling the patient and his dejecta or about boiling water intended for the household: the two procedures the masses could best follow.
>
> (Smith, 1979, p. 233)

John Snow had demonstrated in 1854 that the Broad Street pump was the cause of the cholera epidemic in that area. This was empirical knowledge based on observation. Snow could not explain it although he tried various theories (Pelling, 1978b, ch. 6). It was explained when Robert Koch identified the relevant organism, *vibrio cholerae*, in 1884 (although credit is now given for this to Filippo Pacini, who published his findings in 1854: Pelling, 1978b, p. 3).

At a time when the medical profession was not fully consolidated, medical technology was changing and the social framework was in flux, it is not surprising that there was a lack of consensus which emerged in the pages of the *Lancet* of the day.

THE ROLE OF MEDICAL AND STATE ELITES

The picture received so far from all this confusion is of the élite of British medicine as represented by the Royal College of Physicians adhering to outdated positions and of those in middling positions struggling hard to make sense of new diseases and of old diseases in the light of new knowledge. Of the 1832 epidemic Morris (1976, p. 183) says: 'Contagion was a ruling class doctrine.' It was the doctrine of strong government, although in the end the supporters of miasmatic theories through Chadwick were to have a more profound effect upon the public health, for it was they who initiated public health legislation.

An abrupt change in government policy took place in 1854 when Chadwick was deposed. John Simon, the first medical man to hold government office, replaced him in the new post of Medical Officer and later became head of the Medical Department under the Privy Council. Simon advanced public health legislation and health control measures with policies greatly opposed by Edwin Chadwick, Florence Nightingale and the sanitarians (see Eyler, 1979, ch. 7). Simon shifted the emphasis 'from sanitary engineering to sanitary science' (Lawrence, 1981, p. 154). In 1875 the Public Health Act consolidated Simon's somewhat piecemeal work over the preceding twenty years. The Act established compulsory medical officers of health (MOH) at local government level. Being an MOH was not their only occupation, but in this capacity they had power to control nuisances of all kinds and to impose health regulations upon a locality even against the opposition of local tradesmen and dignitaries. Many of these remained discontented, as did the workers, about the controls imposed upon them. But a long road had by now been travelled from the early attempts at control which had caused riots in 1832. Also in 1875 Cambridge examined its first candidates in sanitary science. By the 1890s public health had emerged as a specialism with its own journal (Lawrence, 1981, p. 161; see also Watkins, 1985). New means of controlling the populace (meaning the working class) were in place, and medicine was in charge of them.

DEVELOPMENTS IN MEDICAL KNOWLEDGE: BIOMEDICINE EMERGES

During the same period when Simon's influence was strong there were important developments in medical science which, although independent of Simon, were used by him. It was in 1864 that Louis Pasteur isolated organisms under the microscope and proclaimed, 'Germs cause putrefaction: do away with germs and you will not get putrefaction' (Poynter and Keele, 1961, p. 62). The next year Joseph Lister made his first experiment in antiseptic surgery, later on developing asepsis, the principle whereby in the operating theatre infection is prevented from entering rather than being controlled during the operation as in Lister's first experiments.

Lister, a surgeon, had seen the correctness of Pasteur's analysis of bacteria and applied it medically in the operating theatre. Pasteur, a chemist, could not make medical applications. From then on a new discipline of bacteriology developed, and the concepts of disease developed in France at the outset of modern clinical medicine were modified. Now disease was seen 'as the reaction of the whole man to invasion by bacteria, not just that of one or two of his organs' (Poynter and Keele, 1961, p. 64). Knowledge that was important for hospital curative medicine, especially for surgery, was also important for public hygiene.

However, it would be wrong to imagine that Simon was able to legislate so successfully on public health because there was now medical consensus on the cause of epidemic disease. This was by no means the case. The conflicts had continued to rage, and it was not until the end of the century that medical concordance upon the correctness and importance of the germ theory was established. As a theory

> it was immensely successful, it had a very high predictive power and the potential for massive technological exploitation as the development of diphtheria anti-toxin showed . . . What might be called the theatrical resources of the theory, its capacity to explain, mystify, amaze and create, fostered public esteem.
>
> (Lawrence, 1981, p. 163)

This consensus of medical view about the cause of infection, the final arrival of biomedicine, did much to help consolidate the medical profession, but that is to run ahead of our story.

SEXUALITY AND CONTAGIOUS DISEASE

Venereal disease in the nineteenth century was (as AIDS has become in the late twentieth) a public health issue, although until latterly VD has not always been included in histories of public health (although see Brockington, 1965, p. 231). Brian Harrison (1981) discusses it in the context of the women's movement and women's health; he does not discuss its scientific or medical underpinning. The issue is, as Harrison recognizes, important in understanding the relationship between medical men and the state and the role of medicine in controlling women. Although crucially important to both men and women, the attempts at state control of venereal disease were directed entirely at women. Medicine, I would argue, was acting for men as a group to help sustain their freedoms and their dominance. Medicine was also defending itself against the incursion of self-help and lay knowledge. For these reasons I would want to modify Morris's conclusion mentioned earlier and say that contagion was a ruling-class doctrine, but also a *male* ruling-class doctrine.

There had long been an understanding that venereal diseases were passed from person to person in the sexual act. With regard to other epidemic diseases disputes between contagionists, miasmatists and others had been about the necessity for quarantine, the contagionists insisting on it. In the case of VD it was not suggested that soldiers and sailors should be confined to barracks or refused shore leave (i.e. be quarantined) until they were given a clean bill of venereal health, although this was the proposed procedure where all other alleged contagious diseases were concerned. Instead it was assumed that women were the source of the contagion and not its victims. None of the erudite debates about contagion or other theories can explain that, nor can arguments about whether actions were in the interests of the rising bourgeoisie or in the defence of the old landed aristocracy. The Contagious Diseases Acts were clearly directed against working-class women (A. S. C. Butler, 1954, p. 73; J. E. Butler, 1910, *passim*; Rowbotham, 1974a, p. 53; Uglow, 1983, p. 152). Any competent explanation of this has to do with the relationship of women to men and in particular with men's understanding of what they wanted women to do and be, since the making of legislation was at that time entirely in men's hands.

The legislation, introduced in 1864 by the Lord of the Admiralty under the title Contagious Diseases (Animals) Act, arose from the wish to control VD in the armed forces. Outside Parliament it was assumed to be to do with the afflictions of cattle, hence the title of the Walkowitzes' article 'We are not Beasts of the Field' (1974). 'On the contrary, it was entirely to do with women; and, in its final form, it was an attempt to rail off prostitutes and keep them under surveillance for the protection of men' (Butler, 1954, p. 64). There were in all three Acts: 1864, 1866 and 1869 (Uglow, 1983). Their introduction can be understood only in the light of Victorian notions of sexuality and of the proper place of women.

Western thought had long included the contradictory notions that women represent the ultimate in either purity or evil and are finally the most subversive force. These notions had been associated with patriarchal (using that word in its technical anthropological sense), male-dominated societies. Woman has been either on the pedestal or in the depths; either the supporter and comforter as well as the life-giver or the destroyer of men. Unsurprisingly neither image in any era has approximated to the empirical reality of what women have been and do. The way in which these images have been invoked and used has varied from one historic period to another, but they have persisted and been espoused by women as well as men (L'Esperance, 1977).

In the nineteenth century this dichotomy was stressed in close relationship with the ideas which surrounded the bourgeois family and strongly influenced the ideas of the burgeoning middling classes. The role of the pure wife and mother was underscored by strong religious faith (Davidoff and Hall, 1987, pp. 114). The degradation of one group of women was inseparable from the false reverence kept for the wife of the bourgeois (Rowbotham, 1974b, pp. 65–6). For the most part the medical profession supported and promulgated this view.

There were thus good women who were virgins at marriage, who suffered but did not enjoy (because women were believed not to have the capacity) the sexual attentions of their husbands. There was a good deal to be said for the celibate woman, but after all the race had to be perpetuated, so the sacrifice involved in marriage and child bearing was praiseworthy. There were on the other hand women who had 'fallen', that is, they had enjoyed (or merely experienced) intercourse outside marriage; one episode would be enough to put a woman beyond the pale of polite society. Having 'fallen' there was little other choice than a life of prostitution. It was hard for the Victorian middle class to understand that a woman might choose to sell her body simply as a means of earning a living. Perhaps it could be understood in the light of extreme poverty, but as a preferred alternative among a variety of health-destroying occupations open to the working class it was incomprehensible. Nor was the way women might drift in and out of prostitution, as common then as now, recognized (L'Esperance, 1977).

This lack of comprehension derived from the notion that women and men were quite different in their sexual make-up and wishes. Men were 'driven' by strong sexual urges. They required an outlet for these. Hence the necessity of the occupation of prostitution; it went along with monogamy and was needed to sustain it. Men were not seen as either pure or impure, in the way that nineteenth-century women were either angels or whores, or witches in an earlier period (Greg, 1979). But men were not let off the Victorian hook of maximum sexual control. Masturbation and night emissions were not only morally wrong, they were also medically pathological. Treatises from medical men such as Acton (1862) made this plain (L'Esperance, 1977). Men were expected to exercise strong self-control over these urges (or submit to regimes to prevent the involuntary wet dreams) and over their urges with regard to women other than their wives. However, the temptations which they experienced were enormous and could be resisted only with the help of women. Thus it was women's fault if men were overcome, and the particular sin of the prostitute was to tempt them. This had always been a problem in Christendom, but with the apparent arrival of syphilis (from where? Variously Italy, Spain, or France depending on your own country) in about the fifteenth century (Poynter and Keele, 1961, p. 89) the punishment for sin became worldly suffering in terms of disease.

Only in such a context is it possible to understand how it might be that the 'state regulation of vice', as it was called, sought to control only women and that the possibility of quarantining men who had the disease was never considered. The threat to the fabric of middle-class men's domestic lives which prostitutes were seen to pose was enough for them to see women as the exclusive object of regulation. As men as well as officers they understood what difficulties their men in barracks or on returning ships faced. They did not focus on the possible spreading of disease that those men might be causing by contacts made abroad and/or homosexual activities on board ships or in garrisons, a charge Josephine Butler laid against sailors and soldiers (Uglow, 1983, p. 155).

That was yet another topic not to be discussed. The Contagious Diseases Acts were applied only in designated areas (garrison towns and ports). Here women were liable to be stopped in the street, asked to sign to say they were prostitutes and to submit to medical examination. The powers of the special police involved were not restricted; they could apprehend any woman in the designated areas. Contrary to normal British justice the onus was on the woman to prove her innocence. Rich men were said to be pleased with the regulations and to travel to designated areas where they knew they could indulge themselves so long as the woman they bought had a recent certificate (Butler, 1954, pp. 72–3). Women who refused to submit voluntarily were brought before magistrates and forced to be examined. If found 'diseased' they were incarcerated in a special Lock hospital or the Lock ward of a general hospital (Uglow, 1983; the term 'Lock hospital' derives from the Lock lazar-house in Southwark, but its origin is unclear: *OED*, 1983).

France under Napoleon had instituted the registration of prostitutes in 1802. (A brief overview of prostitution in France can be found in O'Faolin and Martines, 1979, pp. 302–16; also in Butler, 1910, who deals with France and other European countries and the USA.) Nearly thirty years previously Flora Tristan (Hawkes, 1982) had recorded her view of the degradation and health hazards to which prostitutes were subjected in London and how women and children were ruthlessly snared into the trade. She saw no point in forbidding brothels as English law did, for it 'was an inevitable consequence of the way European society is organized' (p. 93). The London excesses were a consequence of 'The profound corruption of the wealthy classes and the high prices they can afford to pay (which) protect and encourage this obscene trade' (p. 97). Whatever may have been the inevitability of brothels, central regulation on the French model was not the English way any more than it was in hospital provision or the care of the poor. For reasons of this kind the Contagious Diseases legislation related only to certain areas. Wholesale legislation would have too greatly infringed English ideas of liberty.

JOSEPHINE BUTLER AND THE MEDICAL MEN

Protest followed, led by those who had opposed slavery and by other libertarians. The leading role of Josephine Butler is instructive. An evangelical Christian and a philanthropist, daughter of an abolitionist, a 'salvationist feminist' (Taylor, 1983, p. 277), she became the leader of a persistent movement for the abolition of the Acts. She had been involved in rescue work before becoming president of the National Ladies' Association of the campaign. She had a clear understanding, rare in the upper and middle classes, of the privations experienced by working-class women. She saw the regulations as an encroachment on the liberty of women and the compulsory physical examinations as a violation of their very womanhood and one from which poor women, not the well-to-do, would suffer. She did not argue for sexual freedom for women, could not understand prostitutes who said that way of life was their preference, but believed that the purity which was expected of women should also be expected of men. Implacably opposed to the 'double standard', she wished the same restraints and the same liberties to be enjoyed and experienced by both sexes. She took monogamy and the sanctity of the family very literally (A. S. G. Butler, 1954; J. E. Butler, 1910; Taylor, 1983; Uglow, 1983).

The part played by the medical profession is of particular interest to us. Reading Josephine Butler's memoirs (1919, *passim*) it is clear that medical men were to her most at fault in influencing and supporting the passage of the legislation. From time to time she gratefully acknowledges medical men who helped the campaign against the Acts for reasons of religion, philosophy, or politics. She wishes the medical profession could be 'purified' for mostly she sees medical men as arch enemies and the architects of this affront to the person and the liberty of women. They require purifying for they support the 'double standard' of purity for women and sexual licence for men (see also Harrison, 1981, pp. 33 and 45). Butler relied on the primacy of her God and was strongly monogamous. Others supported the campaign against the Acts for more radical reasons. Sharing Butler's belief in her rights over her own body, they included atheists and believers in free love (Butler, 1910; Harrison, 1981, p. 21, 34 and 37; Uglow, 1983).

There is no doubt of Butler's radicalism, however. Secrecy surrounds medical knowledge; it is esoteric, and from this comes professional power and influence, for only the initiated may know and speak of this knowledge. It was also a part of Victorian sexual morality that women were not to speak about sexual matters; but were not meant to know about them, it would offend against their purity and delicacy. It follows they were supposed neither to know nor speak about their own bodies. Josephine Butler, this respectable middle-class Christian, encouraged women to speak in the 'hygiene' sections of Contagious Diseases conferences in defiance of these taboos (Butler, 1910, p. 163). The campaign was therefore not only a challenge to the Acts, it was a challenge to doctors as doctors, developing lay understanding of their esoteric domain. It was also a challenge to doctors as men. The Contagious Diseases Acts were finally repealed after a long campaign in 1886, and England gave up any attempt to adopt the continental system of the regulation of prostitutes, but the Acts had done their work of constituting prostitutes as a class (Walkowitz and Walkowitz, 1974, p. 220).

Above and beyond this particular issue, the evidence is that nineteenth-century medical men used their new scientific authority to support the norm that women were the weak and submissive sex, that they should be passive and confined to the domestic domain, unless they were working women. The medical role in blocking higher education and the professions to women will be referred to in Chapter 6.

Mention may be made here, however, of medical efforts in defining sexuality. Research in the late nineteenth century suggested that any deviation from the heterosexual was abnormal; homosexuality among both women and men was redefined as pathology, to be pitied rather than condemned. Physical measurements as well as analyses of psychological dispositions were made. Same-sex love could in no way be natural. More recent appraisals of these works suggest that they may better be seen as medical assertions of the values of the new mode of male domination than as valid scientific enterprises (see, for example, L'Esperance, 1977; Faderman, *c.* 1980; Lhomond, 1986).

BIRTH CONTROL

Medical men were also less than helpful in another major public health arena. It is now generally recognized (e.g. Cochrane, 1972; McKeown, 1971) that birth control has been a major cause of the improvement in longevity. The spread of birth control information owes nothing to the majority of medical men, although much to a few and to a small band of dedicated medical women.

In the first half of the nineteenth century hindrance, not help, came from medical men. Information about sexuality was among the matters which orthodox doctors left to the 'quacks and charlatans' (see pages 50–1). The sheath, the douche, the sponge and coitus interruptus were discussed as methods of birth control, but not in the medical press, whose 'main response to the issue of "artificial" means of contraception was almost total silence' (McLaren, 1977, p. 95). Silence as a means of rejection is, of course, one of the most potent. It did not prevent the ultimate spread of contraceptive methods, but it did ensure that it took place outside élite medical circles and was slower than it would have been had it received medical help and approval much earlier. Instead part of the early birth control movement took on the form of a self-help movement designed to encourage lay people to have faith in themselves and to control their own lives (McLaren, 1977. See also J. A. Banks, 1954 and 1981; Banks and Banks, 1964).

BIOMEDICINE ESTABLISHED

In a number of important ways biomedicine can be said to have been established by the end of the nineteenth century. Orthodox medicine had a network of hospitals and medical schools at its disposal; its practitioners had become those upon whom the state relied for advice on the health of the nation; they it was who were responsible for monitoring the state of the national health. How they became consolidated as such a powerful occupation is discussed in Chapter 6.

At the outset it was not at all clear that the responsibility for hygiene would be a medical one. The sanitary engineers were after all not primarily medical men. The responsibility for care of the sick in epidemic conditions did however fall to medical men, who also became involved with the attempts to control and regulate epidemic disease. Entrepreneurial capitalism had also by end-century come to terms with the benefits of some state intervention to regulate health.

After 1875 medical officers had adequate powers, but clinicians continued to look upon them as lower forms of medical life (Lawrence, 1981, p. 161), although as registered medical practitioners they had equality with all others so registered. Arguably housing, sanitation, water supply and pure food taken together with improved nutrition and birth control were more effective in improving the health and longevity of the population than all the work of the curative practitioners throughout the nineteenth century (McKeown, 1971).

A price paid for this improvement was an increased control and regulation of the population; moral welfare was imposed upon hospital and workhouse inmates along with the curative regimes they experienced. The public health measures also had their regulative aspects. Epidemics provided opportunities for intrusion into the homes of ordinary people to insist upon fumigation, ventilation and other matters (Morris, 1976). Medical men had become active partners in the control of the population for the good of their health according to the insights provided by medical knowledge and the interests of the profession.

Although agreement was not complete until the early years of the twentieth century, by the end of the nineteenth bacteriology was well on the way to acceptance and with it the triumph of biomedicine. It was already more than a hundred years since the new medical 'gaze' had begun the transformation of medical knowledge. Already according to Armstrong (1983b), even before there was consensus about bacteriology, a new and extended medical gaze was emerging. Before however we can trace medical knowledge and medical practice into the twentieth century we must investigate the major changes which had taken place in the division of health labour in the nineteenth.

6 Organizing the Division of Labour in Health Care

Chapter 5 discussed nineteenth-century developments in medical knowledge, in particular the two modes associated with the hospitals and with public health, the latter being taken over by medicine in the third quarter of the century. Of all the plethora of healing modes and cosmologies which had been available in the sixteenth and seventeenth centuries, by the end of the nineteenth century one mode of healing, itself now being transformed into biomedicine, came to dominate all others. This mode is sometimes referred to as allopathic (literally, treatment by opposites) to distinguish it from other modes, notably homoeopathy (treatment by similarities; see also Chapter 11).

The purpose of the present chapter is to describe and analyse the social and political movements which made domination by this mode possible. In the course of the nineteenth century allopathic medicine became centrally organized, legitimated by the state and male dominated; medical practitioners became the leaders of all other officially recognized health-care workers. In 1858 the General Medical Council was established. By the end of the century the reformed nurses were in place as 'handmaidens' to doctors but with their own hierarchical occupational structure. Medical leaders had accepted that doctors could respectably practise obstetrics, and midwives were accepted within the official health-care division of labour but in a position clearly subordinate to medical practitioners. A hierarchy of health workers had thus developed which was part of the class structure of the society and also of a redefined sexual division of labour in the public domain.

Our first task must be to examine how the central organization and state legitimation of allopathic medicine came about; then to examine how the gender order was redefined as emerging occupations jostled for position, establishing a new division of labour, and how male domination was reinforced; the attempts of women to become doctors, the displacement of the midwives and the 'new' nurses. To understand these processes we need to locate them in the social and economic changes that were taking place and thus creating the necessary opportunities.

Before we can embark on this enterprise however we have to come to terms with the notion of a profession, since claims and counter-claims about professions and professionalism have been of the essence in the creation and the maintenance of the division of labour in health care.

OCCUPATIONS WHICH CLAIM TO BE PROFESSIONS

There has been a good deal of dispute over the meaning and sociological value of the term 'profession' and as to whether there are ways in which professions may be distinguished from other occupations. Eliot Freidson has argued that it is useful to think of a profession as an occupation which has assumed a dominant position in a division of labor, so that it gains control over the determination of the substance of its own work ... it is autonomous or self-directing ... [sustaining] this special status by its pervasive profession of the extraordinary trustworthiness of its members.

(1970a, p. xvii)

A profession is thus a particular type of occupation (p. xvi), of which medicine is one example. It is moreover an 'organized consulting profession' (p. 5). To think of professions as a particular type of occupation is to my mind useful. However, the claims that others in the division of labour have made to be professions and the problems they have encountered have led to the use of such curious notions as 'semi-professions' (Etzioni, 1969). This notion derives, on the one hand, from the claims of organized members of an occupation to professional status and, on the other, to the subordinate position of their occupation in the division of labour. It is for these reasons that I prefer to think in terms of occupations which make claims to be professions (Stacey, 1984). It then becomes an empirical question as to what claims are made, how well the occupational group succeeds in its claim and under what circumstances. These are matters of interactions of groups with each other and of the exterior constraints within which those interactions take place. In the case of nineteenth-century medicine these claims succeeded remarkably well, and we must examine why this was, just as we must examine why the claims of midwives and nurses were less successful.

Freidson (1970a), in the argument quoted, stresses particular characteristics which distinguish professions, namely, their autonomy and control over their work. There have in the past been attempts to enumerate the 'traits' which constitute an occupation as a profession based upon the notion that there is something special and timeless about a 'profession'. Terence Johnson (1972) has shown that this is not very fruitful. He focused on the relationship the professional has with the client. He argues that this is the key, that professions are a particular institutionalized form of client control. Freidson also sees relations with clients as crucial; a profession attempts to define clients' problems and to manage clients. The autonomous position of the profession in society 'permits it to recreate the layman's world' in its own terms (1970a, p. xvii).

Johnson, on the other hand, stresses the *un*specialism (1972, p. 41) of the client; clients who lack exterior sources of power (of which the eighteenth-century noble patron had many) are relatively helpless. The medical practitioner is a specialist, and the generalist consumer is socially and economically dependent, in addition to being considerably socially distanced from her/his adviser. In these circumstances, Johnson argues, the specialist knowledge of the medically qualified creates systematic relations of interdependence but of a kind which the medical person can dominate, thus achieving work autonomy (1972, pp. 41–2). The situation is one in which the uncertainty which inheres in any producer/consumer relation is reduced at the expense of the consumer. Esoteric knowledge is developed from which the patient is excluded.

PROFESSIONS IN THE CLASS STRUCTURE

Johnson stresses the historical specificity of profession, as does Freidson (1986), Johnson seeing the professional/client relation rooted in the conditions of the societies in which they are found. Specifically he argues that the nature of client control changes as societies change; the professional mode of the nineteenth century was possible only because of the development of industrial capitalism and the rise of the bourgeoisie. The relationship of the occupation to the class structure is therefore of the essence for Johnson but not so for Freidson (1977), who sees specific institutional arrangements as the critical feature (1986). In a later paper, Johnson (1977) argues a narrower and more abstract Marxist case that professions in capitalism specifically legitimate the existing class structure by claims to moral neutrality.

Parry and Parry (1976) also see the importance of relating the rise of the professions to the class structure, but their approach is somewhat different. Taking the control which professional associations themselves develop over professional colleagues (p. 248), Parry and Parry argue for a process of upward social mobility on the part of general practitioners; the colleges of physicians and surgeons had always been groups of peers designed to pursue collective ends and not primarily concerned to control clients. Parry and Parry demonstrate well the status considerations felt by the nineteenth-century medical men as social actors (see, for example, 1976, pp. 104–16). Nineteenth-century society was after all undergoing considerable transformations in its stratification system; the changing and expanding division of labour in medicine would have made medical men and their wives sharply conscious of newly emerging status groups and rankings. It was not however simply a more elaborated status system in which doctors and their wives were successfully upwardly mobile. As Johnson argues, the class system itself was emerging (Perkin, 1969; Thompson, 1963). The new kinds of medical practitioner were playing their part in its emergence as well as in the emergence of new status groups.

GENDER AS WELL AS CLASS STATUS

An account of these processes is however inadequate without reference to the sexual division of labour. None of the conventional accounts of professions and professionalization address the genderized nature of the division of labour; indeed, in many the reader might be unaware that there are two sexes in the world. Yet the empirical evidence is that historically occupations which have made successful claims to be professions, which have gained work autonomy and become dominant, have all been male occupations; those which have succeeded less well, Etzioni's semi-professions, have been female or female-dominated occupations.

Recognition of the gender order is as important as of the class structure if one is to be able competently to analyse professions and professionalism. At the outset of this book (see pages 8–9) I indicated that a distinction between public and private domains is necessary to comprehend the division of labour in health care. This differentiation between public and domestic domains is partly an empirically existing and changing one and in part is ideological, an ideology which helps to mould the empirical reality. These ideas have to be specified more closely for the purposes of analysing the emergent health-care division of labour of the nineteenth century.

Eva Gamarnikow (1978) has attempted to do this for reformed nursing. She seeks to understand the sexual division of labour in health care in the nineteenth century in materialist terms, not however in a conventional Marxist way based only on its relation to capitalism but based on the relation of the division of labour to patriarchy. She rejects biologically based explanations which assume that a particular division of labour is in some sense 'natural'. She would thus disagree with the views of women like Josephine Butler, the reformer, Elizabeth Blackwell and other nineteenth-century women doctors, who felt that women could make a natural and special contribution to health care on account of their sex, a view also shared by Florence Nightingale and other nurse reformers (see page 90). Gamarnikow sees the division as social and not biological. Patriarchy she defines 'as an autonomous system of social relations between men and women in which men are dominant' (1978, p. 99). Her use of 'patriarchy' is thus equivalent to my 'male-dominated gender order' (see pages 7–8). Male–female relations are social relations 'which among other things organize biological reproduction, rather than being determined by biology' (p. 99).

Following Delphy (1977), Gamarnikow argues that 'the marriage contract is a labour contract by which men appropriate women's labour power' (1978, p. 100). While men can only expect unwaged services from women they are married to, the sexual division of labour encompasses all women and men. This comes about, Gamarnikow argues, because all women are treated as potential wives–mothers simply because they are biological females. Thus all women are identified as a separate category of worker, and the sexual division of labour then 'situates individuals in jobs and designates jobs as sex specific' (p. 101).

ORIGINS OF MALE DOMINATION OF PROFESSIONS

To my mind there is a great deal to be gained from an analysis which looks at both health care and marital relations as labour processes, as Gamarnikow proposes (although there are obviously other ways in which both should be analysed as well). I would however want to situate the analysis also in other facets of the social structure and to establish the conditions in which the male-dominated gender order could take the course it did. European, including British, society had been male dominated for many hundreds of years before the nineteenth century. From the time the public domain began to emerge as distinct from the domestic domain and its members met in another locale than the household, the public domain had been strongly male dominated. This followed from the patriarchal structure of kinship around the twelfth century (Stacey and Price, 1981, ch. 2).

The public world of the nineteenth century was almost exclusively male, certainly the governing bodies of the state, legislature, judiciary and military were. The corporations had for centuries been systematically excluding women. By mid-century the cult of domesticity was at its height. When in this and previous chapters I have written 'medical men' it is no sexist slip of the typewriter, for they were men – not that women throughout the century were happy to accept that situation. Paradoxically but perhaps also predictably (with hindsight) the struggles began in earnest just as the domestication of women, especially middle-class women, was at its height. Through their command of the public domain as well as their patriarchal authority in the domestic domain men were able to ensure that the occupations which succeeded in their claims to professional status were male occupations. In the nineteenth century women were still non-persons with no legal or public existence.

Medical teaching and research could not have taken place without the poor and powerless people who submitted to the treatment offered in hospitals. Neither could they have developed without the subordinate labour of the nurses in hospitals and of the wives and domestic servants who supported the physicians, surgeons and apothecaries in their households. I shall first look at the professionalizing activities of the medical men and then turn to the sexual division of labour.

ENTREPRENEURS OF HEALING

We spoke earlier of healing knowledge of three kinds: domestic, folk and professional (pages 28–30). The medical entrepreneurship which Roy Porter (1983) discussed (see page 51) developed in the seventeenth and eighteenth centuries outside the domestic sphere and separate from folk medicine, although the latter was widely popular. This entrepreneurship was confined neither to trade nor to the profession of allopathic medicine. Improved communication and the development of advertising and publishing all helped this burgeoning commercialism. Waddington (1984, pp. 24–6) has shown how the upwardly mobile provided many new patients for orthodox practitioners; they also provided clients for those described as quacks.

While these middling classes were not as powerless as the hospitalized poor and were treated in their own homes, they lacked the power of the eighteenth-century patrons which Jewson (1974) described. The development of the market further changed the doctor–patient relationship, giving more power to the medical men. This constituted a further condition making successful claims for status by medical men possible.

A NEW DIVISION OF MEDICAL LABOUR

Changes were taking place too in the hierarchy of the medical élite and the division of labour within it. Three facets must be noted: first, the development of hospital consultants as a social group of influence, the emergence of the general practitioner and the tension between these two categories of medical men; second, the emergence of the concept of a medical *profession*; and, third, its collective organization by mid-century under the surveillance of the General Medical Council. The critical development, however, was the emergence of a self-conscious occupation aiming for control of work situation and client, controlling its own supply and its own remuneration.

We saw at the end of Chapter 3 how medicine had been divided into three segments – the physicians, surgeons and apothecaries – although these were probably less clear in practice than in law. The lines were by no means clear even before the nineteenth century. In Chapter 4 we noted how, in both the old and the new voluntary hospitals of the eighteenth century, the apothecaries along with the pupils did most of the daily and demanding work, while the physicians and surgeons held honorary appointments and visited once or twice a week and sometimes less; how also the tiny minority of gentlemanly physicians educated at Oxford and Cambridge felt themselves superior to the workmen surgeons with their origins in trade. Jeanne Peterson (1978) has demonstrated that in the hospitals these divisions began to be broken down. Physicians and surgeons began to develop a unity of interest as they worked together in the hospitals and co-operated in the medical schools, and also in gaining medical control over against the lay boards of governors and the lay administrators of the hospitals. The differences between them came to be of somewhat less importance than their common interest as hospital consultants. The establishment of medical education in the University of London, which rapidly became popular, can be said to be the beginning of the end of the division between the élite education of the physicians and the practical education of the surgeons (Peterson, 1978, p. 68). They mutually gained in prestige as teaching and research expanded in the new medical schools and hospitals became the centres of medical excellence and purveyors of new knowledge. The medical schools also encouraged a sense of solidarity among the students, primarily with their own school – the pride of being a Guy's or a Thomas's man – but beyond that loyalty to medicine itself (Peterson, 1978; Waddington, 1984). The hospital consultants therefore began to see themselves and to be seen as a collectivity and a superior élite over against other qualified practitioners. This, rather than the breakdown of the historical division into physicians, surgeons and apothecaries stressed, for example, by Holloway (1964 and 1966) and Waddington (1984), may be the critical development of the nineteenth century.

There were many sources of dispute between general practitioners and the hospital consultants. The hospital doctors had available to them a majority of the most wealthy private patients, and could supplement their income from the medical students' fees. In addition the general practitioners believed that the consultants stole their patients. When a local practitioner referred a patient to a hospital consultant for advice he might not get her/him back. This came to be increasingly the case with the establishment of out-patient dispensaries. These provided interesting clinical material for the medical schools additional to the in-patients and a way for the 'deserving' poor to get medical treatment on an out-patient basis. They diminished the general practitioners' clientele, however (Abel-Smith, 1964; Loudon, 1986, *passim*; Peterson, 1978, pp. 226–31).

The new teaching and research centres were not exclusively in London, but London dominated the English scene. (Scottish developments were somewhat different.) In addition to tensions between consultants and GPs there were also tensions between London and the provinces. The medical societies in the provinces were not exclusively composed of general practitioners; many reformist organizations cut across corporate lines (Peterson, 1978, p. 19).

As the nineteenth century proceeded, groups of general practitioners were formed, and the struggles associated with the new division of labour accelerated. Out of these emerged the British Medical Association, destined to be the major champion of general practitioners at least until the College of General Practitioners was established in the second half of the twentieth century. The BMA still remains the GPs' principal trade union, although it represents other medical categories as well. It was from the Provincial Medical and Surgical Association, founded in 1832, that the present British Medical Association emerged. A relatively short-lived and much more radical body, which was London based, had started in 1836, originally with the name British Medical Association. It claimed to speak for general practitioners throughout the kingdom. It campaigned specifically for medical reform, something which the Provincial Medical and Surgical Association did not begin to do until 1840. The Provincial Association's original aims were friendly and scientific. Unlike the BMA, it was led by physicians and surgeons, not general practitioners. The original BMA ceased to exist in the mid-1840s, and in 1855 the Provincial Association took over its name (Waddington, 1984, pp. 69–75; see also Parry and Parry, 1976, pp. 128–9; Peterson, 1978, pp. 24–5). Other societies were formed by Poor Law Medical Officers and the Medical Officers of Asylums and Hospitals, also groups of medical men who felt neither the London élite nor other associations understood or represented their situation (Peterson, 1978, p. 23).

These activities have to be seen, as Waddington (1977, pp. 182–3; 1984, esp. ch. 2) points out, as part of a contradiction between a new occupational structure and traditional corporate institutions which were organized on quite different principles. The struggles were structural in origin and not to be attributed simply to the actions of exceptional individuals (1984). He also indicates, as does Peterson (1978), how great was the range of wealth among early nineteenth-century medical practitioners. The hospital consultants, as we have said, could attain great wealth and also power, both within the medical profession and beyond it. Some of the new general practitioners made comfortable livings, but such evidence suggests that some were in or on the verge of poverty (Peterson, 1978, esp. ch. V; Waddington, 1984, pp. 29–30). It is certainly the case that medical men in the nineteenth century could not all be placed in the same status situation (Davidoff and Hall, 1987, pp. 264–5). It remains doubtful if they even had a common class situation in either the Weberian or the Marxian sense.

MEDICINE BECOMES A PROFESSION

As their occupational consciousness developed and with whatever justification, medical practitioners began to complain that there was an oversupply of their labour. This may seem surprising given the increase in the numbers of people seeking treatment. Waddington (1984, pp. 140–1) suggests that the profession may have been overcrowded in the first part of the nineteenth century when the expansion of medical schools led to an increase in the supply of doctors. Demand was measured, not by the total population, but only by profitable sections of it (Pelling, 1987). From early in the nineteenth century an agitation developed to restrict entry to the profession and to seek state aid to that end. A debate in the *Lancet* in the early 1840s on these lines finally proposed a strategy to impose high standards of entry qualifications. This would reduce the numbers qualifying, 'the character of the profession would be greatly elevated, and the public welfare would be promoted' (*Lancet*, 1842–3, *1*, p. 764, quoted in Waddington, 1984, p. 142). These moves were afoot at the same time as the more entrepreneurially minded were busy touting for trade in the market.

The pro-regulation ideas finally emerged in the 1858 Medical Act which established the General Council of Medical Education and Registration known as the General Medical Council (GMC), but only after seventeen previous Bills had been presented and defeated. The 1858 Act charged the Council to regulate the medical profession on behalf of the state, to oversee medical education and to maintain a register of qualified medical practitioners. It was this Act which finally made a distinction between the qualified and the unqualified. It did not however prevent the unqualified practising healing arts (nor indeed does the 1978 Act by which the present medical profession is governed). What it meant, then as now, was that no one other than a registered practitioner could call himself a qualified medical practitioner (Parry and Parry, 1976, pp. 128–30; Peterson, 1978; Waddington, 1984, chs. 6 and 7).

THE PROFESSION UNITED?

However, the Act left much unchanged:

> The privileges and powers of the corporations were left intact, as was the hierarchical order of the profession. The GMC itself had largely supervisory powers, and its membership was made up of representatives of the Royal Colleges, the Apothecaries Society, the universities granting medical degrees, and a number of Crown nominees. There were no seats specifically designed for general practitioners.
>
> (Peterson, 1978, p. 35)

General practitioners did not gain representation on the GMC until the Medical Act of 1886 (Peterson, 1978, p. 233).

The 1858 Act is often hailed as a great milestone in the successful professionalization of medicine. It reflected a new unity among the practitioners of allopathic medicine by putting them on one register whose members were thereafter the officially recognized healers (Loudon, 1986, pp. 297–301). This official status becomes increasingly important in the successful domination by the end of the century of biomedicine over all other healing arts. From the time of the register, official appointments could be held only by registered practitioners. Thus it was these practitioners who worked for and co-operated with the state in pursuit of the enhancement and regulation of public health, as Chapter 5 demonstrated.

Only in these limited senses can the Act be said, as Parry and Parry (1976, p. 131) suggest it did, to have 'closed' the profession; nor did it instantly unify it. Peterson's (1978) account of the subsequent years makes this plain. Indeed, it increased the distance between the London élites and the mass of practitioners (Peterson, 1978, p. 231). Medical Officers of Health, Poor Law officers and other salaried employees continued to be despised.

CONTROL OF ENTRY?

Did the 1858 Act restrict entry into the occupation? Peterson (1978, p. 238), whose work focuses on London, argues that the corporate rulers of medicine did not recognize the plight of the general practitioners and refused to restrict enrolments or increase standards. She says that these solutions to overcrowding and low pay were not considered in mid-century. Waddington (1984, pp. 148 ff.) on the other hand, using calculations based on the Census figures for 1861, 1871 and 1881, claims that in the twenty years or so after the Act of 1858 the growth in the number of medical practitioners in England and Wales was quite minimal and was far outstripped by the growth of the population. By the 1870s and 1880s there was a clearly recognized shortage of doctors, a shortage which was drawn to the attention of the 1882 Royal Commission and blamed by the Cambridge Professor of Anatomy on the GMC for raised standards in the period 1867–75 (Waddington, 1984, p. 150).

Waddington's thesis in summary is that medical practice had changed in the course of the nineteenth century from being a relatively insecure and often part-time occupation at the outset to being relatively secure, stable and rewarding by the end (although, as we shall see in Chapter 7, not all GPs or Medical Officers of Health would have agreed with that); had developed a strong sense of community at the national level; and was able to assert primacy over the lay world. Medical men (and even by the end of the century, they were still almost all men) enjoyed 'a steadily increasing degree of control over their work, their patients and their own careers'. In his terms they were therefore 'emerging as a profession' (Waddington, 1984, p. 205).

THE DOMESTIC DOMAIN

Kinship remained important in the establishment of a medical career, both in terms of acquiring an education and setting up in practice afterwards; for capital, or access to it, was essential. As Peterson (1978, p. 22) points out, there was a great advantage to be had from joining the practice of a father or an uncle, and such partnerships along with those of brothers or cousins were not uncommon (see also Davidoff and Hall, 1987, p. 263). Furthermore the family of marriage, the service of wives and domestic servants, continued to be crucial to successful medical practice (Davidoff and Hall, 1987, p. 264). In non-medical families women's healing role continued. The establishment of increasing numbers of hospitals in the nineteenth century should not be taken to imply the removal of healing entirely from the domestic arena. In the mid-nineteenth century most healing continued to take place in the home (Peterson, 1978, pp. 90 ff.).

Nor had there been any thoroughgoing separation of home from work place in medical practice. The removal of poor patients to hospital gave practitioners a greater opportunity for treatment and experimentation, and that part of their work was certainly outside the domestic domain, as was the site of the work of those who were medical officers to workhouses. However, the home remained the locus of most medical practice (Davidoff and Hall, 1987, p. 360). The honorary consùltants saw all their private patients at home; general practitioners in London and the provinces also practised from home. The labour contract implied in the marriage contract (see page 81 above) had special implications for medical wives. They were indeed 'married to the job' (Finch, 1983). 'A wife was "almost a necessary part of a physician's professional equipment [sic]" ' (Peterson, 1982, p. 92, quoting Thompson, 1857). Women were reticent to seek advice from a bachelor medical man, but marriage without an assured income was imprudent (ibid.). Wives were critical as part of the medical division of labour. The best sort of wife was one who came from a medical family. Such 'medical wives' knew the rigours of medical practice. Furthermore, such 'an alliance could also be an entrée to medical practice' (Peterson, 1978, p. 107).

The tasks wives performed depended on the success and affluence of their husbands. We may assume that this varied across the range which Patricia Branca (1975, p. 183) has indicated. They may have acted as receptionist, chaperon or nurse depending on their husband's position. Wives were also important in helping doctors place themselves in society. Whether among the wealthy and influential in London, or in a rapidly expanding town like Sheffield, in the life of the local tradesmen and industrialists (Inkster, 1977) these social relations were important for the advancement of medical careers. The division of labour in the domestic domain among clients and potential clients was also important because of the role with regard to health care attributed to women in the home. So wives and mothers were important as clients. 'The favor of women was frequently the target of general practitioners' attention and concern. Such a perspective may reflect the realities of Victorian domestic life and women's role in family health matters' (Peterson, 1978, p. 129; see also Davidoff and Hall, 1987, pp. 339–40).

MIDWIFERY AND OBSTETRICS

The dispute within medicine as to the propriety of medical men undertaking midwifery continued, as did the vilification of women midwives. The conventional upper-class physicians and gentlemen continued to hold the view that midwifery was women's work, inappropriate for gentlemen (Oakley, 1976, p. 31), although their opposition may have been more professional than moral (Loudon, 1986, pp. 92–4). For reasons such as these the newly founded General Medical Council did nothing to require future medical practitioners to be qualified in midwifery, although the Apothecaries' Society had already made this requirement for its diploma in 1827 (Waddington, 1984, p. 45). In the same year that the GMC was founded, men who were practising midwifery founded a new Obstetrical Society (Donnison, 1977, p. 56; Waddington, 1984, p. 45). By this time men midwives had begun to call themselves by the Latinate and presumably more 'scientifically' acceptable title 'obstetrician'. Several had already been elected as Fellows of the College of Physicians, which accepted them before the surgeons did (Donnison, 1977, p. 57). There were two issues: the struggle of women against men, and that of lower-status male doctors against their upper-class colleagues.

General practitioners were anxious to practise midwifery because this was one of the routes whereby they could influence the women of the house and thus gain access to the health care of the whole family and increase their clientele. Women of the new middle class continued the trend started by wealthy women in the eighteenth century, and increasingly called in medical practitioners to attend them in childbirth (see, for example, Davidoff and Hall, 1987, pp. 307–8).

When the Medical Act of 1886 reformed the GMC and allowed for the representation of general practitioners, midwifery was for the first time included as a necessary qualification for registration. Obstetrics was now not only accepted as a medical specialty; knowledge of midwifery was seen as an essential part of the training of a doctor (Donnison, 1977, p. 106). The medical men who had invaded the female domain now had the support of all their colleagues.

It is tempting simply to see those medical men who opposed the reform as old fashioned and conservative. However, the dispute between those who thought midwifery should be no part of medicine and those who insisted upon including it can be seen as a dispute between those men who wished to retain the old gender order and those who wished to transform it. No doubt those who wished for transformation were to a large extent those who had material interests at stake, such as the general practitioners who stood to gain by increased practice.

Somewhat speculatively, one might suggest that in the old gender order there was clear sex segregation supported by strongly held beliefs and notions of pollution which helped to sustain the boundaries. The new gender order transgressed those boundaries, but women were to work for men in subordinate positions, under paternalistic authority in the public domain as they were under patriarchal authority in the domestic domain. There was no question on the part of those who wished to overcome the old order that women should be offered equality of status, with one or two notable exceptions. Male domination was not questioned. *It was its form which was to change.* Clearly also the whole loosening of the religious sanctions associated with the Enlightenment and the new medical knowledge played their part. If dead bodies were no longer sacred, why should women's privates be? Yet women still had to be 'protected'.

WOMEN AS DOCTORS?

That the medical men had no intention of permitting any change in the gender order in the direction of sex equality is clear from their treatment of women who in mid-century wished to become doctors. Elizabeth Blackwell was an early target for attack. She was an Englishwoman who had gone to the USA where, after a great deal of difficulty, she achieved a medical qualification. Returning to England, because she held a diploma from the Irish College of Physicians she was admitted to the medical register in 1858 (Smith, 1979, p. 381), believing it to be a real breakthrough for women (Blackwell, 1977, p. 226). The GMC at once ensured that all those who held foreign degrees were excluded from the register, thus blocking that route for others. Elizabeth Blackwell herself, who had already been practising in New York and London, continued to have great difficulty getting further formal training and qualifications (Blackwell, 1977, ch. VI *passim*).

Much to the ire of the medical profession Blackwell gave a series of lectures on physiology in London in 1859 to encourage other women to become doctors. It was here that Elizabeth Garrett was inspired to become a physician. The opposition of the medical profession continued to be implacable. Having succeeded initially in acting as a nurse at the Middlesex, Elizabeth Garrett was subsequently admitted as a medical student but later removed because of the opposition of the students. The Society of Apothecaries found that it had to accept her application for membership because her private tuition legally constituted an apprenticeship, at that time a qualification for entry. The apothecaries were advised that they could not legally exclude her because their regulations referred to 'persons'. 'To prevent such a thing occurring again the Apothecaries' Society changed the rules. Henceforth education in a recognized medical school was also made a prerequisite for qualification "with the deliberate purpose of excluding women" ' (Newman, 1957, p. 301, quoted in Parry and Parry, 1976, pp. 174–5). Finally Elizabeth Garrett was able to qualify and worked in the Marylebone Dispensary for Women and Children, later founding the Women's Hospital for women patients and staffed entirely by women. The Elizabeth Garrett Anderson Hospital is that same hospital about which a major struggle was fought to ensure its survival in the last quarter of the twentieth century.

The aspirations of women to enter medicine were closely associated with the issue of midwifery, for many women who shared the older medical view that men should have no part of midwifery did so because they felt that for men to examine a woman's body was a violation of her womanhood. Many feminists shared with the male supporters of the old gender order the notion that women were essentially different from men in a way which pervaded their whole life. Male doctors saw the implications of the differences in quite another light and in two contradictory ways at once. First, their biology unfitted women to be responsible for the care of others because of menstruation and pregnancy and, secondly, medical education would destroy their feminity, because it would remove their innocence (L'Esperance, 1977, p. 118).

Women must be sheltered if they were to retain their essential purity. Studying medicine would give them intimate knowledge quite inappropriate for a woman to have. Attendance in maternity wards or lock wards where VD was treated would shock, debase and degrade them. Furthermore it would take women out of the domestic and into the public sphere. In 1875, for example, the Society of Obstetricians again rejected female candidates saying they were 'not by nature qualified to make good midwifery practitioners' (quoted in Smith, 1979, p. 380). Since these doctors were seeking to displace the female midwives the rhetoric was that of *the new male-dominated gender order*. Not only the cult of domesticity but the ideology of the newly emerging social class structure coloured these utterances. 'The work was arduous and required firmness of mind. Only "vulgar females" would be attracted to it and they would only "lower the profession" ' (Smith, 1979, p. 380). Neither the mind nor the body of women were suited for medicine; indeed, medical training would damage them physiologically and mentally; furthermore they would pull down the educational standards. As Lord Neaves said in 1873 when refusing women entry to medical education:

> There is a great difference in the mental constitution of the two sexes, just as there is in their physical conformation. The powers and susceptibilities of women are as noble as those of men; but they are thought to be different, and, in particular, it is considered that they have not the same power of intense labour as men are endowed with ... [They should aim] for the special acquirements and accomplishments ... from which men may easily remain exempt.
>
> (Quoted in Sachs and Wilson, 1978, p. 18)

Not only did the majority of medical men steadfastly oppose the entry of women to the profession, they also used their authority to oppose higher education for women altogether, now basing their arguments not on 'nature' alone but on nature supported by the newer teachings of physiology. Indeed, they argued that education of any kind which would be likely to suit women for anything other than the domestic arts might do much damage. It could even induce 'disease or death', said Keiller, one-time president of the Royal College of Physicians of Scotland (Bauer and Ritt, 1979, p. 251). Emily Davies, great champion of education for women, replying to 'A Physician' in 1861 found herself arguing against a case that women did not have the aptitude for medicine, either 'naturally' or by virtue of early schooling, nor would they be able to find space in which to practise (Bauer and Ritt, 1979, pp. 154–6).

WOMEN DOCTORS FOR WOMEN PATIENTS

The reticence of some women to consult male practitioners was one of the arguments used by those who supported the entry of women into the medical profession and to convince opponents that there would be a clientele for women practitioners.

> 'Is there a proper field for the employment and support of female physicians?' We unhesitatingly reply that all disease to which women and children are liable would naturally come within the province of the female physician, and surely that is a domain wide enough without encroaching on the sphere of men.
>
> (Emily Davies, quoted in Bauer and Ritt, 1979, p. 155)

Emily Davies goes on to argue that women who understand that women physicians are properly qualified doctors prefer to consult them rather than a man. Josephine Butler herself stressed this point, expressing her immense gratitude at having been able to consult Elizabeth Garrett. She clearly felt it debasing to be examined by a man (Lewis, 1984, p. 87). Elizabeth Blackwell is said to have been motivated by arguments of this kind as well as by an intrinsic interest in medicine (L'Esperance, 1977, pp. 119–20).

Among the few men who supported the entry of women these arguments also were used. Thus Thomas Markby supported a limited entry for the practice of pharmacy, midwifery and paediatrics, the aspects of medicine which would be conventionally appropriate for them. However, the women's objections were qualitatively different from those of the men, as l'Esperance (1977, p. 127) has pointed out, based as they were not on the maintenance of the old gender order but on the violation of a woman's sovereignty of her person. Many shared with other mid-century feminists a belief in the moral superiority of women. Blackwell was one such. In addition, women's entry to the profession would modify the gender order quite radically.

Notwithstanding the opposition, women continued determinedly to find ways to train for medicine at the London School of Medicine and the Royal Free Hospital, but by the end of the century they were still few in number. The 1901 Census lists 212 females under the heading 'physicians, surgeons and general practitioners' (Smith, 1979, p. 382). There were over 36,000 registered medical practitioners at that time (General Medical Council, 1901).

WOMEN MIDWIVES

Most medical men were clear that they wished to keep obstetrics, a part of medicine, as a male domain. They were more confused and divided about their attitude to midwives. They had opposed and vilified them. Would it now, later in the century, be right to recognize them and if so in what guise? These were the issues which underlay the debate about the registration of midwives. Midwives themselves came to feel that if they had state registration they would be able to control their occupation and achieve a respected place as a profession. Many medical men opposed this, fearing that registered midwives would undermine male medical practice. As time went on, others came to see that registered midwives could prove helpful and non-threatening. They could watch with women in the long hours of labour and call the medical man at the point of parturition. Thus it came about that the male medical opposition to 'following on' a midwife was gradually replaced.

On the condition therefore that midwives should attend only 'normal' births, a majority of medical men ultimately concluded that midwives could be admitted to an official place in the medical division of labour. The restriction of midwives to normal labour was first recognized by the Midwifery Diploma granted by the Obstetrical Society of London in 1872 (Oakley, 1976, p. 37). This definition of what a midwife could do was finally enshrined in the Midwives Act of 1902. Midwives did not disappear in England as they virtually did in the USA. The Act constituted them as practitioners in their own right. In this the medical men were disappointed. But as Donnison (1977, p. 174) says, the Act 'was like no other registration Act, before or since, and was to put midwives in a uniquely disadvantaged position among the professions'. Not only was their practice circumscribed, but the Board which was to regulate them was not even required to include a midwife. It had a medical majority. The Act exemplified what Larkin (1981, p. 16) has called 'a logic of subordination'; many later Acts delineating the health-care division of labour were to follow this logic.

In this way the medical men of the nineteenth century helped to create a new male-dominated gender order. They had a right of attending any birth; they had secured for themselves the right and responsibility of handling all difficulties and complications in childbirth and had made it the midwives' responsibility to see that they were called in such cases. They had ensured that midwives would be trained in the way they thought right. Women could work in the public domain so long as their work there was appropriately restricted and controlled.

WHAT IS NURSING? HOW IT CAME TO BE DEFINED

Most nursing, like most healing, had always taken place in the domestic domain, although for centuries there had been limited exceptions to this generalization; notably women of religious orders had cared for the indigent sick as well as travellers and others who came to their hospices. Women nursed household members who fell sick; in addition, those who could afford it hired women to come into their homes to nurse sick members there. The monthly nurse who took up residence after childbirth was well established. These tasks (like all those which housewives and their servants performed) were part of the domestic division of labour. The nurses were domestic servants.

The hospitals established in the eighteenth and nineteenth centuries employed women as nurses, largely to do domestic work and to watch the sick. The successive reforms of nursing in the nineteenth century were partly about the increasingly sharp definition of nurses from other domestic and health-care workers; they were also about the assimilation of nurses to the medical division of labour and their subordination to medical men.

Celia Davies (1980a) has shown how the census definition of 'nurse' kept changing throughout the nineteenth century. A nurse might be someone who came to look after the children (what we might think of as an untrained nanny); someone who came to the house to look after the sick; a woman working in the hospital. The enumerators made so many changes that the statistics they developed cannot be used to measure changes in the numbers of nurses employed during the century, but they say a great deal about how nursing as an occupation developed. By the end of the century a nurse might be trained and certified; at its outset such people did not exist.

RECRUITING NURSES TO THE MEDICAL DIVISION OF LABOUR

Abel-Smith (1960) provides a detailed account of the history of nursing, demonstrating clearly the harsh conditions of life of hospital nurses in the early nineteenth century. Hospital nurses were women who might have been employed elsewhere in domestic service, indeed often had been. They were required to sleep in the hospital in spaces in the wards among the patients. Their pay was meagre, and out of it they had to provide their own subsistence. When reading the vilification to which the unreformed nurses were subjected, such as being drunken and taking food and possessions from the patients, it is well to bear in mind their conditions of work, their difficulty in making ends meet and how they were issued with an ale ration as part of their terms and conditions of work.

The way in which nineteenth-century commentators saw the transformation of nursing depended upon their position and interests, as Katherine Williams (1980, pp. 41–75) has shown. She contrasts two accounts given in 1897, the year of Queen Victoria's jubilee ('Sixty Years a Queen'). A doctor ('medical historian' of the *British Medical Journal*) and a nurse (Miss Breay, writing in the *Nursing Record and Hospital World*) agree that the unskilful and untrustworthy 'Sary Gamp' of Dickensian fame had been replaced by the 'modern nurse': clean, sober, trustworthy, efficient and trained in the course of the last fifty years. They disagree however about the characters who had 'done good' and benefited the healing process and about their contributions. Both agree upon Elizabeth Fry's pioneering contribution in inaugurating the Institution of Nursing Sisters to provide reliable private nurses for the well-to-do. However, the medical historian stresses the nurses' womanly characteristics which Elizabeth Fry ensured should continue. Fry learned how to train private nurses from her own experience of the best hospital nurses of the pre-reform days. 'Medical historian' is anxious to see the conventional womanly virtues put at the disposal of doctors in hospital. The women should be trained by doctors and their training kept as distinct from that of medical students as possible. He is dissatisfied because he sees theory as having been developed at the expense of practice.

Miss Breay, on the other hand, sees Florence Nightingale as the 'Chief Pioneer' of hospital nursing and the introduction of nurse training as having excellent consequences. Miss Nightingale has transformed the nurse from a domestic servant to an educated pupil and probationer, a woman who can take her place in the public domain in her own right. All that is now needed, Miss Breay feels, is the acceptance by the state of nursing as a profession. This will set

the seal not only on the profession but on the notion of the independent qualified woman, precisely what distresses the medical historian.

The principles established through the Nightingale fund at St Thomas's challenged the medical view of a nurse trained in a set of practices derived from
medical knowledge. Williams (1980) shows how the Nightingale principles
broke the ward physician/ward sister relationship because the training of the
pupil nurses was ultimately in the hands of the matron. The probationer was a
learner as well as a worker. The ward physician through the sister could no
longer control the workforce just as he wished. Furthermore the expenditure of
the Nightingale Fund could not be scrutinized by the lay management. Nursing
thus achieved at St Thomas's some independence from both doctors and laymen.
It is not perhaps surprising that the men, both medical and lay, were less than
enthusiastic about the new nurses.

CLASS AS WELL AS GENDER

The transformation of nursing in the nineteenth century is however, not only a
matter of nurses versus doctors, or women versus men, for the developing class
structure along with the structure of the bourgeois family of that period also had
much to do with it. We have already noted the increasing domestication of
women which was encouraged by men of the rising bourgeoisie. By mid-
century there was also an embarrassing surfeit of women, the 'spinster problem'.
Women who had not found a husband were not welcome in the households of
their brothers, and had little outlet since the public world was closed to them.
The uncomfortable life of many as governesses or lodgers has been described
(see, for example, Davidoff, 1971, and 1979; Peterson, 1980). Nightingale and
her colleagues in seeking to reform nursing were also seeking an escape for
women, to persuade the middle class that nursing could be a respectable occupation for them, for women of the middle class as well as for the 'better' type of
working-class women. Fathers had to be persuaded that they could trust their
daughters to the care of the hospital matrons; the appalling living conditions in
hospital also had to be improved, but close discipline had to be established (see
also Vicinus, 1985, ch. 3). The tensions which developed among the ladies and
between the ladies and the paid nurses in the Crimean War is well described by
Anne Summers (1983).

What in the event happened was that the upper-class women who went into
nursing were trained to become leaders, the matrons of the reforming hospitals.
There were in fact two classes of nurses; the lady pupils and the probationers
(Abel-Smith, 1960, ch. 2). The ordinary probationers got free training and
maintenance, while the lady pupils paid for their maintenance during their training (Abel-Smith, 1960, p. 23). From the outset therefore 'modern nursing' took
into itself the Victorian class structure. It is also the case that if Nightingale had
not been well connected in the upper class and able to work through prominent
men she would not, despite her personal energy and initiative (exercised from
her invalid couch), have been able to effect such remarkable changes.

NURSING DOMINATED BY WOMEN OR MEN?

Earlier (page 81) we saw that in Eva Gamarnikow's (1978) view the way in
which nursing emerged had more to do with patriarchy than with the capitalist

class structure. She applies her theory to the Nightingale model of nursing as a paid occupation. For her the 'central interprofessional relationship which subordinated nursing to medicine' (1978, p. 102) is crucial rather than the intra-professional disputes which have so exercised nursing historians. Gamarnikow arraigns Nightingale for setting up the new nursing in a way which mirrored the Victorian bourgeois household: doctor-father, nurse-mother and patient-child. The nurse was to have her own sphere, but it was to be one in which she was subordinate to the doctor and bound to take his orders. She would not interfere in diagnosis and would carry out his prescriptions. Undoubtedly this was the outcome, yet, as Williams (1980) has argued, the Nightingale method did give nursing an independence from medicine, which medicine greatly disliked and found threatening. What else a mid-nineteenth-century woman could have done is unclear.

Interpretations of this history vary. Abel-Smith (1960) sees the development of the nursing profession as 'an instalment of the emancipation of women. It gave power – power over men.' No doubt, as Miss Dunbar indicated, it gave them more freedom than domesticity accorded them (1960, p. 30 and n.). Abel-Smith correctly sees some of the lady nurses as wishing to enhance their own status, in this sense part of a wider feminist movement, although one should note the many 'faces of feminism' (O. Banks, 1981). He is no doubt correct to argue (p. 36) that the 'new ladies had to fight the male doctors, the male lay administrators, and the male members of the hospital committees'. Whether the power which the matrons had sought and gained was as great as he argues is more doubtful. Furthermore he sees the (much later) establishment of the nurses' register as anti-masculinist. 'When the women obtained power, they used it to discriminate against men' (Abel-Smith, 1960, p. 114). No man could become a member of the College of Nursing. In this, women were simply following the male example. They had for long been excluded from the Colleges of Physicians and Surgeons and the Society of Apothecaries.

In the context of male domination, the notion of separate spheres and the prevailing cult of domesticity, it is hardly surprising that Nightingale should write in 1867 that 'the whole reform of nursing . . . is to take all power out of the hands of the men, and put it into the hands of *one female trained head* and make her responsible for everything (regarding internal management and discipline) being carried out' (quoted in Abel-Smith, 1960, p. 25, original emphasis). Nightingale was an opponent of orthodox medical men; her association with Farr and her belief in environmental causes of disease will be recalled (see pages 61, 68, 70).

NURSING IN THE WORKHOUSE HOSPITALS AND THE ASYLUMS

The story so far recounted relates to the voluntary hospitals, but a great many more people were nursed in the workhouse hospitals where the sick poor were accommodated. There the history of the division of labour and of the development of nursing is different. For the first half of the century the sick poor were looked after by other paupers. As Rosemary White (1978, p. 86), drawing on contemporary reports, has it: 'In 1867 there were few paid nurses and in 1896 there were some trained nurses; in 1867 there were mostly pauper nurses whereas in 1896 there were paid assistants.'

The reform of nursing happened in the voluntary hospitals, in many of which there were medical schools and in which nursing schools were also established. The reformed nurses were therefore closely associated with the development of clinical medicine. Just as the medical officers had to struggle against the uninformed lay control of the workhouse master, so the paid, and later trained, nurses had to struggle against the supremacy of the matron (Crowther, 1981, pp. 165–6; White, 1978, p. 89). Some Nightingale nurses were employed in particularly enlightened infirmaries, notably Agnes Jones who went to Liverpool in 1865 (White, 1978, p. 31); mostly however the developments in the workhouse hospitals and infirmaries were distinct from those in the voluntary hospitals.

When the Metropolitan Asylums Board was established after the 1867 Act and new infirmaries were opened, the value of employing trained nurses was appreciated. However, great difficulties were experienced in finding appropriately trained women. This was also true of guardians who wished to employ trained nurses. By 1881 the Local Government Board said it was its policy that trained nurses should be employed, but the shortages remained. There were also difficulties in judging the standard of training received. We have seen that workhouse hospitals had no associated medical schools; apart from some hospitals founded under the 1867 Act, they had no nurse training schools. From 1875 the Local Government Board hoped that the new infirmaries would provide appropriate facilities for nurses' homes and nurse training schools. Progress was slow, and a voluntary body, the Association for Promoting Trained Nursing in Workhouses, was established and was itself successfully training nurses by 1885 (White, 1978, pp. 71–5). Nevertheless, according to Crowther (1981, p. 166), pauper nurses, often elderly women, remained the core of the workhouse nursing service until the end of the nineteenth century. The Association could not fill the gap in demand, and nurses trained in the infirmaries often left for private nursing (Crowther, 1981, pp. 176–7).

Dean and Bolton (1980, p. 86) see the voluntary hospitals and the workhouses as sites which represent two distinct 'economies': the workhouse as the place for the least expensive confinement of those who add nothing to society's wealth; the hospital as the place of investment of medical knowledge and practice where those patients were permitted who were 'deemed useful for the research and education of medical practitioners'. Or, as Rosemary White (1978, p. 198) has put it: 'The Poor Law nurses did not voluntarily stay with the incurables ... Whilst the voluntary hospital nurses followed the scientific and technological progress of their doctors and moved further away from the caring role of bedside nurses, the Poor Law nurses remained there.' In the popular mind and in the history books, it is the medical and nursing activities in the voluntary hospitals which have attracted most attention, yet undoubtedly the majority of sick people were cared for in workhouse hospitals. In nursing terms, White argues (1978, p. 198), 'because of the Poor Law nurses, the profession did not lose its caring role entirely'.

The situation of nurses in the asylums was also much different from those in the voluntary hospitals (Carpenter, 1980). Asylum nurses were essentially custodians; most of them were men. The task was a working-class one; the ladies did not seek to enter those occupations. Rejected by the reformed nurses, the asylum workers sought reform through the trade union movement. While their struggle started at the end of the nineteenth century, its locus is even more in the twentieth century than that of the struggles of the general nurses. For women nurses it has had ironic twentieth-century consequences, as we shall see (page 129).

CREATING A NEW CLASS STRUCTURE AND A NEW GENDER ORDER

The account of what happened to nursing as an occupation in the nineteenth century has to be seen as part of the creation of the new class structure and the new gender order. The women who were recruited were encouraged to discipline and teach the sick in the highly regulated hospital environment by which they themselves were also disciplined. It was also a way through which the gender order was transformed to cope with the new circumstances of industrial capitalism and yet retain male domination. It helped to create the 'new woman' who was permitted to move in the public world and earn her own living, not only in a respectable manner, but in one deemed to be praiseworthy. At the same time it committed her to a great deal of drudgery, long hours, low pay and subservience to medical men.

The Nightingale reforms emerged out of the internal contradictions of nineteenth-century patriarchy with its doctrines of domesticity and faced with a demographic imbalance which led to an excess of women for whom no husbands could be found (a situation which undoubtedly made life easier for those who preferred not to have husbands). Lown (1983 and 1984) has argued, for industry, that when Victorian men found it necessary to employ women in the public domain some resorted to an ideology of paternalism. Nightingale was negotiating within such a patriarchally dominated social situation, which led to the outcome which Gamarnikow (1978) so ably describes. Hospital nurses were resident for long periods, as were many of the patients. In this residential setting, in contrast with the day labour of industrial workers, a patriarchal model such as Gamarnikow describes was easier to install. The rhetoric surrounding the creation of paternalistic industry was not necessary. It all seemed so 'natural' that men should command and order cure, women should care, and patients should be subservient and passive. It was after all the order of the Victorian household, where 'the mistress of the servant was herself normally the servant of some master' (Summers, 1983, p. 53). All that was changed, it seemed, was the locale.

CONCLUSION

Thus by the end of the nineteenth century the principal locale of healing begun to shift to a territory in some ways indeterminately placed between public and domestic domains but in others undoubtedly owned and controlled in the public domain. A new division of labour in health care had also been established, one in which medicine had organized an increasing number of subsidiary occupations to serve it. Chief among these, medical men had established themselves in a powerful position and ensured the subservience of the female occupations of nursing and midwifery.

The dispute about blood-letting between the Edinburgh physicians Alison and Bennett in the 1850s had revealed two distinct perspectives on the relationship between scientific knowledge and clinical practice: the one representing the newer tradition of laboratory science; the other, older, based on bedside observation (Warner, 1980). Not only was the germ theory widely accepted by the end of the century, but the importance of laboratory science as a basis of medical practice was widely recognized among the medical leadership. The foundations of twentieth-century biomedicine were well laid by 1900. Medical men were by no means content, however, as we shall see. Furthermore, their therapeutic skills were still of limited efficacy. Their rise to positions of power and authority with government and their rising public reputation had well antedated any great increase in their healing power.

7 Laying the Basis for the National Health Service

This chapter will look at the development of medical knowledge and at changes in the methods and funding of health-care provision and in the division of labour in health care in the first half of the twentieth century. It will show how these changes were all related to and also contributed to changes in the class and gender orders of British society during that period. At the outset Britain was still at the height of empire but no longer safely pre-eminent in industrial production. The United States and Germany were serious rivals. These were not just problems for the captains of industry, they were also of concern to a state wishing to defend the national interest in its far flung and its home territories.

The early years of the century were ones of domestic unrest. A number of the tensions which had been inherent in the change-over to a factory-based economy, sharp divisions between management and labour and tensions also in the structuring of the Victorian bourgeois family erupted in those years. A decade of industrial disputes, of parliamentary challenges from the young Labour Party, of women uprising and demanding a place as voters in the public domain, of violence and threats of violence, ended with the First World War in 1914.

When that war ended there was a brief postwar boom and high hopes for economic expansion and welfare advances, but in the event the interwar period was overshadowed by the Great Depression. At the beginning of the century class and gender divisions had been clear and deep, and ideas about the 'naturalness' of both were still persisting when the Second World War broke out in 1939. Class divisions may have been less visually apparent in the 1930s than they had been in the first decade of the century, but they continued to be profound and were exacerbated by the Depression.

Webster (1980, 1982a and 1985) has reviewed the evidence about the relationship between health and the Depression in the 1930s. He concludes, contrary to the optimistic health pronouncements of officials at the time, and contrary also to recent apologists for the period, that the unemployed and the poorly paid probably were not well nourished and that the Depression did have adverse effects upon the health of sections of the population. Evidence depends largely upon a series of detailed local studies which reveal what the nationally collected statistics apparently concealed. The gender differences in health were underscored by Marjorie Spring Rice (1939). Her evidence for part of London at the beginning of the 1930s shows not only the class differences but the burden of ill health experienced by wives and mothers.

In the first half of the century there were some important changes in the mode of delivery of health care and in the organization of the medical profession. There were, also, interesting developments in medical knowledge. As Chapter 6 indicated, by the end of the nineteenth century medicine had achieved greatly enhanced prestige and status, although it did not have many powerful tools for healing. The increased longevity of the population in the nineteenth century has been attributed more to improved sanitation, nutrition and birth control than to medical intervention (McKeown, 1971). Medicine was, however, well poised to develop better tools. It had resources available, research laboratories and valuable clinical material in the shape of increasing numbers of hospital patients. The three arms of health care – hospitals, public health and general practice – were established. With these and increasing medical knowledge the health-care division of labour became more fragmented, and specialization increased.

THE SOURCES AND STATE OF MEDICAL KNOWLEDGE

By the first decade of the twentieth century bacteriology had come to be fairly widely accepted by medical scientists. This new knowledge, based on microbiology, represented a different understanding of life and disease from that of the early nineteenth-century protagonists of miasma, contagion and their variants. The new knowledge was critical for the development of clinical medicine, along with asepsis and antisepsis, in the area of surgery. The foundations were laid for the advanced microbiology of later in the century. Hospitals became increasingly entrenched as the focal point of healing, the central locus of medical training; they increasingly dominated the medical scene. The bacteriological knowledge, however, was widely applied; an understanding of this led to efforts to ensure that young children were given uncontaminated milk and was associated with the development of milk depots (Rosen, 1958, pp. 354–60) – an important development in the services for mothers and children, other aspects of which are discussed later (see pages 110–15).

In these and other ways the scientific basis had been established on which high-technology medicine was later to develop. The foundations were also being laid for a new phase of biomedicine which was to extend its authority even more widely among those who were not ailing but might ail, and who did not know they were ill but might be so defined. Foucault has argued that the new medical 'gaze' which saw below the surface of the patient had led to the development of the new clinic around 1800, which made the birth of biomedicine possible a century later (see pages 57–9). Around the turn of the twentieth century, Armstrong (1983b) argues, a new gaze was profoundly to reorganize medical knowledge and the nature of medical practice. Armstrong refers to this as the *Dispensary*, following from the organization of health-care delivery with which it was involved but using the term symbolically, in the manner in which Foucault (1973) has referred to the new medical knowledge of the turn of the nineteenth century as the *Clinic*.

Its origins, according to Armstrong (1983b), can be found in the late nineteenth century in Edinburgh with the TB dispensary started by an aspiring specialist frustrated of his wish to found a TB hospital. TB patients referred to the dispensary were visited by a staff of nurses in their own homes to discover their needs, report on their circumstances and their contacts, arrange charity as necessary and teach a healthy way of life (1983b, p. 7). In this way the medical, clinical gaze was extended. Whereas the clinical gaze which Foucault analysed had penetrated the surface of the body to the mysteries beneath, the gaze of the dispensary focused 'not on individual bodies so much as the interstices of society' (p. 9). The gaze now stretched into the homes of the people and sought to trace the spread of the disease there. But it was not only that the medical gaze extended to the social; it accepted 'the "social" … as an autonomous realm' (p. 10).

Although Armstrong does not remind his readers of this, the 'social' was, of course, a realm which others had earlier recognized and explored. What the staff of the Edinburgh TB dispensary did in visiting homes, advising household members and calling charitable help was something which philanthropic middle-class women had themselves done since the mid-nineteenth century to help the poor (Stacey and Davies, 1983, ch 3; Summers, 1979). Some of the earlier out-patient and dispensary facilities had also been involved in home visiting, thereby grasping the social context, if not the social network, of illness and disease (see pages 55–6). What Dr Philip did in Edinburgh was to take these notions and apply them to TB patients. The techniques of the survey which he and later practitioners picked up and used to medical ends had been used before: at the end of the nineteenth century by Booth and later by Rowntree, but before that by administrators hoping to keep track of burgeoning urban populations and to understand how to govern them. These techniques medicine now took to itself.

The change in medical perception which emerged in the TB dispensary also came to apply to venereal disease, about which there was renewed anxiety in the early twentieth century. As early as 1913 a network of clinics to provide free diagnosis and an educational campaign were proposed. However, a continuing norm of silence about sexuality and sexually transmitted diseases prevented the expansion of the idea of the Dispensary to VD until the 1930s, when, Armstrong argues (1983b, p. 13), 'Venereal disease changed from being used as a means of forbidding certain relationships to a mechanism for observing them.' The Contagious Diseases Acts, as we saw (pages 71–5), not only had forbidden certain relationships in principle but had set out to punish only one sex for indulging in them. Armstrong (1983b, p. 13) is correct to say that when the form of the Dispensary became associated with venereology it 'began to create a network of surveillance that monitored the social contacts, values and environment of recorded patients', a form of control which appears to avoid moral judgement and to be gender neuter. The various applications of the notion of surveillance were not gender neuter, however, as we shall see.

The medical concern with the 'social body' came to include the notion of comprehensive health care. The revolution in thinking consequent upon the work of Freud and the psychoanalysts also played its past, as did the links which developed between medicine and the social sciences, particularly psychology and the techniques of the social survey. Once attention could be diverted from the historic infectious diseases, which gradually lost their virulent impact as the twentieth century proceeded (McKeown, 1965), the discipline of the survey penetrated general practice, paediatrics, geriatrics and the other areas of medical practice which developed in the twentieth century.

THE PATENT MEDICINE INDUSTRY

Other scientific developments which were profoundly to affect knowledge and practice within medicine were under way at the start of this period. The large-scale manufacture of pills and potions had already begun by the end of the nineteenth century; it was to achieve massive proportions in the second half of the twentieth century. The remedies which medical practitioners and others used for many years owed a great deal to the empirical understanding of wise women and cunning folk. Housewives went on making potions and lotions for members of their households throughout the nineteenth century, but brand medicines had already been known in the eighteenth century (McKendrick, 1982, p. 185–6). Towards the end of the nineteenth century commercial firms were producing erstwhile domestic remedies as well as doctors' and pharmacists' potions in bulk.

Marjorie Lodge (1985) found that when talking to women who had reared children between the wars they referred to remedies their mothers had made up. These remedies bore a remarkable resemblance to many of the patented remedies such as Owbridge's Lung Tonic and including preparations still on the market today such as Vick. Such remedies were no doubt as effective or otherwise as their predecessors. Scientists, however, were increasingly developing knowledge as to how to improve on these remedies, to synthesize them and later to invent chemical compounds to new effect.

The pharmaceutical breakthrough came with the manufacture of the sulphonamide drugs in the mid-1930s. Their most loudly hailed application was in the control of childbirth fever, the maternal mortality rates in hospitals reducing as soon as they were used (but see Macfarlane and Mugford, 1984, p. 206). Pharmaceuticals advanced remarkably during the Second World War, and thus, almost coterminous with the establishment of the NHS, a new phase of medical treatment began. The availability to medical practitioners not only of the sulpha drugs but also the highly effective postwar antibiotics and mood-changing chemicals was to alter medical practice remarkably, but largely from outside itself. It has also had a notable impact on the health-care division of labour (see pages 216–20).

Medical practitioners at the beginning of the century were not, however, greatly concerned about dependence on non-medical scientists and large-scale industry. They were more concerned with their attempts to gain patients for their practice, subscribers for their hospitals and the support of the state in their enterprises. In particular the general practitioners, as we have noted, were feeling aggrieved.

GENERAL PRACTITIONERS, THE 'SICK CLUBS' AND THE 1911 NATIONAL INSURANCE ACT

General practitioners were perhaps the least contented of medical men around the turn of the century, at all events they were most outspoken about their difficulties. They developed a considerable campaign and ultimately gained support from government. Those who lacked family support or other patronage continued to face serious problems in building up a practice and making a reasonable living out of it. Only well-to-do patients could afford large fees. In some areas general practitioners were able effectively to subsidize the poor by using the method of a sliding scale, charging their wealthier clients more than the poorer. This was not possible in areas where there were concentrations of working-class population.

In any case a fee-for-service burden still fell upon the patient, possibly at a time when s/he was least able to pay. Various voluntary initiatives, generically described as 'clubs', were part of the self-help which developed to fill the gap in primary medical care. Some were societies organized for the workers, to which they contributed money but in whose running they had no say. These included doctors' clubs, provident dispensaries and commercial companies which provided medical benefits either for profit or as part of other subscriber plans. Then there were those societies organized by the workers themselves and run by them usually through a committee. There had been a great upsurge in the number of 'sick clubs' of all sorts from the 1880s, although some had existed from early in the nineteenth century. Central government had encouraged self-help and the friendly societies for some years, an encouragement which continued into the twentieth century. In that period, too, many trade unions also provided friendly-society functions (Earwicker, 1981a, 1981b, p. 39; Eder, 1982, pp. 17–22; Honigsbaum, 1979, pp. 12–14).

The principle on which the clubs ran was that the members paid a small weekly sum, often a simple flat rate, in return for which they, and sometimes their dependants, could receive treatment. Quite how much was covered and whether they also received sick-pay varied, as did the details of running the clubs. What they all had in common was that they were under lay control, whether of industrial management or members.

General practitioners strongly disliked lay control. The *British Medical Journal* commented that to be controlled by a committee of working men 'is not a pleasant matter for an educated gentleman to serve under' (1875, p. 484, quoted in Parry and Parry, 1976, p. 147). General practitioners were employed on conditions which made it impossible for them to choose their patients (all club members had to be treated; the members had no choice of doctor either). The practitioners complained a great deal about levels of pay as well as the conditions of work. In the provident clubs doctors were commonly paid by capitation, i.e. a fixed sum per annum for each club member. Many general practitioners were constrained by the absence of a sufficiently lucrative private practice to work for the sick clubs, as many also found they had to work part-time for the Boards of Guardians providing medical attention to sick paupers under the Poor Law. (Taking full- and part-time doctors together about 3,700 worked in the Poor Law services in 1910, i.e. about a sixth of all doctors in England and Wales: Stevens, 1966, p. 35.)

The discontent of the general practitioners had not gone unheeded. At the insistence of the medical defence unions set up to defend GPs, the General Medical Council held an inquiry which concluded in 1892 that the club doctor 'is, at times, placed in a position of great dependence, inconsistent with the conscientious performance of his duties' (*Lancet*, 3 June 1892, p. 1347, quoted in Earwicker, 1981b, p. 39). In practice, terms and conditions varied. Earwicker (1981b, p. 41) has shown that the extensive service developed in South Wales had pay and conditions which attracted doctors from many parts of the country.

The Boer War had revealed the poor health of much of the population, and increasingly in the first decade of the twentieth century health and welfare measures were developed. As well as increasing recognition of poverty and ill health, the Lloyd George government was concerned about social unrest. In this context the National Insurance Act of 1911 was introduced with provisions for health and unemployment insurance. The idea of social insurance was already quite widespread in Europe, having started in Bismarck's Germany in 1883 (Eder, 1982, pp. 23ff.). Although it was in the end to turn out to be to their advantage, the general practitioners initially opposed the health insurance aspects. Having decided that their opposition would be unsuccessful, however (partly because of the failure of the consultants to help them), the general practitioners' politicians decided to try to get the best deal they could out of government. They had a six-point demand:

> an upper income limit . . . ; free choice of doctor by the patient, subject to the doctor's acceptance; benefits to be administered by local health committees and not by the friendly societies; choice of their method of remuneration by doctors in each district; medical remuneration to be what the profession considered adequate for the work performed; and adequate medical represen-tation among the insurance commissioners . . . , in the Central Advisory Committee, and in the local health committees, with statutory recognition of a local medical committee representing the profession in the district of each health committee.
>
> (Stevens, 1966, p. 36; see also Eder, 1982, p. 34)

In short, they wanted rid of lay control, help for those who could not afford their fees but maximum freedom for private practice, hence the income limit.

THE PROVISIONS AND CONSEQUENCES OF THE 1911 ACT

What the health side of the Act eventually provided was a system of panel practice whereby every worker below a certain wage should be insured with contributions paid by the worker, the employer and the state. The scheme was operated by 'approved societies' which were modelled on the democratic principles of the old friendly societies for mutual insurance and aid. Such societies became approved societies, but so also did industrial insurance companies and trade unions. None were permitted to make profits on their approved society activities. With few exceptions the general practitioners elected to be paid by capitation fee, i.e. so much per annum per patient on their panel. The worker received some sick benefit in cash when ill and off work and free treatment and medicines from his/her GP. Hospital and specialist services were not included. Employed persons earning over the income limit were excluded. This limit was raised from time to time after inflation had altered its meaning, right up to the termination of the scheme when the National Health Service came in in 1948. The limit was always raised against the opposition of the doctors, who were anxious to defend their private practice by keeping as many patients as possible off the panel. The marginal middling classes were excluded in this way; the upper classes could presumably afford treatment anyway. Those who were not gainfully employed, notably wives and children of workers, were also not covered by health insurance. Sometimes they continued to pay into a club – quite often one started by the doctors themselves, who continued to operate a sliding scale of payment for those outside their panel practice. The alternatives were out-patient dispensaries or Poor Law health care. By joining the families of their panel patients into their clubs the GPs increased their private practice (Earwicker, 1981b; Eder, 1982; Honigsbaum, 1979; Lodge, 1985; Parry and Parry, 1976; Stevens, 1966).

General practitioners were on balance much better off for joining the scheme. Their fees were higher than they had been under the various clubs; there was a wider assured clientele to draw upon. Furthermore, through the system of contracting to provide services they had avoided becoming direct employees of the state. At the same time they had succeeded in permeating the administration of the service.

The Act provided for a local medical committee elected by medical practitioners representative of the whole profession in the area and a committee representative of panel practitioners (Honigsbaum, 1979, p. 60 esp. fn.a; Parry and Parry, 1976, p. 193). Thus although the ultimate control in the administration by the approved societies was lay, control relevant to the daily work and conditions of the doctors was strongly influenced by medical practitioners. Gone were the possibilities for consumer control, with a consequent increase in professional autonomy. The constraints on the medical practitioner exercised by the rich patron of the eighteenth century had been evaded when hospital patients from the working class became available to clinicians (Jewson, 1974 and 1976). Now the constraints of lay committees had been overcome also. Notwithstanding their initial opposition, GPs soon supported the NHI strongly. Theirs was a net gain, an assured clientele and better fees. By 1938 90 per cent of all GPs had panel practices, but only 40 per cent of the population was covered (Parry and Parry, 1976, p. 195).

NHI A CONSEQUENCE OF CLASS STRUGGLE?

Navarro (1978) has written a provocative analysis of the establishment of National Health Insurance and the subsequent National Health Service (NHS) based upon the notion that these developments can be understood only in terms of class struggle. He believes, quoting Marx and Engels, that 'the history of all hitherto existing society is the history of class struggles' but he adds not only the societies' histories but also 'their social legislation' (1978, p. xv). He is correct to pay attention to the social and economic transformation which Britain had undergone in the eighteenth and nineteenth centuries, and to challenge the idea that it was simply altruism or a wish for good government alone which led to social reform. Undoubtedly the material interests of the protagonists were also involved. However, in addition to many superficialities and some inaccuracies in his work (see also Reidy, 1984), there are problems with his analysis in class terms. The relationship of medical men to capitalism and their alignment with the upper class is less clear cut than he portrays. Nor is it entirely clear that national interest, which undoubtedly motivated some of government's health measures, can be altogether equated with class interests, or not without resorting to some device such as speaking of fractions of capital being associated with national interest while others may not be – a level of finesse Navarro does not entertain. Nor does he discuss the public health movement and its relationship to the state's and capital's interest, in whatever way one might specify those abstractions empirically.

GENDER AND NATIONAL INSURANCE

Navarro (1978) emphasizes the history of the class struggle but in this work neglects the gender order and tensions within it. There was no woman's voice in the establishment of NHI; nor were women's interests safeguarded in any way. Women who were gainfully employed were covered by NHI, but, as we have seen, wives were excluded along with all other unpaid workers. This cannot be understood in class terms. It has to be understood in gender terms. The principle of the 'family wage' was well established by the early twentieth century: the notion that a man should earn enough to keep his wife and family. Even in those terms, however, it remains illogical to suggest that if he requires free treatment when ill his wife and children do not; it is also dubious to assume that his wage if sufficient to keep them in health is sufficient to cope with illness. The Act was undoubtedly discriminatory against women, although it did not discriminate against them in straightforwardly sex terms. The discrimination flowed, as so much discrimination did and still does, from the assumption that it is 'natural' that a woman should be a wife and mother, and therefore 'naturally' she does not require so large a wage. Additionally women were also increasingly being recruited as unpaid health workers in the first quarter of the twentieth century. An understanding of this phenomenon is crucial to understanding the pre-1945 development of health care. However, before we turn to an analysis of the role into which the unpaid workers were cast by administrators and medical practitioners, it is perhaps important to understand the crucial role of the hospitals in the early twentieth century.

HOSPITALS BETWEEN THE WARS

Whereas before the nineteenth century almost all treatment took place in the domestic sphere, by the twentieth century treatment was increasingly removed to hospitals in the public domain. This transfer had started in a small way (see pages 61–3) with the beginnings of the voluntary hospital movement. Alongside it the Poor Law hospital system had developed, as well as, from mid-nineteenth century, the cottage hospital movement. From the 1880s a rapid increase in hospital provision took place, not only of general hospitals, but of isolation hospitals for those with infectious diseases and of asylums for the mentally deranged (Abel-Smith, 1964; Pinker, 1966; Smith, 1979).

Around 1930 a diverse array of hospital provision remained. At this time the Poor Law was finally being dismantled. An Act of 1929 allocated the Poor Law hospitals to the Public Health Committee of the local authorities, which already had isolation or fever hospitals under their wing. The voluntary hospitals, some of them linked to medical schools and acting as teaching hospitals, and most of them involved in training nurses, were increasingly in financial difficulties. By now they were not confined to the sick poor. Indeed, the latter had been, since the turn of the century, more and more likely to have recourse to the Poor Law hospitals, for the middle class was taking up beds in the voluntary hospitals (Abel-Smith, 1964).

What this might mean to the sick poor is well documented by Bella Aronovitch (1974), who wrote a remarkable account of her hospitalization from 1928 to 1932. The working-class daughter of Russian refugee parents living in the East End of London where she worked as a furrier, she continued to go to work although she felt ill, because one had to work, the money was needed. One day she felt so ill that instead of going home she walked into a nearby hospital, choosing the smaller rather than the larger of two available. She had a ruptured appendix and general poisoning. The wound after the operation remained open for most of those years she was in hospital. She was moved down the status line from one hospital to another, narrowly missing being relegated to the work-house as an incurable pauper. She was rescued from this fate by her mother, who persuaded the honorary consultant of a prestigious voluntary hospital to try to cure her, a final desperate attempt. This he successfully did, although she was left with continuing problems and much pain. Her story also provides insight into the medical hierarchy of the day and the separate and inferior place accorded to women medical students. It tells much of the way in which pain was borne. Nothing could be done about it, so one did not mention it; others knew about the suffering but did not discuss it, for that would not have helped.

INCREASING DIVISIONS OF LABOUR: BOUNDARIES AND SPECIALTIES

A consequence of the increasing influence of hospitals and the changed status of GPs under the 1911 Act was an increasing differentiation between GPs and consultants from the time of the Act. 'Most of the 15,000 GPs who entered NHI [National Health Insurance] found themselves increasingly cut off from their colleagues in hospital' (Honigsbaum, 1978, p. 12). It was from among the ranks of the 5,000 who stayed outside NHI that the GP-specialists arose.

Other features of the developing division of labour around this period must also be noted. The first is the increasing specialization among consultants; the second the establishment of a hierarchy within the occupation of nursing. Associated with these is the way in which other health-care workers were defined into or out of the medical division of labour.

Medical Specialization and Other Divisions
After the First World War, and to some extent stimulated by it, there was

> development of special skills and special interests, particularly in psychiatry, orthopedics, and plastic and thoracic surgery. At the same time, advances applicable to medical practice were being made in non-clinical fields – biochemistry, bacteriology, and endocrinology – and in the social services. Radiotherapy was being adopted in a number of hospitals; diagnostic radiology was expanding. By the early 1920s medical specialization, although deplored by those who saw that medicine was irrevocably disunited, was generally accepted as necessary and inevitable. Many specialties were grad-ually evolving from a peripheral interest in particular spheres of general medicine or general surgery to bodies of knowledge in their own right.
> (Stevens, 1966, p. 38)

There was also the question of what to define in, and how to do that, and also what should be defined out. Eyes, feet, teeth and bones all constituted particular problems, for all had in one way or another been dealt with separately in earlier divisions of labour (not to mention childbirth and 'women's problems', which have been discussed as a special issue throughout this text).

Orthopaedics became a recognized specialty within medicine, but practitioners of osteopathy, with a different knowledge base and refusing to accede the right of diagnosis to medical practitioners, remained outside the orthodox orbit, albeit with their own education, training, entry and control (Larkin, 1978, p. 853). Larkin has discussed the relationship of those dealing with X-rays (1978), teeth (1980) and eyes (1981) with orthodox medicine, as well as their own professionalizing tactics (see also Larkin, 1983). Opticians (Larkin, 1983, ch. 2) have a long history, having had an incorporated guild, the Worshipful Company of Spectacle Makers, as long ago as 1692. But in the mid-nineteenth century they had come into opposition with the medical profession. Disguised in a professional rhetoric a trade battle was mounted which became intense by the turn of the century. While medical practitioners thought they should have charge of the whole field of health and healing, no matter what part of the body was involved, the public voted with their feet (or in this case their eyes) and took their problems to opticians rather than medical practitioners. Intense debates in the 1920s, including attention paid to the issue by the 1926 Royal Commission on NHI, led ultimately to a settlement. This involved state registration for opticians, who were expected to refer to a medical specialist of opthalmology any cases where sight defects might be caused by underlying disease conditions. Referral where disease was suspected was made legally obligatory in 1958 (Larkin, 1983, p. 57). The anxieties of the medical profession, championed at no less a level than that of the General Medical Council, while ostensibly related to the protection of the public, were in practice closely related to their fear of encroachment upon medical preserves by other health-care practitioners. Medical practitioners insisted upon having a major interest on the professional regulation bodies. With regard to ophthalmic opticians as to other paramedical groups, self-regulation was thus somewhat of a mockery for all but the medical practitioners themselves.

Problems with teeth were also something which the public in general had seen as separate from 'physic' and which had attracted specialists from an early period, if only those who attended at fairs and markets and pulled out offending teeth. Here again, notwithstanding the antiquity of a separate occupation, medicine made strong bids to incorporate dentistry. Dentistry itself in its professionalizing tactics behaved much like the medical profession in eliminating or subordinating rival practitioners (Larkin, 1980). Dentists in 1921 became a closed profession, 'with entry only through GMC approved schools' (Larkin, 1980, p. 224) with the exception of dental dressers. Mostly women, dental dressers had done a good deal of the basic care of schoolchildren's dental health under the public health provisions. In deciding for closure, but accepting medical domination, dentists also pursued a policy designed to eliminate dental dressers, while developing an alternative division of labour involving secretarial, mechanical and non-surgical groups clearly defined as subordinate to the professional dentist (Larkin, 1980).

The case of radiographers and radiology is similar in some senses but quite different in that the division of labour which had to be negotiated in this case was a question of how to deal with a new technology rather than one derived from an ancient division of labour based on particular parts of the body. Doctors for the most part knew nothing of the technology upon which X-rays were based. They were in a situation in which they were liable to become dependent on non-medical skills and in which the few of their number who had taken the trouble to understand the new developments could command a new specialty. The upshot of this struggle, as Larkin (1978; 1983 ch. 3) analyses it, was the systematic deskilling of those who took the X-rays, who by the 1930s were predominantly women, relegating them to a position of technicians. Medically qualified radiologists reserved the right and the power of diagnosis and advice. The female-dominated healing skills of physiotherapists and occupational therapists were similarly subjugated. Their experiences were consistent with those of other women in the health-care division of labour who felt the impact of the strongly male-dominated and well-established gender order which had persisted from previous centuries.

Divisions in Nursing

As well as being dominated by men, women were divided by class and status. Thus nursing, a predominantly female profession, had its own internal stratification during the first half of the twentieth century. What Maggs (1983, pp. 26–8) has called the 'occupational imperialism' of general nursing might be seen as a root cause of the nursing hierarchies. At the same time, it is fair to say that this state of affairs resulted, at least in part, from medical imperialism, in part from the male-dominated gender order and in part from the demand for more and more pairs of hands on the part of hospitals with increasing numbers of patients.

Given the realities of a class- and gender-divided society, it is difficult to see what other sets of relationships among the health-care occupations there might have been. (Although one must note that, in the case of dentistry, Larkin, 1980, has shown that New Zealand came up with quite a different solution from Britain.) Celia Davies (1982) has shown that despite differences US nurses, like their British sisters, were also effectively trapped in a subordinate position to medicine and hence, I would wish to add, also to men.

Given this subordination the leaders of general nursing set out to carve as relatively autonomous a role as possible for their members. We have already noted (pages 65, 96) the disciplined hierarchy within nursing and the discipline which nurses imposed upon their patients. Sisters were subjected to the authority of matrons, and probationers to sisters. The discipline was stern and clear; the ward work was routinized; nurses lived in and remained single and celibate or left. General nurses were given a sense of belonging to a corporate body and having the training and the discipline which made them and their skills invaluable anywhere. This sense of collective unity was designed to overcome any differences of class origin, that there might have been among them. Many came from the 'lower orders', but even while admitting this no mention was made of the working class; all came from the 'earnest' class; their earnestness and their training wiped out social distinctions and thus turned all into trained nurses and members of the 'earnest' class (Maggs, 1983, pp. 21–2).

The early attempts by Nightingale to reform workhouse hospitals had not altogether succeeded, however, and by the end of the century there remained more than one type of nurse, experiencing different working conditions and different occupational leadership. Training schemes were by now generally available in the voluntary hospitals and were increasingly being instituted into the hospitals established under the Public Health Act of 1875. The best of these came to offer as good treatment for the patients and training for the nurses as the voluntary hospitals. Workhouse hospitals were also improving but neither in the workhouse nor in the asylums for the treatment of the mentally ill and handicapped did the model of general nursing prevail. Rather, general nurses became the élite of the nursing profession, relegating workhouse and asylum nurses to an inferior position.

The differences between them came to be reflected in their different modes of collective organization. Following a professional pattern, general nurses stressed vocation, selflessness and dedication; they formed a College of Nursing in 1916 (Abel-Smith, 1960, pp. 86–95). However difficult they might find negotiations about wages and working conditions, the strike weapon was not for them. Asylum and Poor Law nurses, on the other hand, perceiving the tasks they had to do as much the same as those of other workers and the way they were treated in similar vein, joined in the trade union movement (Carpenter, 1980).

Later the division between the ladies and the probationers in general nursing was replaced by other distinctions. In the mid-nineteenth century there had been little for women from working-class families to do except domestic service, or for genteel women, governessing. Nursing in its reformed and disciplined mode was a not unattractive alternative for both ladies and women. By the end of the nineteenth century other alternatives were beginning to develop, such as typing, shop work and teaching, and even the professions were beginning to open. From the First World War onwards opportunities for women increased. At the same time the number of hospitals also increased and with it the demand for nurses. During the First World War the problem had been dealt with by the introduction of Voluntary Aid Detachments (VADs), women who were given a minimal introduction to nursing. Their presence caused a good deal of anxiety to the leaders of the trained nurses, just as the notion of 'dilution' did to skilled workers (Abel-Smith, 1960, pp. 83–7, 99–101 and 108–10). By the Second World War, the chronic shortage of nurses, which had been a matter for investigation throughout the 1930s (Abel-Smith, 1960, ch. XI), was finally acknowledged, and the 1943 Nurses Act introduced the Roll in addition to the Register which had been established in 1918. State Enrolled Nurses (SENs) could qualify after only two years compared with the three necessary for entry to the Register. Ultimately therefore there were not only SRNs but SENs and auxiliaries as well. Not only was nursing now stratified within the training grades, as was medicine, but there were also stratifications of skill among the trained and their helpers. From the outset of course the nursing care of the patient had depended heavily on the nurse in training, and it continued to do so.

Distinctions between grades of general nurse remained. Other distinctions had been removed. The ban on men entering general nursing went in 1943, but it remained the case that most male nurses were to be found in the area of mental illness and handicap. General nursing retained its status as superior to fever nursing and asylum nursing: a distinction which reflected the relative status of the hospitals in which the nurses trained.

FURTHER ISSUES IN THE SEXUAL DIVISION OF PAID HEALTH LABOUR

It was not only in the professions supplementary to medicine (as they came to be called) or in nursing that the societal gender order was imprinted on the health-care division of labour. As was noted in Chapter 6, midwives were accorded state registration in 1902, giving them a responsible position in health care but one which was definitely subservient to the medical profession. The register had finally been granted to nurses in 1918, partly in consequence of the work which women had done during the war and partly because of the model which the midwives register had established.

There were by 1900 a limited number of women doctors, as we also saw, such that from now on, although men continued to dominate the medical profession throughout the first three-quarters of the twentieth century, it would be incorrect to use the shorthand 'medical men' for the medical profession. In response to the suffrage movement and impelled by women's war work, all legal bars to women entering the professions were removed by Act of Parliament in 1919. Plenty of *de facto* barriers remained, including the imposition of quotas upon the number of women students which medical schools were prepared to admit.

In 1918 also limited suffrage was granted to women, who could now vote so long as they were over 30. It was not until 1928 that the 'flapper vote' was granted, and women and men were accorded formal political equality (see also Stacey and Price, 1981). It was against this background that the maternal and child health movement developed. This is an instructive example of the way in which the class structure of the society and its gender order shaped the division of labour in health care. Women as mothers were encouraged to rear children more healthily for the nation; they were effectively recruited as unpaid health workers. Paid women health workers, registered medical practitioners and others were recruited to provide health education and health care under the control of predominantly male Medical Officers of Health.

The actions of the state in this development must be understood in class terms, in the sense that the efforts were specifically to educate working-class women to be better mothers. They have also to be understood in terms of the perception by government of the national interest, rather than directly the interests of capital. A healthier and stronger workforce may have been of interest to capitalists, but men fit to fight ('cannon-fodder') were even more important to rulers of the state.

RECRUITING THE MOTHERS

Jane Lewis (1980) discusses how poor health exhibited by recruits for the Boer War aroused the interest of the state. The focus came down on the children; if they were brought up healthily the next generation would be fitter. In this context, free school meals were instituted in 1906, and the school health service was established in 1907, both under Education Acts – partial answers to the poverty that was implicated in the poor health of the adult population. This focus on children drew attention to the mothers' child-rearing practices rather than to the family's poverty and bad housing. Much of the poor national health could, it was concluded, be accounted for by the ignorance and fecklessness of the mothers. Maternal education was the answer. In 1918 the Maternity and

Child Welfare Act permitted local health authorities to provide a range of services for women and children, with central government providing matching grants (see also Lodge, n.d.).

THE PAID CHILD HEALTH WORKERS: WOMEN DOCTORS AND HEALTH VISITORS

A woman doctor, Dr Janet Campbell, with a staff of five women, was responsible for national aspects of the programme at the newly established Ministry of Health in London. The local organizers of the service were the Medical Officers of Health (MOsH) and were almost all men. Child health work itself was however thought of as women's work. This was especially true of the health visitors, who were to visit the homes of the mothers. A disproportionate number of the few qualified women doctors went into child health work with the local authority. Ironically, a service which women, both lay and medical, had worked for because they saw it meeting their needs became an area where women doctors, nurses and health visitors were employed at low rates and from whence they had little chance of advancement, as Davies (1988) has shown by examining evidence about public health work and comparing the careers of women and men doctors in that sector.

Public health was not highly valued. Honigsbaum (1979, p. 84) suggests that a new panel doctor (i.e. an NHI general practitioner) with an income of £1,200 in 1922 would start at a level equal to the highest paid MOH and four times higher than a beginner in the public health service. The salaries for maternity and child welfare officers were hardly more than the income of a woman schoolteacher. Many of the women doctors worked part-time only (as they still do), while some of the men were also general practitioners. Furthermore, maternal and child health was not a branch of public health which led to promotion within that service, let alone led to élite positions in medicine more generally.

Davies's (1983, pp. 30–1) survey of a sample of women and men doctors employed in the public health service from 1921 to 1939 shows that a few stood out who reached senior positions; these included both women and men. Apart from this handful there were big differences between the sexes in the doctors' situations and careers. Twenty-three women but only three men worked in maternity and child welfare out of twenty-nine women and thirty men in her sample. One of these three men was on his way to becoming an MOH; the women stayed as medical officers in maternity and child welfare, where in some authorities they were subject to the marriage bar (i.e. women, but not men, had to retire upon marriage).

In addition to appointing these predominantly female medical officers, the state, through the MOsH, provided mothers with information cards and leaflets, milk depots for pure milk, schools for mothers and classes for schoolgirls. Health visitors had been employed by the Ladies Sanitary Association in the 1860s and 1870s. The work of the health visitors employed by the MOsH 'evolved from the efforts of the late nineteenth century "lady health missioners" who had combined poor visiting and the distribution of religious tracts with sanitary visits and the distribution of soap and disinfectant'. The original lady visitors 'taught mothers elementary hygiene, methods of infant care and management'. They were expected to 'counter the influences of hostile, old fashioned grandmothers and interfering neighbours' (Lewis, 1980, pp. 105 and 106).

From the outset, as Celia Davies (1983, pp. 25–6; and 1988) has pointed out, health visitors were given a contradictory task. They were expected to take the qualities and relations of the private domain and use them in the service of the public domain; they were expected to befriend and gently influence but also to monitor and report. Manuals for health visitors written between 1915 and 1926 which she studied make these points plain. The health visitors were instructed as to how they should cajole and control without being inspectors. One MOH who had set his face 'dead against an inspectoral role' said: 'My practice has been to instil into the minds of my own staff that they go to the house as a friend of the family and not merely [sic] to find cause for reproach.' Another thought that legal rights of entry were not needed because in practice he had never known a suitable visitor who could not ordinarily gain entry by tact alone. The notion of the friendly health visitor is constantly stressed; if they chided they would be unlikely to receive confidences or be able to give advice.

At the same time they were there to improve the manner of life of slapdash mothers. To this end they must keep themselves to themselves. The health visitor must make for herself a way of life that was a class apart; she must behave as if she were in the domestic domain but at the same time follow the more bureaucratic rules of the public domain. She must of course not forget her public-domain responsibilities: 'She must always be open to criticism from her MOH and from her committee [the public health authority]; she must always be extremely accurate in her reports, knowing that at any time they may have to stand the test of a court of law'

Notwithstanding the ambiguities and difficulties of their position, health visitors became established and respected health workers. By 1927 they were sufficiently professionalized to have achieved occupational closure in the sense that only a State Registered Nurse (SRN) could qualify (Davies, 1983; see also Davies, 1987).

LAY WOMEN AND THE CHILD HEALTH PROGRAMME

In these ways did the child surveillance programme begin, mothers recruited as unpaid health workers on behalf of the state and new class and gender divisions worked out in the health-care division of labour. These were all developments associated with the changes in medical knowledge and practice in the twentieth century, discussed by Armstrong (see pages 99–100). His account does not pay attention to the gender order nor to what lay women wanted.

Jane Lewis points out how the arguments for the maternal and child welfare services were made 'in an unimpeachable rhetoric which talked of the need to save lives and improve the quality of motherhood' without addressing the 'real needs of mothers and infants' (Lewis, 1980, p. 219). Working-class women 'approached their instructors with more needs than were met. Problems arising from insanitary living conditions were as pressing as any individual inadequacies' (Lewis, 1980, p. 61).

The Women's Co-operative Guild had collected evidence, published in 1915, about the lives of working women (Llewellyn Davies, 1978). The women told of poverty such that they had to go on working at heavy tasks right up until their confinement and be back on the job and/or servicing the household as soon as they could get up afterwards. There were so often many other children in the house to care for. Many women had totally inadequate diets in pregnancy, stretching inadequate wages round too many mouths and having to try to save for the doctor's, nurse's, or midwife's fee as well. The Co-operative women called for maternity benefit and more competent health care (some of the accounts of supposedly professional attention are most alarming). Their demands were for municipal not philanthropic action, the Guild encouraging women to take part in local government. They wanted improvements for the whole working class as well as specific measures for the mothers (Llewellyn Davies, 1978, pp. 16–17). The Women's Co-operative Guild itself supported the idea of a School for Mothers. Lewis concludes (1980, p. 100) that 'there is no doubt but that the centres provided information, much needed nourishment, companionship and a measure of reassurance for many women', although they did not address all the working-class women's problems.

MATERNAL HEALTH

The national concern was expressed in terms of quality of the population and measured by mortality rates. Initially the focus was entirely on *infant* mortality rates (see pages 161–2) for a discussion of mortality and morbidity rates). It was not until later that attention to the survival and health of infants led to attention to the health and survival of the mothers themselves, and then it was attention to them not as women in their own right but as vessels for the production of children (Arney, 1982, p. 208). The focus was again on mortality rates. The women's movement, although it was composed of a number of disparate groups, was engaged in the debate about maternal mortality at the start of the century and continuing throughout the interwar period. The women themselves, however, were also clear about the pervasive maternal morbidity, the chronic ailments from which they suffered especially after childbirth, and which were not even recognized – nor was treatment accessible to working-class women (Palmer, 1978 and 1987).

THE MIDDLE-CLASS VIEW

Middle-class sections of the women's movement were also concerned about maternal mortality, but their demands were somewhat different, being concerned less with the material base and more with facilities to enable them to learn how to rear their children and to reduce the maternal mortality rate (see Palmer, 1987).

While the 'ignorant and feckless' were the target of the state maternity child health campaign, women from all classes wanted advice on rearing their children. The development of the medical and social sciences had convinced them of the inadequacy of received wisdom; mothers as competent child rearers suffered a special kind of deskilling at the hands of professionals. The state from early century supported an ideology of motherhood which 'persuaded women that their role in the home was of national importance and that motherhood was their primary duty' (Lewis, 1980, p. 224). It has also since persuaded them of the correctness of surveillance and the need to co-operate with it. The upshot has been double-edged for women and their children.

WOMEN TRAPPED AND DIVIDED

The effect of the involvement of women in the maternity and child health services was to make new divisions of women against women. The wives of the bourgeoisie had long played their part in upholding the class structure by their involvement in charitable work. Some had employed working-class women to do the work for them, although others, like Josephine Butler before them, did the visiting themselves. Although reinforcing class divisions, genuine help was given to individual cases. Now women were employed in their own right, using their specially trained skills to help other women but also to monitor and control them. Their task, both as doctors and as health visitors, was to convince mothers that they needed professional help with their children, not only when they were ill but when they were healthy and normal.

There were thus these two ironies; the women's attempts to claim public-domain services for themselves led to the development of an area of medical work in which the paid workers were exploited and which divided women against each other – the women who controlled other women being employed by and reporting to men. In this way this corner of the ambiguous intermediate zone between the public and domestic domains was created. Women recognized that their sisters needed help; they themselves thought that women could best help each other; women thought it was good work for women professionals to go into; because it was women's work, the men devalued it; the whole area of preventive child health work remained something until recently (see page 191) in which 'real doctors' were not interested. When they did it, they passed the work to an inferior such as a health visitor.

CHILD HEALTH CARE IN THE DIVISION OF MEDICAL LABOUR

The bulk of general practitioners (mostly all men still) were not happy about the development of the preventive child health service. GPs in the 1920s were alarmed that the development of the service would 'encroach' on their rights to practise. They themselves had paid little or no attention to the care of working-class mothers and children other than on a fee basis in cases of acute illness. Their campaign against encroachment was successful to the extent that doctors working in the maternal and child health clinics were not allowed to treat, only to examine and advise: a situation which remains to this day. Thus if a clinic doctor in the course of examining a child and advising the mother as to the child's normal growth and development should discover some pathology, she cannot prescribe; her role is to advise the mother to take her child to the general practitioner or refer the child for hospital treatment. In this way the child health clinic and its workers were given low status; the doctors could not practise 'real medicine', and mothers were put to the trouble of taking their child, if ill, for yet another consultation. This did, however, give her the benefit of two opinions.

PLANS FOR A MORE COMPREHENSIVE HEALTH SERVICE

Throughout the interwar period proposals and counter-proposals for the reorganization of health-care provision were made, many edging towards universal and publicly funded health care. These will be reviewed in Chapter 8. What should already be clear is that it would be a service organized by and for biomedicine. By the mid-twentieth century the medical profession was firmly entrenched at the head of an increasingly complex division of labour. It had subordinated to its own service a variety of other health-care workers and was served by an increasingly stratified nursing profession. Access to health care was differentiated by both class and gender; the health-care division of labour was also so differentiated. These features were greatly to influence the structure of the emergent National Health Service.

8 The State and the Division of Health Labour: the National Health Service

Where does the establishment of the National Health Service (NHS) fit into the pattern of health-care development which the mode of analysis used in this book has suggested so far? We have seen that the establishment of NHI in 1911 was part of the Liberal government's answer to social unrest. Blanpain (1978) has suggested that all the European health insurance systems arose in similar circumstances. Does this mean, as Navarro (1978) argues, that whether health provisions are made and how they are made depend on the current score in the class struggle? Does state intervention follow from the logic of biomedical knowledge and the techniques and facilities required to practise it? Does it flow from successful collective organization on the part of the medical profession, as Parry and Parry (1976) propose? Is the NHS the creature of administrators and their advisers anxious to have a rational and controllable structure to undertake what by the mid-twentieth century had come to be seen as an essential service to be provided in any advanced industrial society? Was the NHS the logical culmination of humanitarian moves based on values associated with equity and redistributive justice for which rational planning and administration were necessary (cf. Abel-Smith, 1978)? Or was it, as others suggest, while not denying the humane intentions and personal devotion of many reformers, that the Welfare State, of which the NHS is a crucial element, was developed in response to the internal contradictions of capitalism, of the need to reproduce the labour force and the need which capital shares with the state to maintain order (cf. Doyal with Pennell, 1979; Gough, 1979)? How influential were left-wing interests? Can the NHS be more simply seen as the response of democratic government to the balance of interests in a society with a plural political system (Eckstein, 1958; Klein, 1983; Willcocks, 1967)?

In seeking to sort out these various notions and bearing in mind the task set in this book we should first of all note that there are two questions to address. One is the nature of the societal changes involved, both those which led to the establishment of the NHS and those which flowed from it. The second is the nature of the social interactions which led up to the legislation. Clearly the two are linked, but they are analytically distinct. What the founders of the NHS thought they were doing and what in fact emerged are also two distinct questions, for there were undoubtedly a number of unintended consequences. Subsequent to the establishment of the NHS some profound changes took place in the doctor–patient relationship, in the way health, illness and illness behaviour are conceived and in the division of labour among the health workers. How far these changes may be said to be due to the NHS, how far similar changes are found in other countries where mass biomedicine has been funded and administered on different principles, can only be hinted at in this book. The topic undoubtedly merits closer attention.

THE HEALTH SERVICE A SOCIALIST TRIUMPH?

When the NHS was finally established in 1948 by the Labour government under the 1946 Act, following the Beveridge Report of 1942, the radical feature was that it made health care free at the point of delivery to everyone in Britain. The principle of universalism which characterized welfare and health legislation in the postwar period was perhaps manifested most dramatically in the health service. No more were there to be means tests; no more were some to be eligible for treatment from a general practitioner under the panel arrangements and others not; free medical treatment was available for everyone. Under the parallel social security arrangements, all who paid their flat rate insurance, their 'stamp', poor and rich, women and men, would be entitled to sickness benefit and benefit if unemployed. In addition there was a security net, in the shape of national assistance, to catch those who fell through any unsuspected hole in this supposedly universal coverage.

There was one exception; the quasi-feudal status of married women (see Land, 1976; Stacey and Price, 1981; Wilson, 1977 and 1980) was carried by this legislation into the second half of the twentieth century. A married woman was exempt from National Insurance payments if she so wished but was covered by her husband's payments, always assuming he kept them up. So far as health was concerned the principle of universality was established; workers and non-workers, wives as well as husbands, children and the elderly as well as the working population were included. Persons of all classes, ages, colours and both sexes were henceforth to be treated on the basis of their health need and were in no way to be rationed by the purse. Furthermore, the principal source of funds was to be general taxation; the health component of the insurance stamp was token only. At the same time for those who had money and wished to buy it, private treatment was still available; but such people had to pay their tax and insurance contributions to the state health service just the same. These measures went a long way to remove the stigma which had attached to prewar public provision.

Flowing from this one might suppose that the new health service was one which was designed by and for the people. Among its protagonists this came to be widely believed; by many on the political left it was seen as a socialist health service and a victory for the working-class movement (cf. Navarro, 1978). The whole package of postwar welfare legislation was seen by many Labour supporters as at least a major step on the road to socialism; for many 'social reform became equated with socialism' (Saville, 1983, p. 16). Closer examination of the historical antecedents of the NHS as well as the division of labour and responsibility established within it somewhat temper this left-wing interpretation, as do the subsequent revisions and reorganizations which the NHS has undergone (Saville, 1983).

Such an examination shows that two categories of people played important roles in developing a climate of opinion favourable to a national health service and contributed to the final resolution of disputes among interested parties and thus to the final shape of the NHS. These were the medical profession and senior civil servants.

EARLY STATE INVOLVEMENT WITH HEALTH CARE

When the NHS was established in 1948 it was exactly a hundred years since the state had first become involved in health matters in a major way with the 1848 Public Health Act, the precursor of the great consolidating Act of 1875. From that time the division of labour in health care began to be altered, for the state was now involved as well as the doctor and the patient. State involvement, taken in the interests of what was seen as the common good, was sometimes overt and apparently oppressive – as in the removal of people or their children to isolation hospitals or asylums, in the compulsory fumigation of people's dwellings, or the arrest and compulsory medical examination for evidence of VD of women suspected of prostitution (see Chapter 5).

From 1848 and for the following forty or fifty years the primary health concern of the state had been with public health, with the well-being of the entire population. By the 1880s and 1890s attention had turned more to the curative services (cf. Doyal with Pennell, 1979), and the public health movement to more personal facets of health care. Lloyd George's decision to establish NHI further involved the state. Direct involvement had been avoided by the use of approved societies to administer the scheme and the doctors themselves to run it at the local level. It 'is arguable that 1918 marked the beginning of a conscious attempt to develop modern health services' (Webster, 1984, p. 1); the Ministry of Health was established in 1919 and from that time it was involved on behalf of the state in a general oversight of central and local expenditure in both preventive and curative services and in the formulation of regulations. The ministry set up the Dawson Committee which reported in 1920 recommending an integrated health service and suggesting the establishment of health centres as a focus for the hospital and general practitioner services. Six years later the Royal Commission on NHI in 1926 favoured replacing the insurance basis by public funding as was the case with other health provisions. A civil service view began to develop. The involvement of Janet Campbell, Senior Medical Officer of the Maternity and Child Welfare Department of the Ministry, in maternity and infant services through the 1920s and 1930s is an early example (cf. Oakley, 1984; Palmer, 1987). By the 1930s senior permanent civil servants not only had a view but were active in initiating reform.

THE GESTATION OF THE NHS

Earlier and valuable accounts of the establishment of the NHS (Eckstein, 1958; Stevens, 1966; Willcocks, 1967) were written before the thirty-year rule made hitherto classified documents available and former civil servants, medical and non-medical, such as Godber (1975 and 1983) and Pater (1981) had written their accounts. It is now easier to get a rounded picture of the interests involved and also who was concerned about what (cf. Klein, 1983). The friendly societies and the trade unions (both involved with NHI), the voluntary hospitals (represented by the British Hospitals' Association (BHA)) and the local authorities with responsibilities for hospitals and preventive health care, as well as organized health-care professions and occupations, Civil Service and government all had interests vested in the health-care provisions. Patients and potential patients had important interests, but their organization was partial. Their voice swelled the wartime demand for social reform but was not specifically articulated.

By the end of the 1930s an elaborate and administratively irrational series of health provisions had developed. Not only was the overall pattern muddled, there were problems in almost all the constituent parts as well as in the relations between them. We have already seen that the coverage of NHI was partial, excluding most women, all children and the elderly. The local health authority services did something to make up the gap so far as women and children were concerned, but because of general practitioner opposition could not offer a curative service (Chapter 7; and see Stacey and Davies, 1983). The voluntary hospitals, including the most prestigious, were in continual financial crisis. There were difficulties about delineating the respective tasks of the voluntary hospitals and the local authority hospitals and asylums, which in addition to the infirmaries included the old Poor Law hospitals (Abel-Smith, 1964).

Preparation for the war and the wartime Emergency Medical Service (EMS) gave some impetus to the moves for reform, but the evidence is that these were already under way both within the Civil Service and outside well before the war, when a group of civil servants had begun work which was continued into the war years under the Chief Medical Officer, McNalty (Klein, 1983, p. 7). They worked against the background of depression and working-class ill health described at the outset of Chapter 7.

Outside the Civil Service, but drawing to some extent on those servants' views and experience, bodies such as Political and Economic Planning and the Nuffield Provincial Hospitals Trust (NPHT) were undertaking studies and making proposals for the reorganization of health care and particularly of the hospitals. The NPHT was one of the many of Lord Nuffield's great bequests in the health field and beyond, of which his provision of 'iron lungs' for those paralysed by polio probably received most publicity at the time. Bodies like PEP and the NPHT did much to inform intellectual and administrative opinion before the Second World War.

THE DOOMSDAY BOOK OF BRITISH HOSPITALS

The Ministry of Health undertook a rapid review of hospitals in 1938, when the threat of war came closer, to establish the availability of beds in case of massive casualties. Later, after the Beveridge Report of 1942, a more detailed survey was undertaken, what Godber (1983) has called the Doomsday Book of British Hospitals. This gave useful administrative information, detailing the nature of the problem, and is valuable for us in understanding the preparations that were being made for reform. What we now think of as Health Regions were surveyed one by one. The surveys were not done by 'hired hands' but by leading members of the medical profession, including prestigious physicians and surgeons, as well as local authority MOsH and medical administrators in the ministry itself. It is important to notice how much hard and extra work such people were prepared to put in, even if one might cynically suggest that part at least of what they were after was the improvement of their own working conditions and professional status.

For us also a look at the 'Doomsday Book' can give an insight into the motley array of British hospitals before 1948. Godber himself was responsible for helping to survey what is now the Trent region. His account shows how varied the provision and the standards of hospitals were at that time and also, compared with today, how fluid the medical division of labour was. He visited all the 300 hospitals in the region, which ranged from compulsorily provided small hospitals for smallpox cases which everyone hoped they would never need: 'One was in a quarry on the edge of an operational airfield in Derbyshire; it had two huts, one for each sex, and no fixed sanitary appliance of any kind – the only recourse would have been sheltering in the bushes nearby' (1983, p. 7). There were tiny infectious diseases and cottage hospitals where personalized care was offered. More worrying, Godber found, were the larger hospitals with pretensions:

> the thirty- to fifty-bed so-called general hospitals which we often thought were used far too much for surgery, often done by specialists who visited once a week. It was difficult to decide which should worry us most – the patients who were seen once by a specialist on the wing or those who were confidently treated, usually surgically, by a local general practitioner.
>
> (1983, p. 7)

In this period, using their living in general practice as a base, some GPs developed specialist skills in local hospitals, some going on later to become leading national consultants.

GENERAL PRACTICE IN THE 1940s

We can gain further understanding of the state of national health care just before the NHS from the evidence to the Spens Report, which was set up to look at the remuneration of general practitioners and reported in 1942. Webster (1983) has analysed this evidence. We have already seen (pages 101–4) that, despite their initial opposition, general practitioners had become attached to panel practice under the NHI scheme. Their continual complaint was that the capitation fee was inadequate; they also resisted any raising of the income limits for eligibility to the scheme. Their attachment to the system was so great however that they effectively carried it into the NHS, as we shall see.

There were nevertheless many variations among them (Webster, 1983). Those who negotiated for them in the lead-up to NHS were quite unrepresentative of the hard-worked majority. GP list sizes varied from a few hundred to 5,000; inner-city practice contrasted with suburban practice; and small-town practices varied from those in prosperous to those in depressed areas. Most doctors were single-handed, although some employed medical assistants; most dispensed their own drugs. A cause of complaint towards the end of the 1930s and into the war, as more and more drugs (some useful and some useless) became available, was that their earnings were reduced because of the expense of providing these drugs.

The advantage of NHI to the general practitioners was the 'firm bedrock income' (Webster, 1983, p. 21) which it provided and the opportunities over and above that for private practice. Real chances to make money in private practice varied enormously, as did the chance to do hospital sessions and develop a specialism. Doctors in wealthy areas could have relatively small lists and do well from private fees. Those in poorer areas had no such chances, had to sustain large lists to survive and to work long hours, a 12–14-hour working day being taken as normal by many. Many were poor, and this was reflected in the sale value of their practices. 'In London they were worth 1½ to 2 years' purchase, but in the [Welsh] valleys they only fetched 1 year's purchase, i.e. no more than one year's nominal rental income for the house alone.' Nevertheless the sale of the practice was their 'only and very hard won substantial capital asset' (Webster, 1983, p. 22).

There is no doubt that the affluent practitioners looked down on their poorer colleagues, who not only lacked a chance to earn private fees but had no chance either to develop hospital specialties. Webster concludes:

> General practitioners emerge from the evidence of the Spens papers as less of a mutually supportive brotherhood of equals than as a crowd of individualists in which the class divisions and discriminations of society at large were repeated in a microcosmic form.
> (1983, p. 23)

CLASS AND STATUS DIVISIONS AND ALLIANCES

Whether the differences among general practitioners, and indeed among doctors as a whole, were technically class or status differences is of some interest, especially for those who seek to analyse the establishment of the NHS in Marxian terms (cf. Navarro, 1978). Webster suggests that panel doctors' basic loyalty was to their patients and likens them to the proprietors of corner shops. In these terms they certainly can be seen, in their fierce independence and entrepreneurship, as akin to members of the petty bourgeoisie. Perhaps that was their closest alignment. On the other hand, the prestigious and wealthy hospital specialists with their large private practices were undoubtedly upper middle class in terms of their status and in some cases may have had close affiliations with the industrial and commercial bourgeoisie, as well as among the gentry and aristocracy. Navarro (1978) is in my view incorrect to imagine that they were members of the upper class, if by that he means the traditional upper class (Stacey, 1960). The gentry and aristocracy could never quite bring themselves to accept persons who worked on their bodies as social equals, although they might entertain them in their dwellings and be related to them by blood or marriage. But perhaps these are differences in status rather than class? The élite of doctors were certainly upper middle class and in Marxian terms allied with the bourgeoisie.

The alliance which the British Medical Association struck up with the Trades Union Congress (TUC) in the course of the negotiations about the establishment of the NHS should also not be forgotten. The TUC's interest derived from trade union dissatisfaction with the commercial interests which administered NHI and industrial injury compensation, believing that these worked against the interests of its members. It needed general practitioner support. The BMA, for its part, was being pressed by reformers among its own members: the Medical Practitioners' Union's (MPU) demands for better conditions in general practice; and the Socialist Medical Association (SMA), which was largely based among medical practitioners working in local government hospitals and the public health service. The alliance between the BMA and the TUC developed throughout the 1930s and continued during the war as plans for the NHS were being laid (Honigsbaum, 1979, pt 6 *passim*; Iliffe, 1983, pp. 25–9). The TUC's aims were narrower than those of the SMA with its demands for a full-blown salaried service.

A CONSENSUS OF RATIONAL PATERNALISTS?

In Klein's view a consensus had developed from the early 1940s about the way in which health administration should be reformed which was based on two linked assumptions about the delivery of health care in Britain, namely, that it was inadequate and irrational (1983, pp. 2–3). Inadequacy related to both coverage and quality: to the partial coverage of NHI and the isolation of general practitioners from the mainstream of medical knowledge. The irrationality derived from the dependence of medical practitioners on private fee-paying patients, which led to their crowding in the wealthier areas with a consequent dearth in the areas of greatest ill health and therefore medical need. Voluntary and public hospitals competed rather than co-operating, and the former had frequently ceased to be financially viable.

Webster (forthcoming) has challenged this consensus model with its pluralist or functionalist assumptions, arguing from historical data that there was a good deal of conflict in the run-up to the NHS, the socialist view having been expressed from the early days of the century. From its origins the Labour Party had been opposed to health care under the Poor Law and supported the Webbs' minority report of the 1909 Royal Commission on the Poor Law which argued for the development of a comprehensive state medical service. The insurance principle was disliked, and services such as maternity and child welfare were encouraged, which many opposed as socialistic.

Klein dubs the medical and administrative spokesmen (they were mostly men) of his consensus as *rational paternalists*, 'not so much ... outraged by social injustice as ... intolerant of muddle, inefficiency and incompetence: a tradition going back to ... Edwin Chadwick, via the Webbs' (Klein, 1983, p. 5). Two models, he argues, were available for the resolution of these problems; one followed Lloyd George and was based on the insurance principle, making personal medical care available to all those insured; the other was the public health model of local authority provision.

The Dawson Report (1920) had incorporated both (Klein, 1983; Pater, 1981). It stressed the importance of making both curative and preventive medicine available and stressed also such positive activities as physical culture. All these activities were to be provided in local health centres, leaving hospitals for more specialist activities. Webster (forthcoming) points out that the Labour Party had issued a policy document in 1918 to which 'the Dawson Report of 1920 may be regarded as a counterblast'.

There had been a Socialist Medical League formed in 1908 and a State Medical Service Association in 1912 composed mostly of professionals working for the Minority Poor Law Report. These had lapsed, but in 1930 the Socialist Medical Association (SMA) was formed. It was antagonistic to contributory insurance and in favour of extended public health services (Webster, forthcoming). During the 1930s and 1940s, Webster argues, the SMA exerted an influence disproportionate to its size, even penetrating the BMA's Medical Planning Commission during the Second World War, as well as strongly influencing

Labour's health service plans. Labour influenced reconstruction plans from its position in the wartime coalition government.

Klein seems to see the NHS as an alternative route, following neither the individualistic model of NHI taken in most European countries (Blanpain, 1978) nor the collectivist model of public health. The route had been marked out long before the war (Klein, 1983, p. 6; Pater, 1981). In political terms the NHS may have emerged in the form it did as a consequence of seeking a new model. Certainly the intention was to cover primary health, specialist hospital-based services and preventive medicine. But in the event the NHS came down heavily on the side of curative medicine. This was partly a consequence of the way the residual conflicts were resolved (see pages 124–5).

Klein's discussion also leaves out of account the issue of an occupational or industrial health service, another source of conflict and one which was part of SMA policy (Honigsbaum, 1979, ch. 26). Industrial and occupational health had been a major concern of the TUC, but in the end the TUC did not press the issue because it fell out with the SMA (Honigsbaum, 1979, pp. 272–3; Weindling, 1985, ch. 1).

WHO WERE KLEIN'S 'RATIONAL PATERNALISTS'?

They were civil servants and those academics and administrators who were associated with PEP and the NPHT (see page 119). And who were the people involved in negotiating about the form which the health service should take, in those quiet, behind-the-scenes negotiations which went on until Aneurin Bevan insisted on conducting them publicly? As Klein has it:

The cast-list is as significant for those left out as it is for those included. Among the excluded are the Approved Societies which administered the existing national insurance system: an exclusion all the more notable given the dominant role of these societies in the formation of the system in the period between 1911 and 1913. So, too, are the majority of those actually working in health services: from nurses to floor sweepers.

(1983, p. 9)

So who was included? 'The voluntary hospitals, local authorities and, above all, the medical profession' (1983, p. 9). Klein does not mention the exclusion of the patients and potential patients who were neither involved nor consulted except in so far as general political representations might be said to give them a voice. The interests of the civil servants lay in efficient administration. The doctors had their own interests, albeit somewhat different ones such as the variations between GPs, consultants and local authority doctors; through them too came the SMA influence. The representatives of the voluntary hospitals had vested interests, as had the local authorities interests vested in their hospitals and other health facilities and services. No one spoke for the experience of the patient as such, not even the SMA. Given the capitalist, hierarchical and male-dominated nature of the society in which all of this was taking place, the exclusion of manual workers and housewives is not surprising.

Plans for what turned out to be the NHS were laid by an administrative and political élite of men working with the medical élite. They were mostly men drawn from the upper middle class. By excluding the nurses not only was the single most numerous body of health-care professionals ignored but one which was composed almost entirely of women and led by them. The majority of the patients and potential patients were working class and roughly equally divided among women and men. Their exclusion however derives as much from the professional definition of the patient as someone to whom things are done and for whom plans are made, as it does from their class or patriarchal situation. Lay people among the planners accepted this professional notion; no formal representation in the discussions of those who were later to be thought of as 'consumers' was considered necessary.

So the plans were laid for the reform of health-care delivery by men for women and men, by the middle class for themselves and for the working class, by doctors without consultation with other health-care workers and by upper-middle-class doctors for the rest of the registered medical practitioners. The final enactment was, of course, a political matter; the form it took was influenced somewhat by the presence in power of the Labour government and somewhat by the particular character of Nye Bevan.

MORE MEDICAL THAN SOCIALIST INTERESTS

No doubt the Labour presence meant that the views of the Socialist Medical Association (SMA) were heard more sympathetically than they would other-wise have been. However, what emerged from the negotiations was in the end little influenced by their policies. Apart from the SMA the medical profession was greatly opposed to local government control of the health service; it smacked too much of the hated control of working men over the employment of doctors in the sick clubs (see page 102). General practitioners, furthermore, had no intention of becoming the salaried servants of anyone, local government or other. They argued, successfully, to remain independent entrepreneurs. They settled for a system of payment by capitation modelled on the NHI scheme and controlled by a local committee of doctors with limited lay membership. The major alteration was that all citizens and residents could register with them for primary health care, and for each one to register a capitation fee was received. GPs thus had a large assured clientele. They lost the right to buy and sell practices, something upon which apparently Bevan insisted. This was a loss to older doctors, but clearly made entry easier for the recently qualified and those without capital available.

The Lloyd George model for the GPs was not applicable to public health or to hospital services. Bevan resolved the conflict between the local authorities and the voluntary hospitals and between the advocates of central versus local control by deciding to nationalize the hospitals, a political decision which caused Godber and like-minded administrators great relief (1983, p. 7). It was adminis-tratively tidy and got away from all the old and muddled structures. This was not what the SMA had wanted. It shared Herbert Morrison's preference for local authority control as being nearer to the consumers for whom the service was run. The SMA's strong preference for a salaried service, as opposed to a fee-based system, lost it its influence in the BMA in 1944 (Honigsbaum, 1979, p. 288); and 'there is no evidence that its wisdom exercised any particular charm for Bevan, the Labour Minister of Health' (Webster, forthcoming, p. 22).

The compromises within these overall principles which were made are by now well known. The teaching hospitals were to remain separate from the rest in terms of their government and funding. Consultants would now be paid for their hospital work. Previously, it will be remembered, they had served on an honorary basis in the voluntary hospitals, gaining their income from private fee-paying patients. Their payment would be by salary in the form of sessional fees but they were not required to work full-time. The week was divided into sessions, and by contracting to do a fraction of the total sessions a consultant reserved to her/himself the right to do private practice. Any proportion could be negotiated with the relevant hospital management committee by mutual arrangement.

General practitioners were also accorded the right to undertake private practice, but the conditions were somewhat different. A person consulting a general practitioner privately had to pay not only her/his fee but also the full economic cost for any medicaments, dressings and so forth which were prescribed. The situation for hospital consultants was somewhat different. Having seen a patient privately they could then admit them to the public wards, to be treated at the public expense.

This, along with the provision of pay beds, was something which stored up trouble for the NHS as the years went by. In addition to the great majority of beds, free at the point of delivery, which were available to anyone needing hospital treatment, there were a small number of other classes of beds: amenity beds and pay beds. These beds could be paid for by those wishing greater privacy; but as to amenity beds, they could be let out in this way only if they were not required for NHS patients needing separation, rest, or quiet for medical reasons. Patients in amenity beds were simply buying privacy away from the open ward. Those in private beds were being treated privately.

Some of the later hassle might have been avoided if the same rule had been applied to consultants as was applied to general practitioners, namely, that once a patient had consulted them privately the patient had to 'go private' all the way. This would have made it impossible for some people to get the 'best of both worlds' and to use the private out-patient consultation as a means of queue jumping. This was an area where 'paternalistic rationalism' did not win the day against the insistent demands of the consultants, for such an arrangement would have severely reduced the number of private patients consulting.

CUI BONO?

It is the case that the consultants overall did better out of the negotiations leading up to 1948 than did the general practitioners and that the consultants in the teaching hospitals did best of all. Bevan was correct to claim he had stuffed their mouths with gold (Hart, 1973, quoted in Doyal with Pennell, 1979, p. 327). It is also the case that the doctors overall did better than the nurses, who, as we have seen, were not included in the early consultations. Pater (1981, p. 99) does not mention their inclusion in negotiations until as late as 1944. The ancillary workers were not considered at all. When they went on strike in 1973 many felt that the character of social relations within the division of labour in hospital service has been altered radically in the sense that ancillary workers had ceased to be the docile servants of doctors, no longer accepting that the privilege of working in hospitals justified low pay (Manson, 1977).

In the 1948 settlement the local authorities lost their hospitals but retained preventive and public health, maternity and infant welfare and school health. The general practitioners continued much as before. The nationalized hospitals were to be run by appointed boards upon which local authorities had some seats. These boards were by no means representative either of the population that they were to serve or of the workers in the industry. One might perhaps have expected that upon coming to power a Labour government would have repaired some of the omissions in the personnel involved in the negotiations. But they did not do so. Consumers and all other hospital workers than the doctors remained unrepresented. Nor were they to be included in the administration of the hospital service. Bevan's view of this was expressed in a letter to Sir Walter Citrine (General Secretary of the TUC) where he stressed the great importance he attached to appointing members to Regional Hospital Boards and Hospital Management Committees

> for their individual suitability and experience, and not as representatives or delegates of particular, and possibly conflicting interests. This means that [they] could not be appointed to 'represent' the health workers, and I could not agree (either) . . . that a proportion of members of these authorities should be appointed after consultation with health workers . . . If nurses were to be consulted, why not also the hospital domestics? the radiotherapists? the physiotherapists? and so on.
>
> (Bevan, quoted in Klein, 1983, pp. 21–2)

Why not indeed?

THE NHS AND THE CLASS STRUCTURE

In this way from the outset the management of what was to become the largest British industry not only reflected but was to play its part in transforming the class structure. Alone of all the health workers, the doctors were involved in its management. Nationalized the hospitals may have been; socialized they were not. I say 'transforming the class structure' rather than 'reflecting' it, for the managerial structure of the huge tertiary industries such as health, welfare and education were among agencies creating a new order within the class structure. Their government and administration were for the most part in the hands of an unrepresentative élite, and their multi-tiered managements put many in positions of greater or lesser power over lower-paid workers and patients alike. While related to the economic class structure and through the male-dominated gender order to the patriarchal family form, these new institutions, involving increasing central organization and control, also had the effect of diffusing power. This led often to a sense of alienation and powerlessness among the participants: a phenomenon which Foucault (1979) has sought to analyse and Armstrong (1983b) has applied with effect to the history of health care in twentieth-century Britain (see pages 99–100).

RISING COSTS OF HEALTH CARE

The first problem to assail the NHS arose less from the internal contradictions and tensions associated with the compromise, however, than with the miscalculation that the health of the nation would improve given universally available medical care. The rapidly rising cost of the service at a time of national economic difficulty led to the introduction of prescription charges in 1949 and charges for services to teeth and eyes in 1950.

Rising costs continued to lead to anxiety on the part of governments, the Treasury and therefore also ministry officials. Notions that the NHS was improperly controlled, that the activities of doctors should somehow be curbed and that the administrative structure of the health service was untidy all fuelled the fire of administrative reform. Issues of technical efficiency and managerial reform were raised under the Labour government in the 1960s. The doctors in the shape of the Porritt Committee in 1962 had already proposed that the three arms of the NHS should be unified. This idea appealed to the civil servants because it offered the possibility of more rational administration and greater central control. Details of the plans of the Labour government and the Conservative government which succeeded it and finally presided over the reforms are recorded elsewhere (Allsop, 1984; Iliffe, 1983; Klein, 1983). All the consultative documents however shared the central feature that the reforms were to be administrative. No changes were to be made at the point of delivery, such as the radical change of 1948 to a free and universal service.

THE 1974 REFORM

The reformed service was to have two characteristics; it was to be an integrated service, and there was to be responsibility upwards to managerial authority. The medical profession succeeded in breaching these intentions in two places. First of all, doctors as a whole insisted on retaining clinical autonomy and enshrined in the 'grey book' which was the Bible of the 1974 reorganization a sentence removing them from the managerial authority to which all other health-care professionals and workers were now to be subject.

> The management arrangements required for the NHS are different from those commonly used in other large organizations because the work is different. The distinguishing characteristic of the NHS is that, to do their work properly, consultants and general practitioners must have clinical autonomy, so that they can be fully responsible for the treatment they prescribe for the patients. It follows that these doctors and dentists work as each others' equals and that they are their own managers. In ethics and in law they are accountable to their patients for the care they prescribe, and they cannot be held accountable to the NHS authorities for the quality of their clinical judgements so long as they act within broad limits of acceptable medical practice and within policy for the use of resources.
>
> (DHSS, 1972b, para. 1.18)

This notion, of responsibility only to the patient, is based on a one-to-one doctor–patient relationship derived from mid-nineteenth-century private practice. It bears little relevance to the reality of relationships in large NHS hospitals.

Second, the general practitioners, who had come out less well than the hospital consultants, were by now organized and determined to improve their lot. They had already achieved the 'GPs' charter' in 1965 which improved their pay and status and made possible a restructuring of their working circumstances. (See Jefferys and Sachs, 1983, for a discussion of this process; also Cartwright, 1967, and Cartwright and Anderson, 1981.) The 1974 reorganization created a three-tier health service administered at regional, area and district level. While nominally within this structure, in practice the general practitioners insisted on retaining the structure that they had brought with them into the NHS from NHI. They continued to be run by what were now called Family Practitioner Committees, which were essentially similar to the Executive Councils of 1948. In these ways the medical profession limited the intentions of integration and managerialism (Allsop, 1984, p. 63; Levitt, 1976 and 1979).

THE CHALLENGE FROM THE ANCILLARY WORKERS

The doctors' position in the health division of labour was subjected to strains nevertheless. Manson (1977) has argued persuasively that one of the attempts to increase efficiency, namely the bonus system, actually encouraged the politicization of the ancillary workers. In order to get bonus schemes off the ground, meetings of workers had to be held. These were occasions in which for the first time workers realized that there were numbers of others in similar positions to themselves. Ironically, Manson argues, these meetings encouraged the transformation of workers from a category in themselves to a category for themselves, to paraphrase Marx; that is, they became a self-conscious group and no longer merely a category of personnel (see also pages 125–6).

Without a doubt this period saw a remarkable increase in union activity, not only among the ancillary workers but also among the nurses and the junior hospital doctors (JHDs). The latter's industrial action in 1975 led to an overtime agreement for hours worked in excess of forty a week. The case presented to the public was one of the inappropriateness and danger of doctors working such long hours in hospital. The upshot was not to decrease the hours worked so much as to dent the image of the professional person as one who, so long as sufficiently well paid to compensate for the sacrifice, will respond to the call to alleviate human suffering at any time without any further counting of the costs (cf. Iliffe, 1983, pp. 43 and 96; Klein, 1983, pp. 113–14).

This upshot was the consequence of yet another contradiction within the health division of labour. We have already discussed the tensions between consultants and general practitioners in which initially the consultants did so much better than the GPs, and how the latter became more organized and demanding as the years went by. In hospital employment all medical grades below consultant (with the exception of medical assistants and certain sessional appointments) were training grades. But the incumbents of these grades are qualified and registered doctors. They are expected to do a great deal of what is nominally the work of the consultant. It is in fact an elaborated apprenticeship system. The settlement of 1975 revealed that the careful management of medical unity by the consultants had once again broken down; the upshot began to change the definition of what it was to be a professional.

THE CHALLENGE FROM THE NURSES: SALMON

A further challenge to the dominant position which the senior clinicians had established came from the nurses. We saw how the original arrangements for the NHS were made without reference to the nurses. Two developments here are worthy of note. The first is the introduction of managerialism into nursing, and the second the unionization of much of the nursing rank and file. The first followed the report of the Salmon Committee in 1966 which elongated the managerial hierarchy in nursing (Ministry of Health, 1966) and had the effect of further dividing nurse leaders from the great bulk of the nursing rank and file (Austin, 1977; Carpenter, 1977). In 1974 the most senior of these nurse managers were given an equal status in planning the health service with doctors and administrators.

One might be forgiven for thinking that this move would not only equalize the relationship in the health-care division of labour between the nursing and medical professions, but would furthermore go some way to reduce the male domination, given the female majority in nursing. In the event this was not so. We saw earlier (pages 95–6) that the predominantly female general nursing had adopted a somewhat superior position in regard to asylum nurses. The latter ultimately found that recourse to a trade union model rather than a professional model was the appropriate way for them to organize and to try to gain some control over their situation. We also saw that asylum nursing was the only place in which in the nineteenth and early twentieth centuries any significant number of male nurses were employed. Matrons and sisters in general nursing had been powerful managers of their realms, but had always played this role in subservience to doctors. In the generality of the male-dominated society, furthermore, it was the general experience that a manager was a man. Job descriptions of managers in the 1960s and 1970s (and indeed even in the 1980s) tended to evoke the image of a man. Consequently male nurses applied for the managerial jobs in numbers quite disproportionate to their representation among nurses as a whole. The upshot is that by 1985 a situation had arisen in which a still predominantly female profession at one time led and managed by women was coming increasingly under male management.

While only one Regional Nursing Officer out of fourteen in 1985 was a man, 92 out of 202 other chief officers were men (i.e. 46 per cent) according to national data supplied by the National Staff Committee (nurses and midwives) to Rosemary Hutt (1985, p. 8). Hutt also quotes a King's Fund survey of 1982 which showed that 33 per cent of District and Area Nursing Officers were men. These proportions must be set against those of qualified nurses as a whole, less than 10 per cent of whom are men. There are considerable regional variations in the proportion of male nurse managers, being highest in Yorkshire (82 per cent) and Trent (75 per cent) and lowest in Wessex (19 per cent) and South-East Thames (13 per cent). The overwhelmingly female nature of nursing as a whole seems likely to continue, judged by the numbers of nurses in training in December 1985, of whom 7,382 were men and 77,699 were women; of these 3,855 men and 9,642 women were training for mental nursing (UKCC, 1986, Table 1 (iv), p. 83; see also Davies and Rosser, 1985, p. 21). Although these trends towards male management of a predominantly female profession have been going on for some time, nurses have only recently begun to recognize just what has happened to their occupation (for example, Carpenter, 1977; Nuttall, 1983a and 1983b). Sex segregation in nursing there was from the outset. There is now vertical segregation developing whereby women workers are managed by men (Hakim, 1979).

The second consequence of the introduction of the Salmon structure was to reward managerial skills in nursing and make career prospects available there but to offer no enhanced opportunities for clinical nursing. The only route for upward mobility was to leave the bedside. Medical practitioners were not happy about the Salmon structure any more than they were about any of the rearrangements in nursing which reduced their ability to command 'their' sister (as shorter working hours for nurses also did, for example).

As we saw (page 92), Williams (1980) suggests that nineteenth-century doctors preferred to think of the origins of 'modern' nursing as lying with Elizabeth Fry rather than Florence Nightingale, because the training arrangements of the latter gave some control over the ward to the matron, at least so far as oversight of nurses in training was concerned. Doctors in those circumstances could wield less authority than formerly, for there was someone else with an intimate oversight of the ward's activities, namely the matron. In a remarkably similar way twentieth-century doctors objected to the authority of line managers in nursing who had authority over 'their' sisters. In these circumstances, and in view of the extent to which consultants get junior doctors to do their boring or 'dirty' work (Hughes, 1971), one should view with caution the comparison they made between themselves and post-Salmon nurses. However much they are involved in management, the doctors argued, they still have clinical responsibility; the most senior doctors are clinicians. In their view it was a grave mistake to make the most senior nurses managers rather than clinicians. Despite possible medical self-interest in these judgements, an arrangement which sought to achieve parity of status between doctors and nurses at the managerial level and in so doing failed to reward clinical nursing did have certain inherent contradictions (Allsop, 1984, p. 59; Carpenter, 1977).

In thinking about this problem it is important to remember some essential differences between medicine and nursing in the health-care division of labour. Florence Nightingale made opportunities for women in the nineteenth century, using her class position to influence hospital authorities and re-creating the domestic division of labour. In doing so she trapped nurses in a gender-determined subordination to doctors (Gamarnikow, 1978). It is also true that medical practitioners have been able to maintain their scarcity value by restricting entry to their occupation. Nurses were not able to do that. There was always need for more 'pairs of hands' (Davies, 1976 and 1977). This need became particularly acute later in the twentieth century when increasingly many other occupations became available to women.

A solution to these problems was found in creating in 1943 the Roll in addition to the register which had been established in 1919. In the absence of enough State Registered Nurses (SRNs), who had a three-year training, or State Enrolled Nurses (SENs), who had two years, it was always possible to employ aides or auxiliaries in one form or another. The VADs of the First World War had been seen as a serious threat by trained nurses, although they could not deny the need for more help in caring for the increasing numbers of hospital patients.

We have seen that by 1975 doctors had found it difficult to sustain the rhetoric that all qualified doctors were equal; their use of trainee consultants as hired hands had led to the JHD settlement whereby overtime was to be paid (page 128). How much more difficult for the nurses where a good supply of womanpower was as important as highly trained technical skills. The inappropriateness of applying the medical clinical model (in terms of the division of labour) to the nurses can be seen. There was irony however in so far as there was a grain of truth in the doctors' gibes. The more recent strategy of introducing the nursing process (see Kratz, 1979) can be seen in part as a response to that problem. One can understand how Celia Davies in her comparative study of UK and US nurse education spoke of 'a constant casualty' (Davies, 1980b, pp. 102–22).

The state's search for control, cost containment and increased efficiency continues. It is not yet clear what the final upshot of the Griffiths reforms initiated in 1983 may be in terms of changes in the health-care division of labour. What is clear however is that nurses, women and men, have lost managerial control over the nursing workforce. The service is now to be managed rather than administered. Managers are appointed as such and may come from administration, industry, medicine, or nursing, although few have been appointed from the last. How far doctors will submit (be forced to submit) to management remains unclear.

PATIENTS AND POTENTIAL PATIENTS

But what of the patients and potential patients in the administration of the NHS? We have seen that at the outset they were not consulted at all. The Hospital Management Committees and Executive Councils had some lay members, but they could hardly be said to have been representative. There was not even an adequate consumer complaints procedure (Stacey, 1974). It was not until the 1974 reorganization that they were given a voice. Community Health Councils were set up, charged with the responsibility to see that the services in their area were appropriately provided.

Elsewhere I have argued that the entire managerial model, based on notions of consumers and producers, consumption and production, is less than appropriate for the nature of the activity involved in health maintenance and health care. Nowhere is this more the case than in the matter of 'consumers' of health care. Sociologically this can be said to be a misnomer, since the patient is a producer as much as a consumer (Stacey, 1976; and pages 6–7 this volume).

In this context it is interesting to note that Pelling's arguments (1987 *passim*, especially pp. 102–7, and see page 43 of this volume) imply that the frankly commercial approach of sixteenth-century medicine may have yielded a more honest representation of what practitioners were offering than did the later, more 'professional' mode. Under the sixteenth-century arrangements, she argues, lay people in general, not just the rich patron of Jewson's (1974 and 1976; see also pages 42–43 this volume) analyses, had more of an equal footing with their practitioners.

'Consumer rights' were having a considerable vogue (perhaps more vogue than power) in the late 1960s and early 1970s. In this context the Community Health Councils were set up. They were however the last part of the new administrative apparatus to be established and they were given budgets which were totally inadequate for the watchdog and investigative functions they were charged with. (For an early study of their working, see Klein and Lewis, 1976.)

What was being introduced into the service was a notion of managers and consumers, with the medically qualified providers still in command but increasingly circumscribed. The doctors, through the rhetoric of responsibility to the patient (see page 127), may have come nearer to workers' control than any other group of workers (Doyal with Pennel, 1979), but attempts by central government to undermine that control were continual; challenges also came from nurses and ancillary workers.

The clear definition of social problems as distinct from medical problems can be seen as another aspect of this process. From the time of the Seebohm Report not only were large departments of social services set up in every local authority, but it was clearly established that the diagnosis of social problems was a matter for social workers and not doctors, although it was appropriate that they should work in concert. While good working relations have subsequently been established in many cases (see, for example, Huntingdon, 1981; Jefferys and Sachs, 1983), there has been a great deal of antagonism between doctors and social workers, perhaps reaching its most bitter dimensions in the case of child abuse (see Dingwall, Eekelaar and Murray, 1983).

From this account of the intentions which led to the establishment of the NHS, and the manifold problems which it has run into, it can be seen that the compromises of 1948 reaped difficult harvests notwithstanding the consensus among the élite upon which it was based. In speaking of this consensus Klein (1983) leaves out of account one most important and largely unspoken consensus, that about the efficacy and primacy of medical knowledge itself. It is to this and to the nature of this knowledge and of other types of knowledge which are current that we will turn in Part Two of this book.

H	Surname
J	First
M	Four
A	Letters

N	Initials
E	

1	Card No.
3	Last
1	Four
2	Digits

Take your book to the Issue Machine in the Self Reservation area.
Follow the on-screen instructions to issue your book.

Check your receipt for the date that the book should be returned. It will be renewed automatically unless someone else has reserved the item.
Check your library account through StarPlus.
If you have any problems with your account please speak to a member of staff.

DATE:

Surname	
First	
Four	
Letters	

| Initials | |

Card No.	
Last	
Four	
Digits	

Take your book to the Issue Machine
in the Self Reservation area.

Follow the on-screen instructions to
issue your book.

Check your receipt for the date that
the book should be returned. It will
be renewed automatically unless
someone else has reserved the item.

Check your library account through
StarPlus.

If you have any problems with your
account please speak to a member of
staff.

Part Two

9 *Introduction and Biological Base*

The second part of this book will focus on health and healing in the latter part of the twentieth century. To do this we will move away from a chronological discussion to one which, building on the comparative and historical knowledge already gained, will take a more analytical approach.

We begin, in Chapters 10–12, with concepts of health, illness and healing, covering the main alternative healing systems in existence in contemporary Britain; lay concepts; and the nature of biomedical knowledge, the challenges to it and changes in it. Then follow four chapters (13–16) which deal with various aspects of the division of labour in health care. Chapter 13 looks at the social organization of health care, the division and locale of paid health labour, and the nature and future of the medical domination of health labour; it includes discussion of how the NHS is organized, social relations in the hospital and the relations of health occupations and professions to each other. In Chapters 14 and 15 attention is focused on the unpaid workers, potential patients, patients in and out of hospital and their unpaid carers, including kin members and health-service volunteers. The following chapter, 16, looks at health care in a capitalist society, paying particular attention to the hospital-supplies and pharmaceutical industries, but not forgetting the health food industry. The role of the state in these areas is also discussed.

Finally, in Chapter 17, the conceptual framework which has been used throughout is applied to human reproduction in the late twentieth century; the medical control of childbirth and of fertility including issues of contraception and artificial fertilization; the control of sexuality; the challenge of AIDS; and the challenges of genetic engineering.

Before we set forth on any of these discussions, however, it is well to look at the biological base in the contemporary UK, a base so different from England of the sixteenth or seventeenth century and from Africa, Latin America and the Indian subcontinent today. Thus the social organization of health care in Britain has to deal with remarkably different problems in the latter part of the twentieth century from those of the nineteenth and earlier centuries. It has been the argument of this book throughout that while a variety of different arrangements may be made to cope with the same set of problems, nevertheless any society in making health-care arrangements has to take account of its biological base.

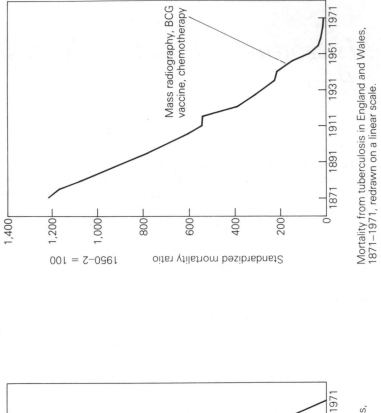

Mortality from tuberculosis in England and Wales, 1871–1971, redrawn on a linear scale.

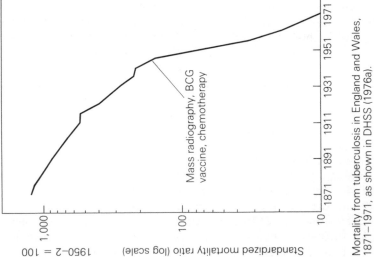

Mortality from tuberculosis in England and Wales, 1871–1971, as shown in DHSS (1976a).

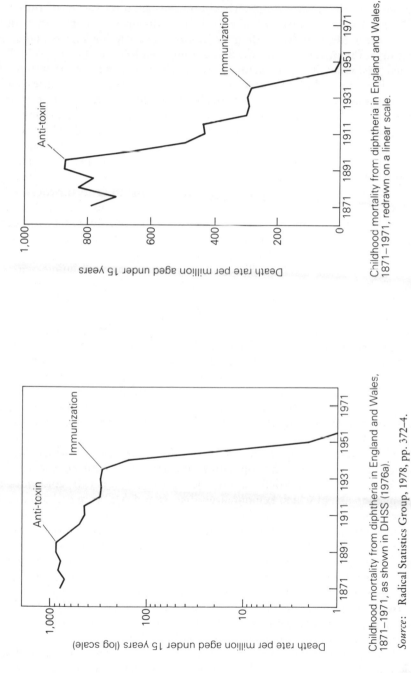

Childhood mortality from diphtheria in England and Wales, 1871–1971, redrawn on a linear scale.

Childhood mortality from diphtheria in England and Wales, 1871–1971, as shown in DHSS (1976a).

Source: Radical Statistics Group, 1978, pp. 372–4.

Figure 9.1 *Two ways of presenting immunization data.*

THE BIOLOGICAL BASE IN THE LATE TWENTIETH CENTURY

It is characteristic of biomedicine that the healthiness of a population is measured by the amount of disease from which it is suffering and from the number of deaths at various ages. These concepts are discussed more fully in the following chapters (see pages 160–2). For the moment we will take them at face value as the mode of understanding the biological base in our society at this time. Looking at the problem biomedically, Thomas McKeown (1976, pp. 26–7) has divided diseases into four main groups. The first two are determined at fertilization and include (a) genetic diseases, i.e. inherited abnormalities, and (b) 'conditions associated with the genetically programmed wearing-out of organs at the end of life'. The second two are conditions which occur only in an appropriate environment, either (a) prenatal or (b) postnatal. The prenatally caused diseases are, McKeown says, attributable to unknown influences acting on the uterus, such that the child is born damaged or distorted. The final category (2b), diseases which are caused postnatally, includes all the infections and also those non-infective diseases not attributable to gene disorders.

Deaths from infectious diseases have declined dramatically, mainly because of improved water supply, sanitation, adequate food supply and birth control. Immunization programmes have played a part here, although just how important a part is in some dispute. Graphs produced by the Department of Health and Social Security (DHSS, 1976b) show these diseases declining before the immunization programmes began, but much more rapidly thereafter (see Figure 9.1). The DHSS consequently lays stress on individual responsibility to take up vaccination or immunization for oneself or on behalf of children. The Radical Statistics Health Group's (1976 and 1978) critique indicates that the effect of these programmes has been exaggerated by the use in the graphs of a log scale. The Group redraws the graphs on a linear scale which stresses the early decline in the rates rather than the acceleration of the fall consequent upon immunization. Its critique implies that the fall was to do more with socioeconomic changes and less with the immunization, although the Group does not wish to decry its efficacy (see Figure 9.1). We shall return to the implications of this dispute in Chapter 13.

What is clear is that the epidemics of infectious diseases which killed or maimed large numbers of the population appeared to be a thing of the past in the third quarter of the twentieth century. Recently new forms of epidemics have been introduced, of which Legionnaires' disease and AIDS are perhaps the most outstanding. Both so far lack effective preventive measures such as immunization or any definitively effective treatment. Although neither so far has killed in the quantities of the old epidemics, and AIDS not with the speed, they have come as something of a shock to many people who thought the scourge of uncontrollable epidemics was a thing of the past. They have helped to diminish the therapeutic optimism of the 1960s. Nevertheless, McKeown believes that diseases in his fourth category, those which are caused postnatally, are controllable, although not all are under control. Furthermore, we do not yet in all cases understand causation in biomedical terms fully or at all.

A consequence of the reduction of deaths from the former infectious diseases which were mass killers has been that the population is living longer. The weaknesses and diseases of old age, and the dependency which is so often associated with them, constitute health-care work which has been increasing throughout the century and particularly in its second half. Chronic diseases, those which kill slowly often over a very long period of time (multiple sclerosis, for example), disabilities, both congenital and those acquired through accident or disease, and mental illness, which appears not to have moderated over the years, constitute the main problems which now have to be dealt with. Whether they are largely caused by individual behaviour, as McKeown (1976) believes, or by the constraints imposed upon people by the organization of industrial life, work hazards and the like – as, for example, Illich (1975) and Navarro (1975) in their very different modes suggest – these are the conditions which the health-care system has to contend with. The task is remarkably different from that of the eighteenth and nineteenth centuries when modern hospitals and professions of medicine and nursing were founded.

Inequalities in the Biological Base

Statistics suggest that all sections of the population are a good deal healthier than they were at mid-century. However, they also suggest that these benefits have not been spread evenly throughout the population. The Black Report of 1980 (Townsend and Davidson, 1982) demonstrated that there are continuing social class differences both in expectation of life and in healthiness. Using mortality as the best available indicator of health (see Chapter 12, pages 160–1) and the Registrar-General's occupational classes as an indicator of social class, they show that

> Mortality tends to rise inversely with falling occupational rank or status, for both sexes and at all ages. At birth and in the first month of life twice as many babies of unskilled manual parents as of professional parents die, and in the next eleven months of life four times as many girls and five times as many boys, respectively, die. In later years of childhood the ratio of deaths in the poorest class falls to between one and a half and two times that of the wealthiest class, but increases again in early adulthood before falling again in middle and old age.
>
> (Townsend and Davidson, 1982, pp. 63–4)

In 1987 the Health Education Council published a review of work on inequalities undertaken since the Black Report (Whitehead, 1987). The evidence presented confirms that 'serious inequalities in health have persisted in the 1980s' (pp. 1 and 9–34). We have to conclude that, while there may be a generally higher level of health than there was forty years ago, the differentials between classes are, for most measures, as large as or larger than they were (see Figure 9.2)

The Black Committee (Townsend and Davidson, 1982) looked at possible explanations for these differences, dividing them into four categories: artefact explanations; theories of natural or social selection; materialist or structuralist explanations; cultural/behavioural explanations. The first kind of explanation suggests that the correlation between class and ill health is an artefact of the statistics or the categories that are used in the classifications. The second proposes that there is more ill health in the lowest classes because the less well

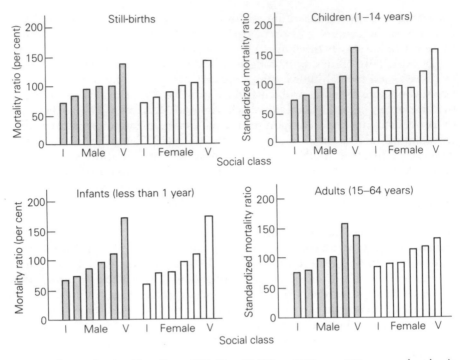

Source: Occupational   Mortality   1970–72   HMSO,   1978,   p. 196,   reproduced   in
Townsend and Davidson, 1982, p. 52.

Figure 9.2   *Mortality by occupational class and age. Relative mortality (%) is the ratio
of rates for the occupational class to the rate for all males (or females).*

drift downwards, being unable to hold down good jobs. The third suggests that
it is features of the socioeconomic structure which cause the differences, being
associated with relative wealthiness or poverty. The fourth kind (cultural or
behavioural explanations) suggests that differential life-styles between the
classes are the explanation for the continued differences.

While conceding that the issue is a complex one and that causation may
possibly vary over the life cycle, the Black Report comes down strongly on the
side of materialist explanations, as does the more recent Whitehead study (1987,
pp. 69–73). The recent health and life-style survey (Cox *et al.*, 1987) 'shows a
remarkably steep and regular association' of self-assessed health status with
income which, the author says, 'may perhaps be seen as summarizing all the
social inequalities in different aspects of health which [the survey] noted'
(Blaxter, 1987, p. 7).

The 'culture of poverty' thesis, with its implications of individual responsibility, had been severely criticized before the Black Committee reported. Since
then the series of research commissioned to investigate the hypothesis has been
published and does not lend it any credence (Blaxter, 1981; Madge, 1983).

What is unclear and remains unclear are the mechanisms whereby these
structural features are translated into systematically differential ill health.
Recent in-depth studies are, however, helping to unravel this mystery, particularly in terms of the relationships between low income, life-style and health

(see Whitehead, 1987, pp. 71–3, for a useful summary). Furthermore, the large and continuing levels of unemployment seem likely to introduce a further factor, for evidence is increasing of the association between ill health and unemployment (U 205 Open University Course Team, 1985b, ch. 11; Whitehead, 1987, pp. 19–23).

Sex and Gender Differences

There are also differences in the disease and illness experiences of women and men. Some of these arise directly from the different reproductive function of the two sexes; others appear to be linked to other aspects of the different female and male genetic constitutions; some to different exposures to hazards at work or in the home associated with gender roles and sex-typed occupations; others to the different illness behaviour and concepts of health associated with masculinity and feminity; others again to the way in which professional health practitioners view gender roles. While the first two sets of differences mentioned may in some sense be biological givens, the remainder – occupation differences, concepts of masculinity and feminity and of gender roles – are social constructions.

Furthermore, as Rose, Lewontin and Kamin (1984) have pointed out, one should not see the biological as distinct and separate from, or opposed to, the social; minds and brains are simultaneously biological and social (p. 284). There are obvious physical differences between the biological form of women and men, yet, when one looks at a wide array of human beings, they are not as clearly divided into two biological forms as our social understanding of two sexes would lead us to believe. The central characteristic of each group must be the difference in sexual and reproductive activity, yet not all women are capable of bearing children nor all men of being their progenitors. The shape and size of breasts and genitalia, shoulder and pelvic girdle shape and the like are not consistently divided between women and men in an ideal-typical way.

As a geneticists' account has it (Roberts, 1976, pp. 13–34), it also appears to be the case that there are certain diseases which are biologically sex-linked and others which have a marked bias to one sex or the other. Differences which are believed to be due to recessive genes on the X chromosome are masked in women by the other X chromosome. In a male they cannot be so masked, and he will show the disorder. Hence geneticists understand such sex-linked recessive disorders to be characteristic in that they appear in males only. Examples are severe Duchenne muscular dystrophy, haemophilia and red/green colour blindness.

In addition, geneticists recognize sex-limited diseases, that is, diseases which are found more often in one sex or the other. Some of these are complex and puzzling. For example, males are much more likely to suffer from pyloric stenosis than females. Cleft palate is predominantly experienced by females; cleft lip with or without cleft palate shows a preponderance in males. Some congenital heart disorders are predominantly found in males. Club feet occur twice as often in males as females, while congenital dislocation of the hip is found more often in females than males, as is anencephaly (Roberts, 1976, p. 17).

When one moves from these congenital conditions other differences in the incidence of disease between the two sexes are less clearly genetically determined or even influenced. The greater incidence of lung cancer among men, for example, was associated with the greater incidence of smoking among men. Now that smoking is increasing among women one may expect the incidence of female lung cancer to increase (see Lopez, 1984; Whitehead, 1987, p. 45). Other differences appear to be more associated with the different gender roles which normatively women and men in our society play. The work hazards which women and men experience differ because a majority of occupations are gendered and undertaken predominantly by women or by men (see also Whitehead, 1987, pp. 74–5).

A puzzle remains as to why it should be that women report more illness but live longer than men (Nathanson, 1975 and 1977; and see the review of recent work in Whitehead, 1987, p. 24). To what extent this has to do with gender roles (such that women are more prepared to resort to the doctor because medicalization of childbirth has familiarized them with medical services) or to what extent it has to do with concepts of masculinity and femininity (such that healthiness and masculinity are seen to go together, making men reluctant to report illness) has yet to be fully resolved.

Juanne Clarke (1983) in a useful review of work in this area, which she appropriately calls 'Sexism, Feminism and Medicalism', has suggested that there are two errors which run through the majority of sociological work; one is a confusion of sex and gender, the other confusion about the conceptualization of health and illness. As she points out, gender role is not coincidental with sex. Studies of androgyny, role reversal, cross-sexuals and transsexuality all show this. She concludes: 'Both gender and sex, as historically defined by male sociologists in male-dominated societies, are conceptually problematic' (p. 66). Furthermore, the distinction between physical and mental illness has been accepted by sociologists, as for example Gove and Tudor (1972–3). In addition, Gove and Tudor exclude from their definition many problems which people take to psychiatrists. Clarke (1983) quotes Dohrenwend and Dohrenwend (1976, p. 1339), who complain that the Gove–Tudor definition is not consistent with the definition which psychiatrists and psychologists would use, as well as not being consistent with the practice of lay people seeking help. All these authors ignore the point made by Dorothy Smith (1975) that the defining of people as mentally ill takes place within a power structure (the psychiatric hospital or clinic) in which men are dominant.

There are other methodological problems, among them the frequency with which data are collected from women about the health experiences and behaviour of themselves and the male members of their households. Clarke (1983, pp. 72–5) gathers together evidence which suggests that women may under-report men's ailments in comparison with their own. Other problems include a failure in many studies to relate admission rates to hospital, for example, to the population at risk, which may be different for women and men. As she concludes:

> When we do not know whether men or women view the same things as symptoms of illness, when we do not know to what extent physicians diagnose the same symptoms differently in men and women, when we do not know about the differential effects on men and women of the hospital experience, how can we theorize about sex differences in illness?
>
> (Clarke, 1983, p. 77)

It is plain that we have been inclined to work with much too simple models of the relationship of sex differences, illness and illness behaviour. One might, for example, imagine that the much greater incidence of early death from heart disease among men was genetically determined. However, since the causes are not fully known, it is impossible to say to what extent the differences are due to genetic characteristics and what to socially created gender differences. In part these simplistic models come from a distinction we tend to make, and to which medicine is a party, between the organism and its environment. As Rose, Lewontin and Kamin (1984, p. 272) point out, this is 'simply wrong, and every biologist knows it'. It is not only that organism and environment interact, they argue, but that they are simply not distinguishable in that dichotomous way. It is undoubtedly clear that the differential disease and illness experiences of the sexes cannot be explained or predicted simply in biological terms; the biology is important but it is inextricably intertwined with the social. It is to facets of these social arrangements, specifically to concepts about health, illness and disease, that we now turn.

10 Concepts of Health and the Nature of Healing Knowledge (1): Lay Concepts of Health and Illness

The ways in which medical knowledge and the popular response to it changed from the medieval period up to the mid-twentieth century have been discussed in previous chapters. In the next three chapters we will look at what has happened to concepts of health, illness and healing in the second half of this century, starting with lay concepts. (Concepts associated with reproduction will be dealt with later in Chapter 17.) This was the period when the Welfare State was established and biomedicine came to be provided on a mass basis throughout all advanced industrial societies, albeit the mode of its financing and administration varied.

One problem in assessing the data about lay health concepts is that much of the early research assumed not only the primacy of biomedicine but the correctness of its understandings. Interest was in how much lay people knew or understood of what biomedicine taught as appropriate health behaviour. Where lay views did not coincide with the biomedical, they were thought to be ignorant or to be clinging to outmoded, useless, or even dangerous ideas. (The safety of biomedical ideas was implied.) Much of the biomedical interest was in how to persuade people to comply with treatments.

The approach taken here, in contrast, is that people think about and explain to themselves in their own way – ways which they may share with others – the misfortunes which happen to them, the ailments which afflict their bodies and the disorders which enter their lives. Their ideas are taken as logical and valid in their own right, although they may not be consonant with biomedical science or any other organized healing system. Ordinary people, in other words, develop explanatory theories to account for their material, social and bodily circumstances. These they apply to themselves as individuals, but in developing them they draw on all sorts of knowledge and wisdom, some of it derived from their own experience, some of it handed on by word of mouth, other parts of it derived from highly trained practitioners. These lay explanations go beyond common sense in that explanations beyond the immediately obvious are included (cf. Horton, 1970, discussed in Chapter 2).

CONCEPTS AS SOCIAL REPRESENTATIONS

Studying middle-class people, mostly Parisians but some Normans, Herzlich (1973) found that popular conceptions of the causation of illness and disease were variations on the themes also found in medical theories.

On the one hand disease is endogenous ... the ideas of resistance to disease, heredity and predisposition are ... key concepts. On the other hand, illness is thought of as exogenous; [human beings] are naturally healthy and illness is due to the action of an evil will, a demon or sorcerer, noxious elements, emanations from the earth or microbes.

(1973, p. 19)

It is not so much that the lay have followed the medical but that both draw on a common stock of understanding. Herzlich shows, using the Durkheimian notion of social representation, that it is possible to extract from lay accounts of illness and health what these concepts are. 'The endogenous theme is represented by the individual and his part in the genesis of his condition. The exogenous theme is the way of life of each person' (1973, p. 19). The way of life is the unhealthy life of the city which is strongly related to the incidence of illness. Factors relating to the individual consist of things like predisposition, constitution, temperament, nature, resistance and self-defensive reaction. Health and illness emerge as the outcome of a struggle between an individual and the way of life. Herzlich concludes:

If illness arises from a conflict between the individual and society, the unhealthy arises in the last resort from the antagonism perceived to exist between what is felt to be the nature of [human beings] and the form and product of [their] activities.

(p. 38)

Individuals feel responsible for their health because, good or bad, they are defined by it. They feel guilty for having, in the conflict, allowed their health to be impaired or undermined; not for having caught an illness, but for having lost their health (p. 50). Herzlich makes plain that there is not only an interior logic to the concepts of health and illness held by ordinary people, but there are also social representations; the concepts are shared by numbers of others and derive from the society in which they all live. Furthermore, the essential logic of people's understanding of and explanation for their health becomes plain.

Recently, with Janine Pierret, Claudine Herzlich has amassed further evidence for this general thesis through a survey of illnesses and ill people from ancient times until today (Herzlich and Pierret, 1984, 1985, 1986 and 1987). In their work they insist that a person's experiences and conceptions can be properly understood only if related to the macrostructure. Part of this is the nature of sickness during any particular period (what I have referred to as the biological base). There may be threat of death from infectious diseases occurring in epidemics. However, nowadays with infectious diseases far less threatening in *mass* terms, chronic illnesses have assumed greater importance, and sickness has become a way of life, not a way of dying (1985, p. 149). Herzlich and Pierret's (1984, 1985, 1986 and 1987) data are derived from writings by historians and from publications, especially diaries and letters, in which sick people described their illness or first-hand observers recorded their impressions, and also from twentieth-century surveys. From these they have shown how lay understandings of illness go well beyond the medical, taking other considerations into mind, and how also certain ideas, about causation for example, persist over the centuries, albeit new ones are introduced to handle new phenomena. /

In their chapter on causation (1986, pp. 71–96) Herzlich and Pierret show how both lay people and medics have long attributed importance to air, climate and seasons; how in the eighteenth century strange biological events, such as eclipses and earthquakes, were added; they discuss the disputes about contagion and infection which raged from the seventeenth to the nineteenth centuries. While settled in biomedical terms in the nineteenth century by the discovery of bacteria and the enunciation of the germ theory (see Chapter 5), Herzlich and Pierret find that such ideas still worry people – the cancer patient who is shunned, for example. Later other ideas come in such as the 'modern way of life' as a cause of illness, and diet too, which changes from not having enough food to eating too much, or the wrong thing. From the Industrial Revolution bad working conditions began to be seen as causing illness: an outstanding example of an impact of the changing macrostructure. As well the social structure/health ideas link, Herzlich and Pierret see a two-way relationship, still continuing today, between biomedical and lay views. This relationship is found in other studies, as we shall see.

TRUST IN THE BODY, HEALTH AND PHYSICAL IDENTITIES

While it is the case that our ideas about health and illness are undoubtedly closely associated with our societies and the social relations we are involved in, it is also the case that each individual has to make sense of her/his health and sickness experiences for her/himself. The ways in which this comes about are only now beginning to be unravelled. To further this kind of understanding, Virginia Olesen, Leonard Schatzman and their graduate students in sociology and nursing are exploring what they call 'mundane complaints' and how people think and act about them (Olesen *et al.*, 1985). They have been looking at two groups of people: ostomates, that is, people who have had surgery such that 'the elimination of bodily wastes, either faecal or urinary, was no longer accomplished through body orifices' (p. 9); and secondly a group of younger people who have easy access to health care since they are linked with Health Maintenance Organizations (HMOs), access as near to that available under the NHS as can be found in the USA.

Olesen *et al.* had expected that the ostomates would have had to make some transformations of the meanings they ascribed to mundane complaints. However, they found that this was not the case, but that the 'self' was profoundly changed. Olesen *et al* had started with a concept of the 'health self' but found that the self the surgery had changed was more than that, it was what they came to call the 'physical self'. A new theme emerged of 'trust in the body' which for some had been lost and for others gained as a result of their operation. The mundane complaint was linked with the dynamics of the self and the shifting views of whether the body was deemed trustworthy (p. 4). They draw attention to how the interaction of person, body and ailment in the individual intersects with social interaction, the latter having been much more frequently addressed in the literature.

Their findings did not only apply to the ostomates. Another group of younger people who had not had such surgery had come to understand their physical selves in the course of their lives in handling ailments and had developed personal theories of prevention and treatments. It seems likely that it is this kind of understanding that the grandmothers Mildred Blaxter (1983) has written about felt it important to convey to the physician when they consulted with an ailment which they felt required expert attention. As she put it, 'people have to inhabit their bodies, and their physical identity is part of themselves' (p. 69). When they consulted, these women wanted their doctors to give them a cause for their symptoms as well as a diagnosis; they felt the cause must be connected with life events and they despaired of being able to convey all the history they thought relevant in the course of a brief consultation. Unless the doctor really understood, how could he help them properly?

When respondents to the Cambridge (England) survey on health and lifestyles were asked about the concept of health it appeared that health in others was described differently from health in oneself.

> Described in another person, three basic concepts emerged, singly or in combination. Health can be seen as positive fitness, as strength and energy, as having an efficient or athletic physical body ... as the ability to work or perform one's normal roles ... [as] 'not being ill' ... Health in oneself ... was very predominantly thought of in psychological terms ... respondents were less likely to emphasize physical fitness *or* lack of disease, but rather to say that health is defined as being unstressed and unworried, able to cope with life, in tune with the world, and happy.
>
> (Blaxter, 1987b, p. 141, original emphasis)

Here is evidence from a large-scale survey of about 9,000 people that personal perceptions of health may be different from general perceptions. The survey also showed more specific ways in which personal experience might modify concepts. While those with a chronic disease were not conspicuously less likely to define health in terms of physical fitness, they were less likely to define health for themselves as 'not being ill' (Blaxter, 1987b, p. 141).

CONCEPTS AND SOCIOECONOMIC CIRCUMSTANCES

Concepts of Working-Class Women
The grandmothers Blaxter (1983) was writing about were drawn from a sample which she and Elizabeth Patterson (1982) had studied, a study which included women's ideas about health and illness. The sample, which was of Scottish women, had been deliberately selected from women who had been neither geographically nor socially mobile and among whom an identifiable subculture might be expected. The women could generally be said to come from social classes IV and V. In writing about their ideas Blaxter is specifically concerned with how they think about disease.

The women distinguish between illness and disease: 'illness was weakness, "lying down to it", being functionally unfit, giving in to diseases' (1983, p. 60). Furthermore, they had clear models of disease which were part of their conception of illness. The names they used for diseases were for the most part ones also used by biomedical science. The categories of cause most often used were infection and agents in the environment, heredity and family susceptibility. 'Germs' could be battled against, but 'viruses', 'a new word', could not. External agents, such as damp housing, caused disease; damp or changeable weather could make one more susceptible; bad working conditions could cause disease, as could poisons in the environment. Heredity and family tendencies were somewhat double edged; they might imply a slur on the family, on the other hand they did account for diseases which would otherwise have to be accepted as random or haphazard. The women were very conscious of the mind–body link, so psychological factors, 'stress and strain', were popular causes of disease and had sophisticated theories associated with them. Behavioural causation was understood but was not usually taken to involve responsibility; in the circumstances of poverty in which they had lived they did not see how they could have done differently. The diseases which were seen as the most frightening were those which 'just happened', they were random and unpredictable. When TB was common and untreatable in these women's youth it came in this category; now cancer was most dreaded. It was frequently mentioned but without discussion of cause.

It is at this level of individual susceptibility that the link can be made with the notion of trust in the body which Virginia Olesen and her colleagues (1985) have come to recognize. However, a difference of emphasis is that in that study, except in so far as the age of the two samples varied, as did ease of access to health care and whether or not the respondents had had major surgery, the understandings recorded were not related to social situation and certainly not to social structure. Mildred Blaxter (1983), on the other hand, pays attention also to socioeconomic conditions and concludes that the way in which her respondents thought of disease and its causation was closely linked to their living and working conditions.

This is a conclusion which Cornwell (1984) also reaches. Her sample was also of very ordinary people in Bethnal Green, many of whom would be categorized as social classes IV or V. They had all, women and men, had hard working lives. She found that the way they thought about their health was much the same way as they thought about their work. They were preoccupied with the moral aspects such as hard work. So far as health and illness were concerned, 'the moral prescription for a healthy life is in fact a kind of cheerful stoicism, evident in the refusal to worry, or complain, or to be morbid' (1984, p. 129). There were however two accounts, the public and the private. Private accounts are not the ones given to an interviewer on first acquaintance.

> Public accounts are selective and partial. In general, they exclude experiences and opinions that might be considered unacceptable and not respectable . . . to members of the medical profession . . . The place where medically unacceptable and incompatible opinions and values are stated is in private accounts [which are] no less selective and partial.
>
> (Cornwell, 1984, p. 205)

Class Variations in France
Alphonse d'Houtaud (d'Houtaud, 1976, 1978 and 1981; d'Houtaud and Field, 1984 and 1986), writing of people in Lorraine in France going for a medical

check-up, has also noticed the way in which people's life circumstances affect their concepts. He focused particularly on how health, rather than illness or disease was conceived. His sample may be self-selected to particular points of view simply because these were people who were reporting for a regular health check. Nevertheless some very interesting differences were found when he classified his respondents by occupational classes.

D'Houtaud's work follows Herzlich's but looks at a broader spectrum of the population and uses survey techniques. In his first study he used an open-ended question to arrive at definitions of health and finally grouped these into ten. He found that the managerial and professional classes (*cadres supérieurs, cadres moyens*) expressed the first four health concepts, namely, that health was a hedonistic way of life (a life without constraint, benefit from life, not thinking of illness, seeing the doctor as little as possible), health was equilibrium (of body, mind, family, or in general), it had reference to the body (that one should not feel it, it should be good, etc.) and it was vitality (able to face problems, optimistic, not afraid for the future and so forth). This last theme was shared with his category of non-manual workers, who used three other sets of definitions of health as well. The first was to do with psychological well-being (joy of living, happiness, good morale, good humour). The second d'Houtaud labels hygiene, which includes notions of regularity, sobriety, avoidance of excess, open air and exercise. The final one was simply to define health by its own value: the essential thing, the greatest of riches. The middle two, i.e. psychological well-being and hygiene, were shared by his category of manual workers. In addition, the manual workers defined health in terms of prevention (health is to have a regular medical examination, to look after yourself, to know yourself well, 'better to prevent than cure', to live as long as possible). They also defined it in terms of physical aptitudes (to be in good form, to be able to work) and finally negatively, as not being ill. The agricultural labourers shared in these three – that is, prevention, physical aptitudes and absence of illness – but they also shared with the non-manual workers notions about the value of health itself.

Reducing these categories further, d'Houtaud distinguished two main tendencies: the manual workers who think of health in terms of use or service, of the collective and the social; the *cadres*, the professional and managerial classes, who think in terms of enjoyment, of the individual and the personal. Looking at the data another way one finds that, moving from manual workers through to the middle and higher classes, the concept of health moves from absence of sickness to psychological well-being and then to the hedonistic way of life; from prevention to hygiene to equilibrium in terms of access to health or improving health. When d'Houtaud repeated the work (1986) using closed-ended questions, the same general tendencies appeared.

CLASS VARIATIONS IN BRITAIN, BUT ALSO AGE AND GENDER

The sample of about 9,000 people whose health status was biomedically measured and to whose health concepts reference was made above has yielded some evidence about the aggregated notions of people living in England, Wales and Scotland as to how health beliefs vary by class and also by sex and age. The notion of health as positive fitness was found more often among men and among the better educated; as functional fitness among older people. Contrary to previous assumptions that the 'never ill' category was characteristic of the disadvantaged, this survey found it equally in all social classes, although more among women than men (Blaxter, 1987b, p. 141). In so far as education measures social class, it seems that those in higher classes feel they have more control over their health than those in lower (Blaxter, 1987b, table 14.9, p. 145).

CONCEPTS, AUTONOMY AND CAPITALISM

Taken together, works such as those of Blaxter (1983, 1987a and 1987b), Blaxter, Fenner and Whichelow (1987), Cornwell (1984) and d'Houtaud and Field (1984 and 1986), and one must add that of Pill and Stott (1982 and 1986) on Welsh working-class mothers, encourage us to hypothesize that, within limits set by individual experience of health and illness, concepts of health may vary according to the immediate material circumstances in which people find themselves and which constrain their action. The extent to which people are dependent on their own physical labour, the extent to which they can command their own daily lives and the lives of others (and possibly also broader features of their social class situation), appear to bear a relationship to what they think health is, as well as the ways in which they think about illness, disease and suffering and what to do about it.

Some interesting further evidence comes from the United States. Robert Crawford (1984) discussed ideas of health with sixty adults living in Chicago, two-thirds of whom were 'white, middle class, under forty and female' (p. 63), although he had tried to achieve a sample covering all social classes, races, ages and both sexes. (Cornwell, 1984, also had trouble in getting men to talk about health.) Crawford made the assumption that talking about health is talking about US cultural notions of well-being or quality of life. In the interviews he found that health 'clearly represents a status, socially recognized and admired and therefore important for our identities' (1984, p. 64); furthermore, much more was ordinarily encompassed in the conceptions of his respondents than biomedicine encompasses. It emerged that health was seen as both discipline and release.

To achieve and maintain health required disciplined work, it did not just happen. Respondents perceived a similarity between occupational work discipline and health work discipline, a concordance which is reminiscent of the symmetry which Cornwell found in Bethnal Green. The Chicagoans themselves commented on the similarity. They also commented that sometimes their work commitments left little time for the health work. Manual workers expressed to Crawford, as they did to d'Houtaud, the importance of a healthy body for work; the body is seen as the body of a worker. However, notwithstanding the strength of their beliefs (consonant with the American ethic of self-reliance and individualism) in working for their health, a number of Crawford's respondents felt there were health-denying attributes in the environment about which they could do nothing, so 'why worry?'. They had acquired a sense of 'somatic vulnerability' (p. 74). Chronic diseases not amenable to medical amelioration, cancer, toxicity all around, were all outside individual control. This understanding had developed along with a new health consciousness.

'If health is a metaphor for self-control, body weight is the metaphor within the metaphor.' Thinness is seen as coincident with health; 'fat is a confirmation of the loss of control, a moral failure, a sign of impulsiveness, self-indulgence and sloth' (p. 70). Unfortunately, Crawford (1984) does not analyse his data on this issue by sex, so we are given no insight as to whether women and men perceived the issue differently. It is one area, however, where the opposition to health as discipline, namely health as release, emerges clearly. 'The releasing motif suggests pleasure-seeking rather than ascetic self-denials, the satisfaction of desire rather than the repression of desire' (p. 81). Eating good food is an obvious self-satisfaction liable to contravene the health goals and health work.

In neo-Marxian mode, Crawford relates these contradictions, which he found not only between people but within individuals, to the contradictory demands made upon Americans by the capitalist society in which they live. Employers require disciplined workers, at both managerial and 'blue-collar' levels. The stress on health as discipline consonant with work discipline fits in workers' minds as well as managers' minds with holding down jobs and producing goods and services. At the same time industry requires market outlets for its goods. Therefore advertising effort is put into encouraging people to spend, which includes encouraging self-indulgence and 'release'. High self-discipline in the working week and the satisfaction of desire at the weekends: is this the way balance is to be maintained?

The issue of balance certainly arises, and Crawford poses it as if it were specific to US capitalism. No doubt its form is, but, as we have seen, the idea of balance as essential for health is a very ancient one. It appears in the Chinese *yin* and *yang*, in European medieval thought, among the twentieth-century French and now again among US citizens. Notions of balance in health matters are often expressed as a requirement to achieve the appropriate harmony. This is not Crawford's position. Rather, he sees the possibility of the body being a site for resistance. he suggests that 'our bodies are both the metaphor and the substance of our struggle against domination' (p. 97). Although he does not refer to it, this has been a feminist understanding in the conflict about gender domination; Crawford's argument relates to class domination. He is talking about the way in which, as he sees it, capitalism is 'using' health concepts to its own ends, and how, in the ways described above, the contradictions in capitalism are experienced in the bodies and minds of individual human beings (see also Crawford, 1980).

LAY AND BIOMEDICAL CONCEPTS

Crawford notes, as have others who have examined lay beliefs about health and illness, that to some extent people talk in the prevailing biomedical idiom but also that their ideas go beyond matters with which biomedicine deals. Cornwell (1984) discusses how over the years the ideas of her respondents have been influenced by biomedical ideas and practices, they have become 'medicalized' as she puts it. Blaxter (1983) also indicated that her respondents used many biomedical concepts and ideas, although their logical framework, like that of the Bethnal Greeners Cornwell spoke to, followed a different model from the biomedical.

The 'Folk' and the Physician
Cecil Helman (1978, 1981, 1984 and 1986) in a justly famous paper has also shown how what he calls the 'folk model' differs from the biomedical model and

is influenced by it and by practitioners' behaviour; also how the biomedical practitioners are influenced by the folk model. He describes and analyses the beliefs of general practice patients on the edges of London about health and illness and specifically about colds and fevers. He shows that the patients shared a clearly established model, or system of classification, of certain illnesses which rests on distinctions of 'hot' and 'cold', 'wet' and 'dry'. However, although they are bodily feeling states, 'hot' and 'cold' do not relate to the biomedical definitions of body temperature. This reminds one somewhat of certain medieval notions about health, illness and balance. Those ailments in which the patients feel hot are the fevers: divided into wet, when there is fever plus congestion or discharge, for example from the nose, or fever and diarrhhoea, and dry, when there is fever plus a dry skin, dry throat, flushed face, non-productive cough. Those ailments where the patient feels cold are described as colds or chills; they are wet when there is, for example, cold with nasal congestion, watery eyes, a non-productive cough, or cold with abdominal discomfort and abdominal pain. They are dry when the cold is accompanied by shivering, rigor, *malaise*, muscular aches.

Colds and chills are explained as 'being due to the penetration of the environment – across the boundary of the skin – into the human organism' (Helman 1986, p. 218). Damp, rain, cold winds and draughts can do the damage. Colds are not caused by people, and there is a strong element of personal responsibility; thus one can get a cold by not dressing properly or going out after washing one's hair, for example. Furthermore, it is one's own responsibility to treat colds; they are not a matter for the doctor.

Fevers, on the other hand, are more serious, more long-lasting and a matter for the doctor. They are thought to be 'due to the actions of entities known as "Germs", "Bugs", or "Viruses". These terms are not used in a strict biomedical sense ... [they] remain a hypothesis, a theory of causality' (1986, p. 221). Germs are all bad, they are single, you only get one at once, they come from other people, and you can pass them on to others. In this sense, although they are external, they are social rather than environmental. People cannot help getting germs; they are not morally responsible. Fevers should be taken to trained practitioners for cure.

CHANGES OVER TIME?

Helman's younger patients compared with the older ones classified more conditions as fevers to be taken to the doctor. He also noticed that with the increase in the number of ailments caused by 'germs', illness has become more social and dangerous, requiring more professional attention and the prescription of antibiotics. Both Blaxter (1983) and Cornwell (1984) also noted an inter-generational difference. The older people attached more significance to moral fibre compared with younger ones, who placed more emphasis on germs, viruses and social stress. One cannot, of course, know whether these differences are to be accounted for by the consequences of having lived a longer life or whether they represent changes in the mores from one period to another, i.e. represent a change over time. Helman notes that between the two generations of his older and younger patients two historic events had occurred: the arrival and use of antibiotics and the establishment of the NHS.

Other evidence (for example, Seabrook, 1973 and 1986; and see the discussion in Stacey, 1986b, p. 15) suggests that in former days greater stress was placed on moral control among those for whom professional health care was not readily available. Some evidence of mine obliquely suggests that the availability of health care may be a factor as between members of roughly the same generation. Over a period of ten years I asked third-year British undergraduates at the outset of their medical sociology course to replicate the question Irving Zola (1966) had asked his students. This was to write down how they would explain an illness or accident to a child. Zola's students' explanations included many moral notions about illness causation of the kind, 'I caught cold because I went out without a raincoat.' My British students did not include these moralistic explanations; they were much more matter of fact and empirical (even one who described a hangover was not self-blaming).

I suspected that the difference between the UK and the US students might be related to the former benefiting from treatment free at the point of delivery, which the US students would not experience. This would also lend some support to Helman's notion that the NHS was a factor in the generational differences he observed.

The young Welsh mothers whom Pill and Stott (1982 and 1986) talked to had ideas which fitted with Helman's younger patients, Cornwell's younger respondents and my students. Blaxter and Cornwell both draw attention to the materially hard lives which their older respondents had experienced in their youth and the greater difficulty then of access to medical care. The younger people, the postwar generation, have grown up not only in the NHS antibiotic generation, they have also grown up in the Welfare State. Whatever may be the bureaucratic rigours involved in claiming benefit, the welfare arrangements have prevented the kinds of privation which Blaxter's and Cornwell's older respondents had experienced in their youth.

Changes in professional behaviour over time may also have an effect. Blaxter (1983) suggests that the women's concepts of what were serious ailments and how they should be treated had been confused by the undifferentiated way in which general practitioners prescribed antibiotics. Helman also noted that some general practitioners prescribe antibiotics rather loosely both for viruses and for bacteria. Professional influences, including those of health educationists, may be part of the explanation for the finding in the Cambridge study of health and life-styles where questions asked about attitudes and beliefs about health and ill health consistently showed differences between the old and the young; the views of the former were further from the professional wisdom (Blaxter, 1987a and 1987b).

However, the traffic is not all one way. Lay health beliefs can also affect professional practice. Helman (1986) suggests that general practitioners collude with the folk model; they negotiate with their patients on the basis of it – agree, for example, that there is a 'bug going round', hardly a scientific biomedical explanation. The diagnosis also tends to be couched in the folk idiom, which is thus professionally reinforced. The treatments offered could not be 'fully justified in scientific biomedical terms ... It is almost as if, in some cases, the patients are treating themselves, using the doctor as a source of folk remedies – rather than the pharmacy, or a supermarket' (1986, p. 229).

CONCLUSION

We have seen that the beliefs of lay people, the concepts of the folk, about health and illness are various and may differ from those of health-care professionals. Nevertheless, the beliefs have their own logic, a logic which can be seen when the believers are located in their social context. Individual concepts vary systematically with their holders' own health experiences (Blaxter, 1987b; Olesen *et al.*, 1985). Lay concepts may be seen, as Herzlich and Pierret and d'Houtaud see them, as social representations expressing values of the society, while Crawford sees the concepts as expressions of societal conflict. Certainly a good deal of evidence suggests that aspects at least of lay concepts vary from one social class to another in ways that appear to relate to the material differences between the classes. There is also some evidence that, as material circumstances, including mode of health-care delivery and welfare arrangements, change over time, so have health concepts changed. As well as lay concepts being socially situated, so is professional practice socially contextualized such that it is itself influenced by lay modes of conceptualization. Nevertheless patients may run into difficulties in consulting biomedical practitioners because of the differences in the concepts each uses (Blaxter, 1983). Biomedicine, however, is not the only healing mode practised in Britain today; let us now turn to the alternatives that are available to patients seeking treatment.

11 Concepts of Health and the Nature of Healing Knowledge (2): Alternative Healing Systems

As we have seen, one of the remarkable features of the development of the health service in the UK was the unanimity about the value of biomedicine. There may have been disagreements between trade unions and employers' organizations and between middle-class and working-class women's organizations about what the emphasis should be in health-care provision. But they were agreed that achieving better access to biomedicine was the issue. With hindsight we can see that not all the implications of this reliance on biomedicine were understood. By the 1980s it has become a fashionable and familiar quip to refer to the National Health Service as the National Sickness Service. Not only has any consensus that the NHS is organizationally the best way to provide biomedical care been broken in the 1980s, but there are increasing doubts about certain facets of biomedicine itself. However, although biomedicine may have become strongly dominant, it was not the only healing system available either before or after the Second World War. Not everybody was so attached to biomedicine as its success might lead one to imagine.

What were the alternatives? When the foundations of the NHS were laid, homoeopathy, imported from Germany (and still espoused by the British Queen in the 1980s, although the Court is also attended by biomedical physicians and surgeons), osteopathy, various herbal systems, Christian Science and other spiritual healing modes were also available. Richarda Power (1984) has documented the problems encountered by practitioners, clients and supporters of these other modes. Particularly she has examined the problems experienced by naturopathy faced with a state-supported biomedical system and the issues of professionalism which were also involved.

The establishment of the NHS was a considerable blow to all healers who were not registered medical practitioners. When only one system (in this case the biomedical) is free at the point of delivery, albeit paid for through taxes, any alternative system has to have a great deal to offer to be able to compete, or the 'free' system has to make a great many mistakes. In addition, the established and state-supported healing system has, as a consequence of its privileged position, a large amount of capital as well as revenue at its disposal. One is entitled to wonder whether, if they had had a similar endowment of material resources, privilege and prestige, some of the alternative healing systems might not have emerged as similarly powerful and effective as biomedicine, albeit in different ways and perhaps with regard to different aspects of suffering. It partly depends upon what one counts as efficacious.

In Britain the establishment of the General Medical Council in 1858 did not have the consequence of preventing healers who were not registered from practising. They were merely prevented from announcing themselves as *registered medical practitioners*. The increasing popularity of biomedicine, especially among the bourgeoisie, had the effect of proportionately reducing the clients of other modalities. It did not banish the other healers. The state may proscribe, but it cannot prevent citizens' beliefs and practices (Caplan, 1984, pp. 81–2; Chow, 1984, pp. 132–4; Coulter, 1984, pp. 73–7; Taylor, 1984, pp. 193–4).

ALTERNATIVES IN EAST AND WEST GERMANY

Unschuld has written about the 'structured coexistence of independently conceptualized therapy systems' (1980, p. 15). He compares East and West Germany. In the former only biomedicine is permitted; in the latter, all systems are available. In both parts of Germany people have resort to a variety of systems: homoeopathy, anthroposophical healing and phytotherapic continue to be practised.

Homoeopathy was established at the end of the eighteenth century in Germany by Samuel Hahnemann, a physician (see also Coulter, 1984). It comes from the same ancient roots as biomedicine, but from that time 200 years ago it developed differently. Whereas allopathy, from which biomedicine developed, worked on a principle of opposites, using procedures, medicines and surgery to oppose, kill off and get rid of the disease or pain, homoeopathy worked on a principle of similarities. It is a systematized body of knowledge for which training is required. Diagnosis and healing proceed by establishing the unique features of the individual sufferer and by the administration of small doses of substances which produce the symptoms from which the patient is suffering. The relevance of treatments for various ailments was established by Hahnemann by a system of tests or trails known as 'provings'. In other respects, such as a passive patient consulting a qualified practioner, relationships within homoeopathy are similar to those within biomedicine. Despite the original methodological opposition between allopathy and homoeopathy, some biomedical practioners nowadays use homoeopathic remedies for their non-toxic, non-invasive properties.

Anthroposophical healing was established by Steiner (whose practices are also found in the UK). Steiner's healers in Germany were MDs. He acknowledged science, e.g. chemistry and physics, but also an 'ethereal' and 'astral' body and 'ego-structure'. He practised eurhythmics but also used drugs. According to Unschuld, a 'significant portion of the German population' share Steiner's world view (p. 16).

Phytotherapic is botanical healing. This system relies on drugs of plant origin, and we would perhaps call it herbalism. Looked at from the point of view of modern pharmacology many of these drugs are now seen as obsolete, either because chemotherapeutic drugs do the same job more efficiently, or because the active ingredients have been synthesized, or because no active ingredients have been found. Yet, Unschuld tells us, enough people still use these drugs to support a multi-million-dollar industry.

In Germany from the 1860s there had been a universal right to be a healer, but in 1939 the Nazi government passed a Health Practitioner Law to regulate the 'occupational practice of medicine without a licence' (Unschuld, 1980, p. 17). Initially the Nazis had said that it was not the business of physicians to cure disease but to treat the people. At first favourable to alternative healers, they nevertheless did not intend to sustain a variety of systems. It had been their initial policy to integrate 'natural healing' into 'school medicine'. All were to be university trained.

Since the war and the partition of Germany, the development of medicine has been quite different in each state. From 1945 in East Germany the government began to regulate drugs; later it legislated against self-medication and the avoidance of expert treatment. The aim was to move towards a health service based on scientifically trained personnel and scientifically justified therapy. Homoeopathy cannot be taught in medical or pharmaceutical schools in the German Democratic Republic; homoeopathic drugs still circulate and are permitted, although the number produced and consumed has significantly decreased. Government policy aims to phase out alternatives and rely entirely upon biomedicine.

In the Federal Republic of Germany, on the other hand, while there is food and drug legislation the right to be a healer is retained. (In contrast with East Germany, homoeopathy enjoys some public funding.) EEC regulations have required proof of the efficiency of a drug before it can be legally admitted, but drugs other than biomedical pharmaceuticals are admitted. However, the legislature applied the notion 'scientific' to homoeopathy and anthroposophy, thus avoiding the testing of those drugs by biomedical procedures; they are tested by their own criteria (see also the discussion on page 175).

Unschuld draws attention to the differences in the political economies of East and West Germany in relation to their respective treatment of differential healing systems. The unitary political and economic system of East Germany restricts practice to biomedicine, while the liberal capitalist West German regime permits pluralism.

Two points about the concepts involved may be noted from this example. The first is that there is more than one elaborated system of health maintenance and healing alternative to biomedicine. The second is that some of these alternatives are rooted in systems of thought or cosmologies which are conceived logically but in a quite different mode from biomedicine. It is therefore inappropriate to test them in biomedical terms; they can logically be tested only in their own terms. However, to some extent a common denominator can be provided by the recipients, who will judge upon the basis of their experience. (See page 175 for a fuller discussion of these points.)

MANY HEALING SYSTEMS

Because of the dominance of biomedicine, and perhaps because of a human tendency to dichotomize, many people speak and write incorrectly of 'alternative medicine' in the singular. The World Health Organization has called 'traditional medicine' all forms of health-care provision that 'usually lie outside the official health sector'. As Ruth West (1984, pp. 341–2) points out, this has created difficulties in countries where by now biomedicine is thought of as 'traditional'; it further creates a sort of dustbin including items of miscellaneous type and worth.

There are problems with categorizing the range of contemporary healing systems in advanced industrial societies, just as there are in categorizing the many healing systems of former times and other parts of the world. The sixty or so therapies in the UK could perhaps be divided, Ruth West suggests, into three categories: physical, psychological and paranormal. The category paranormal is itself, of course, a judgemental term derived from the natural science mode. The tripartite division suggested also follows that conceptualization and includes the Cartesian mind–body dichotomy. Ruth West proposes an alternative, a division between those systems which

> require a high degree of professional training and those that are at heart variations on first aid, do-it-yourself, and self-care techniques. Osteopathy, chiropractic, medical herbalism, homeopathy, naturopathy and acupuncture would fit under the first category [as would biomedicine]; and everything else, barring a few psychotherapies, under the second.
>
> (West, 1984, p. 342)

The plurality of healing modalities which Ruth West indicates (see also Salmon, 1984a) and her attempts at classification remind us of both the Amhara (Young, 1976a and 1986; and see Chapter 2) and England in the sixteenth and seventeenth centuries (Feierman, 1979; and see Chapter 2). How far is the division into externalizing and internalizing systems which Allan Young proposed relevant to an understanding of the array of alternative medicines which are available? Young (1976a and 1986) suggested that externalizing systems looked outside the body for explanations of suffering, while internalizing systems looked to what was happening within.

He suggested that all internalizing systems required a great degree of formal training for their practitioners, as is true of ancient Chinese medicine, Unani, Ayurveda and biomedicine (see also Chapter 2). As Ruth West (1984) says, it is also true of such systems as osteopathy and homoeopathy among others. Many of those contemporary healing systems which she refers to as 'paranormal' would fall into the externalizing mode, believing that something injurious or evil has entered the body from the outside. In addition, among the Amhara there were various healers who worked at an empirical level and with a particular part of the body – bone setters, teeth pullers and the like. They and their counterparts in Europe who deal with only one part of the body seem to fall somewhat outside the externalizing/internalizing dichotomy, perhaps into a category of empirics.

EPISTOMOLOGICAL DIFFERENCES

In the UK and the USA, and doubtless in other advanced industrial societies, some of the alternative modes, some psychic healing for example, can only really be described as externalizing systems. Others, such as chiropractic and osteopathy, focus on the crucial importance of particular parts of the body, in this case the spine; iridology stresses the iris; the Ingham technique focuses on the feet (Taylor, 1984, p. 195). Some accept part or all of the precepts of biomedicine but feel they have a complementary and special skill. Some, like chiropractic, while feeling that biomedicine may treat them as subsidiary, insist that they have a different fundamental theory. Thus osteopathy and chiropractic take the view that misalignments, 'sublaxations', of the spine can be the cause not only of muscular-skeletal disorders as such, but also of a wide variety of conditions such as peptic ulcer, diabetes, high blood pressure and even cancer. Like biomedics they have however ceased to believe in monocausality. They believe that correcting the sublaxation will permit the body to heal itself, but in cases where the disease has become widespread in the body before treatment, they will refer to a biomedical practitioner (Coulter, 1984).

Where underlying epistemological differences between healing systems are large they can be seen most clearly. Traditional Chinese medicine is one example. It is currently practised in part or in whole in both the USA and the UK (Chow, 1984; Lu and Needham, 1980). Western interest in Chinese medicine has perhaps always focused mostly on acupuncture, an interest which began in the eighteenth century and which has recently been revived. This revival is in part associated with Chairman Mao's reinstatement of traditional Chinese medicine in 1949. It had been banned in the nineteenth century in favour of allopathy. Mao also instructed that the traditional healing system should be integrated with biomedicine.

As Chow's (1984) brief and useful account makes plain, acupuncture is only one part of a sophisticated healing system which conceives of the body in ways quite different from those of biomedicine and which also sees the body in relation to great forces of the world. 'The overriding theme of the ancient life style was the harmony of the human microcosm with macrocosmic laws' (Chow, 1984, p. 121). Emphasis was on maintaining health, or prevention as we might more negatively put it. In the briefest outline, medical thinking was predicated on three major principles: the complementary interaction of the *yin* and the *yang* on which much of the theory was constructed; *chi* or vital energy; and the doctrine of the five phases or elements (wood, fire, earth, metal and water). Based on systematic observation, analysis, deduction and interpretation, Chinese medicine was already highly developed centuries before Christ. An extensive herbal had been developed three thousand years BC; and by 200 BC Chinese healers not only had an extensive understanding of what we would call internal medicine but also practised sophisticated surgery and anaesthetics, although Confucius later banned surgery (Chow, 1984, pp. 48–9).

THE INCREASED INTEREST IN OTHER MODES

Over the last ten to fifteen years, there has been a widespread revival of interest in older healing modes, which have continued to develop their understanding and practices. New modes have also been developed using concepts from contemporary science or new technologies – for example, biofeedback, which claims 1,750 members in the Biofeedback Society of America (Taylor, 1984, p. 192, quoting Rubin, 1979). Increased interest in a variety of healing modes has arisen in the USA with its largely free market economy in health care and in the UK alongside the NHS.

Ruth West (1984, pp. 343–4) reports inquiries which show that consultations other than with biomedics were increasing by 10 to 15 per cent a year and that the numbers of practitioners and consultations were increasing five times more rapidly than in biomedicine. One per cent of the UK population say they use an acupuncturist, 2 per cent homoeopathy, 3 per cent practise meditation, 7 per cent use 'natural' medicine, and 16 per cent buy health foods. In February 1986 *Which?* asked nearly 28,000 of its subscribers whether they 'had used any form of alternative or complementary medicine during the previous 12 months. About one in seven said they had.' These figures, like those West quotes, are small, but in a society where biomedicine is free at the point of delivery they cannot be ignored. In a random sample of those who had used some form of 'complementary' medicine *Which?* found that 42 per cent had consulted osteopaths, 26 per cent homoeopaths, 23 per cent practitioners of acupuncture, 22 per cent chiropractics and 11 per cent herbalists (*Which?*, October 1986, p. 443). More than 86,000 people were out-patients at the six homoeopathic hospitals under the NHS in the UK in 1977 (Taylor, 1984, p. 192, quoting Stanway, 1982, p. 157). The British Holistic Medical Association was formed in 1983. Stung by remarks from Prince Charles, and with some champions of alternative therapies in its midst, the BMA set up a committee on alternative medicine (West, 1984, pp. 342–3), an action which alternative healers found threatening. Their fears were justified in so far as the BMA's report was largely antagonistic (*British Medical Journal*, 24 May 1986, pp. 1407–8). However, in a 1985 survey of 145 GPs in Avon more than half said they thought osteopathy and chiropractic, acupuncture and hypnosis were useful, while well over a third thought that homoeopathy and healing were (*Which?*, October 1986, p. 445).

Why are more people going to alternative healers? It seems patients are not just opting out of the NHS with its rushed consultations and queues for hospital appointments. Those who wish for more attention and can afford to pay (either by insurance or directly) may consult biomedical practitioners privately. It must be more than time and attention that is looked for, although these may be involved. Those who spend their money consulting an alternative healer are opting out of biomedicine, not just out of the NHS.

Many biomedical practitioners would like to believe that it is only 'incurable' cases who go to alternative practitioners, and to some extent this is correct. According to *Which?* (October 1986, p. 443), 81 per cent of those who had consulted alternative healers had done so after they had consulted their own GP about the problem; 81 per cent had been dissatisfied because they had not been cured, got only temporary relief, or could not be treated. Of those who had received some form of alternative treatment, 31 per cent said they were cured, and 51 per cent improved; 74 per cent said they would definitely use this form of medicine again, 69 per cent that they would recommend it to someone else with a similar complaint. Only 14 per cent said the treatment was ineffective, and 1 per cent that the problem got worse. Such responses suggest that much alternative treatment is effective in patients' terms.

We have already previously mentioned how, other than by patient reports, one might test the effectiveness of healing systems which conceive of the mind and body quite differently from biomedicine. Some interesting controlled trials have taken place in which relevant alternative healers have co-operated with biomedics and in which the latter have assumed an appropriately humble and questioning scientific approach. One such was a randomized controlled trial of acupuncture for disabling breathlessness. Twelve matched pairs of patients with chronic obstructive pulmonary disease received traditional Chinese acupuncture or placebo acupuncture. After three weeks' treatment aimed at reducing disability the traditional acupuncture group showed significantly greater benefit in terms of 'subjective' scores of breathlessness and six-minute walking distance than those having the placebo acupuncture. This suggests that the benefits patients experience from acupuncture are not, as some have claimed, merely placebo effects (i.e. an effect where the medication has no physiological consequence and the patient merely imagines an improvement). 'Objective' biomedical measures of lung function were unchanged in both groups. That some healing, not understood in presently measurable terms, took place is agreed by all the authors of the trial (Jobst *et al.*, 1986).

In another trial (Fung, Chow and So, 1986), a prospective randomized single blind study comparing real and sham acupuncture to attenuate exercise-induced asthma showed that real acupuncture was more effective than sham acupuncture (at statistically significant levels), although both had some effect. Discussion of the results seeks to explain the way in which acupuncture works entirely in biomedical terms, an approach which is echoed in the *Lancet* editorial of 20/27 December 1986.

Traditional acupuncture is holistic in that any treatment for a specific condition is given in the context of the patient's present total mental and physical state as the practitioner judges it by the patient's appearance and her/his subjective account. The precise treatment given is determined by the assessment, made every time the patient presents, including each time during a course of treatment for a condition. Biomedical scientists have difficulty in coming to terms with both these facets; in their mode it is the already diagnosed disease condition which is to be treated rather than the total person. Traditional Chinese medicine can account for why the treatment works, the release of vital energy being an important part of the explanation. To biomedical practitioners it remains mysterious and therefore suspicious unless it can be reinterpreted within conventional biomedical knowledge.

In the trials cited, traditional Chinese healers have worked with biomedical healers. What in the longer run may be the relationship between biomedicine and not only acupuncture but other alternative healing modes is something to which we shall return. In the meantime let us turn to a discussion of some of the essential concepts of biomedicine itself; at the end of that chapter we shall come back to the relationship of the other modalities with biomedicine.

12 Concepts of Health and the Nature of Healing Knowledge (3): Biomedicine and Beyond

FAITH WITHOUT SCIENTIFIC EVIDENCE

In Part One we saw how by the twentieth century biomedicine had come to dominate over all other healing systems. This was generally believed to be because of its greater efficacy. But hindsight suggests that this was a matter of faith rather than a proposition wholly based on good scientific evidence. It may seem strange to speak of faith in relation to a scientific enterprise, but it appears to have been just that; for the consensus, which had its roots in the nineteenth century as we have seen, seems, when looked at from a population point of view, to have been based on remarkably slender evidence.

Thomas McKeown (1965 and 1971) has claimed that the improvements in the nation's health, the improvement in what I have called the biological base, in the nineteenth century and up to the mid-twentieth, had relatively little to do with allopathic medicine or later with biomedicine. It could best be accounted for, in this order of importance, by 'increase in food supplies from the mid-eighteenth century, hygienic measures from 1870, and limitation of numbers from about the same time'. McKeown goes on: 'Effective prevention and treatment of disease in the individual were delayed until the second quarter of the twentieth century and have been less significant than any of the other major influences' (1971, p. 45).

Before the twentieth century effective surgery was limited, and there were few effective drugs – mercury, iron, quinine and digitalis were among the few (McKeown, 1971, p. 6). Some of these – for example, digitalis for the treatment of heart trouble – derived from the knowledge of the wise women and men of ancient times.

DEATH RATES TO INDICATE HEALTH

McKeown's arguments, although generally taken to be about the improvement in the health of the population, are really about the rise in the population over the last 300 years. The statistical analyses undertaken by McKeown and his associates were complex and sophisticated (see, for example, McKeown and Brown, 1955–6; McKeown and Record, 1962). His principal indicators have to do with birth and death. Using data from 1838 when births and deaths began to be registered, they show that the growth of the population was due to an excess of births over deaths and later to a decline in mortality; the increase was not due to a rising birth rate. Indeed, the birth rate declined during the period he reviews.

McKeown examines death rates from specific causes and shows that the principal cause of the decline in mortality was the reduction in deaths from communicable disease. Except in the case of smallpox after 1800 when vaccination was introduced, this was not due to medical intervention. He examines carefully hypotheses relating to possible changes in the invaders which cause infectious diseases or in the host which alters the response. Many organisms coexist with hosts, most commonly causing no trouble to the host. Sometimes this changes, such that the host becomes disabled, dies, or develops an ability to cope with a previously disabling invader. His analyses lead him to conclude that family limitation, improved food supplies from home and abroad, an improved environment, clean air and water and better housing were the principal causes of the population increase.

From his analysis of the rise of the population McKeown *infers* that people were more healthy. Webster (1984) has more recently shown how the healthiness of one section of the population may improve while that of another declines. Epidemiologists find it most useful to work with indicators of birth and death, because, of all the indicators about the biological base, these are the least equivocal.

MORTALITY AND MORBIDITY RATES

The great authority on medical statistics is Bradford Hill (1962 and 1971), but their construction and use is well explained by Alwyn Smith (1968). Absolute numbers are of limited use for comparison over time and space because populations may vary in size. The notion of a population at risk of becoming ill or dying is therefore used, and one population is compared with another in terms of the number per 100, per 1,000, or 100,000 who experience the illness or die. The *incidence rate* is distinguished from the *prevalence rate*. The *incidence rate* is the number of cases per so many (often 1,000) of the population who died or contracted the disease in a given period, say a year. The *prevalence rate* on the other hand is the number of people in a given period per, say, 1,000 of the population who are suffering from the disease. Incidence rates are more commonly used when illnesses of short duration, such as influenza, are being considered, and prevalence rates when chronic sickness or handicap are in question. Incidence and prevalence are linked by disease duration.

The notion of a *death rate* may seem reasonably simple, but again if one wishes to compare populations it is necessary to be careful. There are problems here about using the *crude death rate*, which is derived by dividing the number of deaths during a year by the number of the population at risk during the year, which is usually approximated by the number of the population at mid-year. The crude death rate will be affected by the age and sex of the population. For this reason a number of more sophisticated measures have been developed. To overcome these problems *age-specific death rates* may be calculated, i.e. the number dying at a particular age divided by the number in the population at that age. Age-specific rates may be calculated separately for women and men. This produces a considerable number of rates for any one population. For this reason the *standardized* death or *mortality* rate (SMR) is ordinarily used when a summary about the total population is required.

Calculation of the SMR involves calculating, for each population under comparison, the number of deaths that would occur in it if, at each age, it experienced the age specific death rates of a suitably chosen standard population. The actual number of deaths is then expressed as a percentage of this calculated number. This ratio expresses the relative mortality experience of the real population compared with that in the standard population and corrects for differences in age composition between the real population and the standard.

(Smith, 1968, p. 47)

Other rates which are commonly used are the *infant mortality rate*, which refers to children under the age of a year, the *neonatal mortality rate*, which refers to infants under 28 days, and the *perinatal mortality rate*, which includes stillbirths and infants who died aged less than 1 week. The last is thought to be particularly affected by the circumstances surrounding the birth, while the first is thought to be more affected by the social, economic and other living circumstances of the child after birth. (See Macfarlane and Mugford, 1984, for a detailed exposition of these and other rates relevant to birth and its sequelae.)

What rates do is offer a way of describing and comparing the frequency with which people die or become ill, are chronically sick or disabled in defined populations. They derive from aggregating data relating to individuals. Mortality rates are somewhat more reliable than morbidity rates, because when someone is finally agreed to be dead the state is a definitive one. Morbidity data, on the other hand, depend upon persons thinking they are not well and upon doctors making a diagnosis and it being reported. There are, however, problems about tables which attempt to analyse causes of death, because although the International Classification of Diseases may be used, physicians might not always agree what was the primary cause of death or may not make an accurate record.

THE USE OF RATES

Rates measuring mortality and morbidity have been extensively used in attempts to influence health policy and to compare the healthiness of one population with another. The position of a country in the league of tables of various death rates is taken to reflect on national prestige.

Maternal mortality rates were used in this way in the interwar years; neonatal mortality rates have been used in the postwar period to justify changes in the locale of childbirth and in the management of labour (see pages 238–9). These are the techniques which have also been used to try to ascertain the causes of the very different health experiences of sections of the British population, in particular the relationship between social class and ill health (Townsend and Davidson, 1982). Such statistical associations have also been used as part of the search for the causes of particular diseases.

THE MECHANISTIC MODEL

Thomas McKeown's lifetime work on the reasons for the improvement in the health of nations was undertaken as a professor of social medicine rather than as a clinician; he wrote as a doctor in the tradition of the public health movement and looked at medicine from a population point of view. He contrasts his approach to the mechanistic model which developed from the seventeenth century. This mechanistic model, following Descartes, separates the body from the mind, but also separates the body from its environment.

> Nature was conceived in mechanistic terms, which led in biology to the idea that a living organism could be regarded as a machine which might be taken apart and reassembled if its structure and function were fully understood [and in] medicine . . . to the belief that an understanding of disease processes and of the body's response to them would make it possible to intervene therapeutically, mainly by physical (surgical), chemical, or electrical methods.
>
> (McKeown, 1971, p. 29)

This physical model led to what McKeown describes as an engineering approach. In contrast he focuses not on individual bodies as clinicians do, but upon populations. His is an epidemiological approach. In part therefore he restores medicine to the social, but there is no real evidence that his ideas in any way fundamentally deny or challenge the Cartesian mind–body split (see also pages 164–6). This he has in common with many clinicians; the distinction between them is that the clinician is concerned with the ailments, the pathologies, experienced by any one person with the aim of intervening and treating – and treatments nowadays are often successful. The epidemiologist, on the other hand, is concerned with the healthiness of the population as a whole. The intra-professional disputes between clinicians and epidemiologists may have exaggerated the differences between them.

In so far as the indicators which the epidemiologist uses are those relating to disease conditions as clinically defined, this amounts to an aggregation of individual clinical data. Such an aggregation puts the circumstances of any one individual into a new perspective, a perspective it would not be possible to achieve by reliance on clinical cases alone. This perspective can help the analysis of the multifarious causes of disease. It can also provide useful guidance for the allocation of scarce resources. If we know which sections of the population are especially likely to suffer from particular pathologies, then, in any rational system of resource allocation, we may concentrate our resources upon people in that category. There is also the question of where to concentrate our efforts if the aim is to reduce mortality from a particular disease condition. Epidemiological studies are also used to test the efficacy of clinical treatments, as we saw in the randomized controlled trials of acupuncture referred to in Chapter 11 (pages 158–9).

ESTABLISHING ILLNESS CAUSATION

The problems of establishing causation and thus moving to preventive action are interestingly illustrated in the case of lung cancer. The history also draws out the close association between clinical medicine and epidemiological surveys. Ann Cartwright (1983, pp. 24 ff.) has discussed this story of the discovery and acceptance of the association between smoking and lung cancer. The method she is describing is what Denzin (1970) would call triangulation and Burgess multiple methods (1982, p. 163).

The first step was clinicians' suspicions from their observations of the patients they were treating that smokers might be more liable to the disease than non-smokers. Note that the disease entity under question is in any case a clinical category. Then a statistical association was established in a survey population (in this case of British medical practitioners) between smokers and sufferers by Doll and Hill (1950, 1952, 1954, 1956 and 1964). This, as Cartwright (1983, p. 31) points out, did not of itself establish causality; other possible explanations had to be ruled out, and such searches can never be entirely exhaustive. Laboratory work was important. This showed that tobacco contained elements which had been shown to induce cancer in laboratory animals, i.e. they were carcinogenic agents.

In the end, of course, it is not claimed that smoking is the only cause of lung cancer. The days when medicine relied on monocausality have passed. Non-smokers may get lung cancer, and smokers may not; what the measures show is that the *chances* are different. Cartwright (1983) discusses the factors associated with the acceptance of the research evidence about the relationship between smoking and lung cancer. She speaks of the economic, political and other factors which led people to be cautious. The association has now been accepted by government, by the leaders of the medical profession and by many ordinary people. However, there are those who remain unconvinced by probabilistic arguments and are more impressed by what they have witnessed themselves and by the alleged eyewitness accounts of others. For people who follow such evidence and its associated logic the cases of the non-smokers who contract the disease and the smokers who do not loom large. Such people no doubt also subscribe to other constructs about illness causation.

Furthermore, believing in an association between smoking now and lung cancer later does not necessarily help individuals who smoke to overcome their addiction. The recent survey on health and life-styles has again shown there is no straightforward association between what people believe about ill health and how they behave (Blaxter, Fenner and Wichelow, 1987, p. 121). Those who stand to gain from continued addiction to tobacco are unlikely to welcome measures to reduce smoking. Prime among these, of course, is the tobacco industry, which is likely to belittle the research findings. Governments may be less vigorous also if only because of the loss of tax revenue that decreases in smoking entail. To achieve effective treatment for smoking, as opposed to treating lung cancer, takes us far beyond the realm of the strictly biomedical.

CARTESIAN DOMINATION STILL?

The issue of the causes of lung cancer is a good example of the way medicine has come to take in new concepts and methods while at the same time the focus remains on cells and the cell changes which constitute disease. Blaxter (1983, p. 68) may be right when she considers 'very narrow and outmoded' a view of medical theory which supposes that medicine 'still prefers single causes, views psyche and soma dichotomously, has a narrow definition of heredity, or regards disease and behaviour as discrete'. Salmon has put it another way: 'the conceptual framework utilized by modern medicine is highly complex and contains many paradigms' (1984a, p. 5), and this is undoubtedly so.

Nevertheless, Berliner is still able to claim that in its most simple formulation biomedicine

> maintains that each cell in the body functions solely on the basis of its genetic instructions and that external influences have little effect on the behaviour of the cell, except in so far as they can alter the cell wall and do damage to the cell. Given this operating principle, it is difficult for [biomedicine] to explain any relationship between mental states and physical functions.
>
> (Berliner, 1984, p. 49)

Some theorists have not been deterred from making such links, however. The whole school of sociobiology proposes that all human life, the behavioural and social as well as the biological, derives from the programme in the DNA which is responsible for transmitting genetic information. (For a critical review of this position, see Rose, Lewontin and Leonikamin, 1984.) Furthermore, as we have already noted, Armstrong's (1983b) analysis suggests that from the later years of the nineteenth century, through the work of TB and VD clinics, medicine began to claim the social as well as the individual body as an arena for its understanding and research (see pages 99–100). He also shows how this attention to the social increased through the twentieth century, particularly through the use of surveys. Around mid-century interest was directed to understanding what might be the state of affairs in the 'normal' body or mind. The pathological then came increasingly to be set into this framework. Clinicians, while still treating individuals and not populations, more and more came to see patients' presenting symptoms within the range found in a population, of which the individual was one member. The knowledge used is thus extended beyond the experience of any one clinician, not only by anecdote but systematically, using statistics.

WHAT IS NORMAL?

There are, of course, problems about the concept of the normal. Are we referring to a statistical average, or a range, or to standards which are normatively accepted? In the use of surveys, it is the former, although the norms of particular groups in the society may well influence what is measured in the first place.

In some branches of medicine the normatively acceptable remains dominant. This is the case, for example, in much cosmetic surgery, where there is no pathology present but the shape of a person does not conform to the preferred and most acceptable body images current in the society at the time. This is no trivial example, but one where medicine is implicated in maintaining dominant norms and where temptations to exceed reasonable ethical standards abound.

The use of a statistical norm provides guidelines suggesting which deviations are such that action should be taken. These become particularly important in cases where certain symptoms may be taken to be the precursor or indicator of an underlying disease. Raised blood pressure is an example. A wide range of blood pressures are found in the population at large for persons of similar age and sex. The cut-off points for treatment to avoid life-threatening episodes – for example, of heart problems – are necessarily arbitrary. The same is true of the 'milestones' in development which children are expected to achieve; failure to reach them by the average age on the part of an individual child may or may not betoken an underlying disability.

A CHALLENGE FROM GENERAL PRACTICE?

Another challenge to the simple version of biomedical understanding described by Berliner has emerged from within general practice since the establishment of the NHS in Britain. Generally speaking the specialisms which developed in hospital-based biomedicine followed from the divisions in the systems of the body as biologically defined, for example, the gastro-intestinal tract, the cardio-vascular system. Specialists are concerned with that part of the body only, while being aware of how that system relates to others, and when to refer the patient to another specialist. Only two specialties, paediatrics and geriatrics, divide their patients among them other than by a part of the body. In those two cases the division is on the basis of age, the belief being that the nature of disease is specific to the age group (cf. Armstrong, 1979).

General practitioners are characterized by their claim to treat the whole person and indeed the whole family. Subsequent to the settlement in 1948 which gave them an assured place but lowly status within the NHS, British general practitioners have paid attention to their knowledge base, as part of a general move to enhance their status. Initially deriving from the teaching of Balint (1956), they began to develop a new way of looking at the relationship of psyche and soma. General practitioners were encouraged by Balint to look beyond the patient's presenting complaint and to recognize that the doctor–patient relationship itself contained elements of therapy. Since Balint, there have been further moves to make a virtue out of their generalness and to treat the 'whole patient' and not only the disease condition itself (Armstrong, 1983b; Jefferys and Sachs, 1983).

Their training, however, remains based on hospital medicine and upon the specialist divisions of advanced clinical medicine. This is now extended by compulsory vocational training. Organizationally, and somewhat ironically, their bid has been to get general practice accepted as a specialty along with others, their specialism being their very generalism.

Over the last three-quarters of a century, therefore, through influences derived from the social survey, used in epidemiology and influencing clinical medicine, and through psychological influences on general practice, some modifications have occurred in the medical paradigm. Increasing attention has been paid to ailments which are thought to be of psychosomatic origin, that is, originating in or associated with mental disturbances and eventuating in somatic or physical illness, the name itself reflecting the original Cartesian distinction. However, this group of illnesses remain among those with which biomedicine is less able to deal successfully.

Not only does the biological model remain powerful; both modes, the clinical and the epidemiological, remain essentially individualistic. Three features should be noted. The first is that the individualism of epidemiology marks it off from a sociological approach in the sense that it is concerned with population aggregates rather than with social systems or social interaction. Second, the biological approach does not lead to any very positive definitions of health, defining, as it does, the normal through the absence of pathology or malformation. Third, the mechanistic model has led to remarkable feats of 'high-tech' medicine but has also brought its own problems in the late twentieth century. Each of these will be discussed in turn.

CONSTRASTING CONCEPTS IN SOCIAL MEDICINE AND SOCIOLOGY

At this juncture it is appropriate that we should be quite clear what it is that social medicine is about, the concepts upon which it is based and how it contrasts not only with the enterprise of clinical medicine but also with the sociological enterprise. While social or population medicine offers a different and more collective perspective from that of clinical medicine, it nevertheless, as we have seen, does not go much beyond the aggregation of individual data and their subsequent statistical manipulation. In so far as epidemiologists think in terms of collectivities, the collectivities are structured from statistical categorizations; they are not composed of interacting social groups.

Groups and Categories

There is a distinction between the allocation by an administrator, researcher, or statistician of an individual into a statistical or administrative category and individuals themselves knowingly and consciously joining a group. To take an example, 'single parent' is a category invented by administrators or data collectors. They have derived it negatively from the normative notion (at one time adhered to more closely than nowadays) that children should have two parents who in their turn should be monogamously married. In statistical analysis, having identified a category 'single parent', aggregations of such parents are then juxtaposed against parents in heterosexual couples according to certain individual attributes or perhaps according to certain characteristics of their children. Inferences are then drawn about the state of single parenthood and about their children, who may be thought to be 'at risk' in certain ways. Any such risk, however (that their children will be less fit, develop less satisfactorily, do less well at school, for example), relates only to a statistical possibility or probability, not to the actual life circumstances and behaviour of any one parent and her/his children.

Contrast such a category with membership of a Gingerbread group. Here we have a group in the sociological sense: a number of people who are aware that they share certain social attributes, that they share certain life circumstances, in this case single parenthood and all that may mean; they have defined themselves and have come together for common ends. Not all persons in the administrative or statistical category 'single parent' will recognize these commonalities with others in like situation or wish to interact with them in a more or less formally organized group. (Graham, 1984, p. 31, discusses some of these problems well.)

The distinction between a group in this last sense and a category derives from Ginsberg's (1934) analysis and bears some relationship to Marx's notion of a class for itself and a class of itself. The sharing of common attributes in the last case is noticed by an outsider (in our case statistician or administrator) who composes a statistical category. This category becomes a group, a class for itself, only when persons in that category join together in interaction. When the attributes of individuals are counted and correlated against each other, we are at a very considerable level of abstraction from daily life; we are furthermore dealing only with probabilities and not with what has happened or will happen to an individual or group.

In sum, we need to distinguish two difficulties that can arise from the application of analyses such as these to real life situations. The first is that because statistical associations can speak only of probabilities, of likelihoods or risks, they cannot predict individual experience or behaviour. The second is that category allocation, unlike group membership, does not necessarily imply anything about social action.

Under the first heading there is a danger of a slippage from administrative or statistical categorization to daily life situations which turns associations between variables back on to individuals as if, because they appear in a certain statistical category, particular people will exhibit certain social characteristics. This can merge into stereotyping.

An example may be taken from the area of screening for cervical cancer. Epidemiological studies, establishing associations between attributes of individuals, have shown that women in certain age groups and in lower social classes are more likely to develop cancer of the cervix than either younger women or those in the Registrar-General's categories I and II. Where resources are scarce (and they are never infinite) it makes good sense in Benthamite terms to concentrate screening upon those age groups and those social classes in which women as a category are shown to be most at risk. Because risks are low in some age groups and among higher social classes, it does not of course imply that no cases are ever found in those categories. It is thus mistaken to infer, as physicians have been heard to, that, for example, 'social classes I and II do not get it', for occasionally a well-to-do woman may contract the disease. The thought of being the one in several thousand is no consolation to a sufferer. Hypothetically, a well-to-do woman who had been denied public screening because of a policy decision to concentrate on the most at risk might well be expected to seek the service privately if she felt her anxiety reasonable. To accept a risk of a potentially lethal but preventable disease on behalf of the 'greatest good of the greatest number' may well be unreasonable in individual terms. A reasonable public policy which concentrates scarce resources on high-risk groups may not only save taxpayers' money but also save the maximum number of lives. The low-risk but well-off woman who consults privately would nevertheless be consuming the same stock of clinical and laboratory services by another route. The personal, moral and social meanings and consequences of different conceptualizations of risk are thus revealed.

A more poignant and difficult example of the problems, which derive from the differences between epidemiological concepts of populations at risk and individual and personal conceptions about life circumstances, may be found in the case of genetic counselling. Here the translation of statistical risks to social action is fraught with difficulty. What does it mean to parents to tell them that genetically they have, say, a one-in-four chance of producing a child with a particular disease or deformity? Are they to have no children to avoid the deformed one and thus deny themselves the possibility of conceiving any one of the three who might be fit and joyous human beings? How does the risk apply to them as a particular couple? Strong moral judgements are sometimes made about those who take the risk, on the grounds that such parents have no right to risk bringing a handicapped child into the world.

At another level, a commonly heard example is the misuse of findings from the Registrar-General's occupational class classification when patients or their parents or other relatives are referred to, for example, as 'typical social class V, what else can you expect?'. Analytic categories, useful in their place, then become weapons with which to stigmatize the unfortunate.

The second point, that allocation to a particular group or category does not imply anything about group membership or other social interactions, requires clarification of concepts about social structure and social action. Sociologically, in so far as one can think of a social structure beyond individual and face-to-face relationships, it is composed of individuals and groups, small and large, in interaction and who have particular kinds of relationship among them. Some will be superordinate, having more resources and power over others, who will be variously subordinate. It is the systematic patterning of intereactions and relationships which can be said to amount to a social structure or social system. Understanding the distribution of such resources among the population as an aggregated set of individuals can help us to understand the sociological structure of a society but does not by itself describe or explain that structure. It is what my colleague Richard Startup used to refer to as 'pre-sociology'. A hazard is that the analyst infers social structure from the very categories s/he has invented, in other words reifies – that is, regards the relationships in the analysis as the social reality. Observations of social relationships and of groups in social interaction are necessary in order to approach closer to social knowledge; neither social survey data nor epidemiological data alone are adequate.

Associations among attributes of individuals cannot tell us about individual or group behaviour nor about the social relationships among them. A statistical aggregate is thus not a social group, nor does allocation to a statistical category imply either particular individual attributes or group membership. Such matters can be inferred only from data which are more direct and multi-dimensional than the statistical. It is perhaps unfortunate that there is no agreed convention in either epidemiology or survey sociology to reserve the word 'group' for persons with some commonality they recognize and for a number of people with this and possibly other shared characteristics, like common membership, and to distinguish these from 'categories', which are nominated by some outside observer on the basis of a predefined individual social attribute.

So we should note that statistical associations can speak only of probabilities, of likelihoods or risks; they cannot predict individual experience or behaviour. Nor can allocation to a category, unlike group membership, necessarily imply anything about social action. These distinctions become important when one is thinking about the collectivistic or individualistic orientations in health and illness concepts. They have led sociologists to think of health and illness in ways somewhat different from both epidemiologists and clinicians.

POSITIVE OR NEGATIVE DEFINITIONS OF HEALTH

Both epidemiology and clinical medicine approach the biological base in much the same way. Health is the absence of disease or death. There are many who like Tillich (1961; discussed by Jago, 1975) feel that one cannot think about health without the reality and possibility of disease. After attending a biomedical clinic or surgery a person who emerges from a health check feeling s/he has been given a 'clean bill of health' has in practice emerged from the investigations with a series of statements relating to various parts of the body 'that nothing adverse has been found'. Similarly the healthiness of a nation is tested by a series of tables which refer to the incidence of diseases among the citizens or the frequency with which they die from various conditions. Dubos (1979 and 1985) showed many of the limitations of this approach.

The most famous attempt to go beyond a conventional disease model is probably the definition of the World Health Organization (WHO). 'Health is a state of complete physical, mental and social well-being, not merely the absence of disease or infirmity.' Such a definition can be used as an ideal state, a goal towards which people are oriented rather than an empirical possibility (cf. Twaddle, 1974, p. 31). This could be said to be the case of the WHO programme 'Health for All by the Year 2000' (known as HFA 2000 by those working on it). All WHO regions of the world are working towards this goal, knowing that the only real achievement possible can be an improvement in health, rather than its total attainment. WHO has also come to realize that it lacks indicators of health; all the indicators are of disease (see, for example, Holland, Ipsen and Kostrzewski, 1979).

Sociological Concepts of Health, Healthiness, Health and Illness
To start with, sociology tended to follow medicine in thinking of illness and disease rather than health; the latter has come in more recently. However, what characterizes the sociological approach is that it is derived from a social interaction or social systems point of view; the abstractions used do not relate to individuals alone but to individuals in interaction. Some begin from the small group, face-to-face situation; we have discussed the study by Olesen *et al.* (1985), for example. Others begin from a more systemic point of view.

Parsons (1972, p. 117), for example, defined health 'as the state of optimum *capacity* of an individual for the effective performance of the roles and tasks for which he [*sic*] has been socialized'. Parsons (1951) was concerned with the maintenance of equilibrium in the social system, and 'from the point of view of the function of the social system, too low in general level of health, too high an incidence of illness, is dysfunctional' (Parsons, 1951, p. 430). Since illness constitutes a 'cost' to society it must be kept in check; 'it is clear that there is a functional interest of the society in its control, broadly in the minimization of illness' (p. 430). It is in this context that Parsons's definition of health, along with his definition of the sick role, is developed (see page 196). Medical practice is the mechanism whereby the system copes with the illness of its members. Illness in this sense is deviance.

Twaddle (1974), following Parsons, argues that health and illness are normatively defined, constituting standards of adequacy relative to capacities, feeling states and biological functioning needed for the performance of activities expected of members of society, expectation which may vary by sex and age. He opposes 'perfect health' to 'death', an opposition which seems logically problematic. To oppose health – even the unattainable ideal 'perfect health' – to illness, disease or suffering seems more logical. Death is not an ideal concept, it is the final transition from life and, through the process of dying, is opposed to living. A life may be more or less healthy in its living. The normal are not always healthy, since at least some morbid episodes may be expected, and all at last will die.

There is an implication in conceiving of health as functional fitness in Parsonian terms, or indeed in the terms proposed by Sokolowska, Ostrowska and Titkow (1975). If the aim of the health service and of other health maintenance activities is to produce a healthy workforce, then there is an allied danger that all those who cannot work or who are no longer fit for work, the physically disabled, the mentally handicapped, the chronically mentally ill, the elderly, will be devalued, and health services for them will be devalued. There is little space here for the concept of health as welfare, which is at the basis of the WHO definition.

Parsons was not critical of the medical system in North America as he researched and analysed it in mid-century. He saw it as functional for the maintenance of the society, a society of which he made no radical criticism. Others, such as Berg (1975), while arguing for a definition of health as functional fitness, and in this way avoiding the grosser difficulties of attempting to define health as an abstract good, are led from this to criticisms of modern medical practice. Thus Berg proceeds to criticize contemporary medicine for the way in which concentration on disease inevitably leads to fragmentation. He argues for a holistic approach. This, as we saw, is something which general practitioners are attempting to move towards (see page 166). It is also a facet of some alternative therapies, although it is certainly a mistake to imagine that all alternatives take a holistic approach (see Chapter 11 and also Salmon, 1984a; West, 1984).

Illness or Disease?

We have noted that what is measured to assess the effectiveness of treatments or health policies is disease rather than health; it is also disease rather than illness. This is a distinction which can be readily made in the English language. We learned (page 145) that Blaxter's (1983) Scottish respondents made a clear distinction for themselves. The distinction cannot be made in all languages, however. Polish is one example (Sokolowska, Ostrowska and Titkow, 1975).

In the sociological literature illness and disease are commonly distinguished as follows. Illness is the subjective state which is experienced by an individual, a feeling of ill-being. Disease is a pathological condition recognized by indications agreed among biomedical practitioners (cf. Field, 1976, p. 334; Helman, 1981, p. 548; Unschuld, 1986, pp. 51 ff.).

The pathological condition is indicated by a set of signs and symptoms. Illness has to do with how a person feels and how s/he responds to that. It is possible to be diseased without feeling ill. This conceptualization leads to the notion of screening programmes, the examination of the apparently well for the signs of disease, the covert cancer, for example. It is also possible to be ill without having an identifiable disease. Furthermore, a person may experience a condition which is recognized as pathological in one healing system but not in biomedicine. *Mal ojo* (evil eye) or *susto* (a sort of terror) in Spanish America are examples (Saunders, 1954). We have already seen that what lay people in Europe or America experience as illness may go beyond biomedical conceptualization.

Blaxter (1987a, p. 5) adds a third dimension. She accepts that, if 'disease' is defined as biological or clinically identified abnormality and illness as the subjective experiences of symptoms of ill-health, 'then it is obviously possible to have disease without illness and to have illness without disease'. She goes on

> The functional consequences of disease or illness usually distinguished by being called 'sickness' are a third dimension, measured by altering one's life style, being absent from work, retiring to bed, consulting a doctor and so on.
>
> (Blaxter, 1987a, p. 5)

Locker (1981) objects to the dichotomy between illness and disease used in this manner. He uses instead the notion of disorder. What people experience is disorder. They then have to decide what to do about it, whether it is an 'illness' and if so whether it is one they should take to the doctor, who may or may not decide that a disease is present.

In biomedicine, deriving from the division between psyche and soma, feelings of illness without apparent disease are often thought to be 'in the mind'; mental problems are felt as physical discomfort, that is, they are somatized. From time to time biomedicine finds a way of fitting lay experiences of disorder or illness into the disease model after all; that is, a pathological condition, a disease, which accounts for hitherto unexplained feelings of ill-being is found. A senior medic once described to me his relief when the diagnosis of 'slipped disc' began to be used. Now he and other sufferers knew that there was 'really' something the matter with them; previously he had had no diagnosable disease and he felt the status of his suffering to be in question. Now more specific treatment could be attempted, although with what limited success and short-lasting effectiveness in some cases those who suffer from slipped disc will be aware. He was comforted simply by the recognition that there was an empirically understood basis for his condition. 'Reality' in the biomedical mode lies in the material, not the mental.

SUCCESSES AND LIMITATIONS OF BIOMEDICINE TODAY

There is no doubt that biomedicine, like the sciences from which it developed, has achieved a great deal in the last half-century. The model is a powerful one, as the dawn of the space age bears witness. In medicine, many people have had their suffering relieved by chemotherapy or by surgery. In part it has been the very success of clinical medicine which has led to challenges to it and the 'generalization of doubt'. Being so successful in some arenas, being falsely attributed with health improvements which had their origins elsewhere, notably in improved socioeconomic conditions, more came to be expected of biomedicine than it was able to offer. At the same time, in the heroics of transplants, replacements, pacemakers and the like it has made great claims. There are, however, limitations to modern clinical medicine which come from the limitations imposed by its conceptual framework as well as from its mode of organization.

Challenges have been presented to biomedicine from within and without. We have discussed the challenge from epidemiology and the attempts of general practice to extend the compass of medicine. Among other challenges from within have been those to psychiatry from practitioners such as Laing (1968),

Laing and Esterson (1973) and Szasz (1961), which Busfield (1986) and Pearson (1975) discuss. Others, of whom Navarro, himself medically qualified, is an outstanding example, have challenged the individualism of clinical biomedicine and its involvement with profit-making capitalism and imperialism (1978, 1979 and 1982).

A major critic from outside the profession, Ivan Illich (1975, 1976 and 1984), writes from a particular moral stance (he trained as a priest) which stresses the virtue of responsibility for self and group members. He upbraids medicine for making us all dependent on professionals and unable to handle pain and suffering. Illich argues that, so far from healing, biomedicine is iatrogenic; that is, it creates illness. Readers will be familiar with the terrible damage done by the thalidomide drugs and the many risks that surgery inevitably involves, hazards of brain damage from misapplied anaesthesia and so on (see pages 215–6 and 224–5 for a discussion of drug hazards). For Illich health is a process of adaptation which includes responsibility; it is a task, not a physiological balance. He distinguishes three forms of iatrogenesis: clinical, social and structural or cultural. Clinical iatrogenesis

comprises only illness which would not have come about unless sound and professionally recommended treatment had been applied ... In a more general and more widely accepted sense, clinical iatrogenic disease comprises all clinical conditions for which remedies, physicians or hospitals are the pathogens or 'sickening' agents.

(1975, p. 22)

Social iatrogenesis relates to the medicalization of life, the continual reinforcing of the tendency for people to become patients, an expropriation of health. Structural (1975) or later (1976) cultural iatrogenesis 'is the ultimate backlash of hygienic progress and consists in the paralysis of health responses to suffering' (1975, p. 27). Much of the evidence Illich uses was collected by biomedics wishing to improve their understanding and their practice and by sociologists wishing to add a further dimension to the healing arts, a dimension which would help them to meet patients' problems better.

Another challenge, which also used a great deal of data similarly collected (but initially at least with less acknowledgement) came from a lawyer. Ian Kennedy (1983) 'unmasked medicine' in the Reith Lectures of 1980 in the sense that he wanted to demystify it and to reach a new relationship between doctor and patient, one in which patients should take responsibility for their lives. He also argued for an increase in the accountability of doctors and a greater respect developed between doctor and patient.

His challenge is more to the organization of the profession of medicine and its methods of health-care delivery than to its conceptual foundations – to the passivity which medicine has expected from patients. While this passivity has derived in part from the mystification used by the occupation to protect practice, it has also derived from the concepts which underlie biomedical science. The scientific mode objectifies the material it is studying. The scientist examines, analyses and concludes what the substance is or the processes are. The application of these ideas to the practice of biomedicine encourages the passivity of the patient, for the scientist knows; the patient, not being a scientist, does not know. In addition, the scientist is apt to treat the patient as an object, again encouraging passivity.

The medical practitioner, however, has always insisted that medicine is art as well as science. We have also seen (Chapter 10) that the patient has her/his own mode of ordering ideas about health and illness, life and death, and in this context is an actor in the health-care system, not simply a passive recipient of care. In these ways concepts lead to practice, a practice which, like the concepts, is socially constructed.

One of the most searching challenges which biomedicine received in the 1970s came from feminism. As well as complaining that they were not getting the care they required from biomedicine, feminists also argued that biomedicine was actively involved in sustaining a male-dominated gender order. These were partly questions of the organization of health-care delivery. They were also questions about the nature of medical knowledge (see, for example, B. and J. Ehrenreich, 1978). Differences between lay and professional views – for example, those described by Graham and Oakley (1981 and 1986), where pregnant women and their obstetricians have quite different notions of what childbirth is all about — are also differences between women and men. The mode of science is claimed to be a masculine mode (Rose, 1982, 1983 and 1987) and to deny the knowledge which women have of the world of health and healing, a knowledge constructed and transmitted in an alternative but viable mode. In earlier chapters we have noted the exclusively male public domain and the secondary role accorded to women in healing. The different perceptions which medical men have had of women and men as to their strengths and weaknesses appear to have had as much to do with the gender order of society as with the different biological constitution of the sexes. Some of these issues we shall return to in Chapter 17.

BEYOND BIOMEDICINE?

There is a question as to whether, in consequence of these challenges and the changes in the biological base and hence in the healing work that is to be done, there will be a major paradigm shift in biomedicine. A proposal from within advocating what appears to be a major paradigm shift comes from Arthur Kleinman, a psychiatrist and medical anthropologist (for example, 1980, but see also 1986). He proposes an integration between the biomedical framework and the ethnomedical framework (i.e. our understanding of the healing systems of other cultures and of lay people). This integration 'would reshape the medical model to include social and cultural questions and methods and would radically alter the program of health sciences and the professions that carry it out' (1980, p. 382). Kleinman distinguishes clinical sciences, i.e. those which relate to the hands-on practice of biomedicine, from biomedical sciences, arguing that the former are as much social as biological. He poses various alternatives for the future, but in the end what he proposes is the co-option of the social sciences (which should keep their own paradigm separate from biomedicine). Medical anthropology would be a social science in medicine, distinct from biomedical science yet an integral part of clinical science (p. 380). His proposal is not to co-opt the social science understanding of healing to biomedicine, but to clinical medicine. (He correctly indicates that the phrase 'healing' is threatening to biomedicine: p. 312.) By abandoning the biomedical paradigm, the (biomedical) clinicians will remain dominant. Otherwise these clinicians may be abandoned in favour of other healers for failing to handle the problems which people experience.

Kleinman's visionary propositions can properly be understood only in the light of the dominance of biomedicine in contemporary society and of the way medical leaders may move to respond to the challenges from within and without. His proposals are to strengthen the clinical-professional sector, as I understand it, even at the expense of biomedicine as presently understood. He himself has indicated that about 80 per cent of healing happens outside the professional sector, but he does not appear to propose anything which would strengthen either the lay ('popular' in his terms) sector or healers from other modalities (his 'folk' sector).

Another possibility is that contact or conflict with a quite different healing modality will lead to the emergence of a radically revised healing system. For example, will Chinese attempts to develop new healing knowledge and practice based both on traditional Chinese medicine and on biomedicine present problems only soluble by such a shift? That seems a distinct possibility. In that case the knowledge base of the new healing mode would be neither that of biomedicine nor that of traditional Chinese medicine.

Or will biomedicine simply annex acupuncture and a few other procedures to itself? It certainly seems likely that biomedicine will seek to co-opt the more popular of alternative healing modes, making them subservient to biomedically trained practitioners. Those modes would then be called 'complementary' not 'alternative', as indeed the *Which?* (October 1986) report does call them. How strongly will alternative healers resist becoming complements (handmaidens?) of biomedicine? Or will they be so anxious for recognition that they will propose such an answer themselves, as the spiritual healers organized in the Confederation of Healing Organizations appear to be doing in offering themselves as a complement to medicine? That they will be divided on such an issue is suggested by the title of the umbrella group which some of them have formed: the Council for Complementary and Alternative Medicines.

Awareness of the methodological and epistemological problems of testing the efficacy of their healing modes and of individual healers within the mode seems to be variable. The Confederation of Healing Organizations were perhaps unaware of these difficulties when they offered to have their healing powers tested in a trial according to the tenets of biomedicine (*The Times*, 14 August 1985). Do they understand that there may be more than one kind of wellness which patients experience and that the disease orientation may not be the appropriate way of deciding their effectiveness? The upshot of the trial was not encouraging for the healers (*British Medical Journal*, 24 May 1986, pp. 1407–8). We have already noted (page 155) that in West Germany homoeopaths insist on having tests undertaken within their own mode and this is permitted. There are other problems; in the trials reported on pages 158–9 it was pointed out that a thoroughgoing double-blind trial of traditional Chinese medicine is not possible because the healing knowledge and understanding require that the healer assess each case; it is not a matter of simply applying a routine procedure to all patients in the trial, for within a general pattern of treatment what is offered to each patient on each occasion is tailored to their needs, as was explained (page 159).

There is also the question of how biomedicine is reacting to the increased interest in alternative medicines. There appears to be a range of response from the hostile to the respectful, summed up by a *Lancet* leader which says: 'The *Lancet*'s forays into fringe subjects such as homoeopathy and acupuncture have been described by some as courageous. Others have used less kindly adjectives' (20/27 December 1986, p. 142). Many still take the view that difficult patients are the ones who resort to alternative healers. For example, three physicians in a thoughtful and enlightened approach to irritable bowel syndrome advocated what they called a 'holistic' view. They suggested that there were three aspects to the syndrome; there might be an identifiable physical cause; the cause might be adverse life events; or, finally, the patient's personality. The first two the authors had treatments for; the third they apparently found difficult. They conclude that such patients 'will often find it more agreeable to undertake alternative forms of therapy and explanations for their symptoms' (Eastwood et al., 1987). There are those biomedical practitioners who are sympathetic and respectful towards healing traditions other than their own – for example, those in the acupuncture trials cited earlier (pages 158–9). There are those who practise either homoeopathy or acupuncture in association with their NHS practice; there are also those who themselves go to osteopaths.

The tone, however, of most leading biomedics is hostile, as reflected in the BMA report of May, 1986 (see pages 158 and 175). The hostility suggests not only what is protested as to the lack of standards and control, for example, but fear of rivals, fear of being toppled from a secure position. This seems hard to imagine for the alternative healers, who, as we have seen, have none of the privileges of 'official' medicine, nor are they embodied in the elaborate organization of the NHS. Taken together, the evidence suggests, as Berliner (1984, pp. 52–4) believes, that co-option is more likely than a paradigm shift. If the latter is to occur perhaps it could be only in China itself. Quite apart from questions of ideas and their acceptance or rejection, any possible changes in the base of medical knowledge have to take place within and around the organization of health care and the institutions which sustain it. It is to these questions and the contemporary division of labour in health care that we now turn.

13 Social Organization of Health Care and the Division of Paid Health Labour

Most health care happens at home; the most expensive health care happens in hospital. Hospitals remain the core training locale for biomedicine and for nursing. There are however a number of intermediate locales where both treatment and training take place. As Armstrong (1985) has pointed out, the modern GP surgery or health centre nowadays has been removed from the domestic domain, but its purpose is to treat patients who will follow the regime prescribed in their own homes. Alternatively they may be referred onward for specialist consultation and possible treatment in hospital. But large numbers of people treat their ailments themselves, at least in the first instance, often acquiring over-the-counter medicaments for the purpose. In the UK something like two-thirds of drugs used in people's homes are bought over the counter (Dunnell and Cartwright, 1972; Wadsworth, Butterfield and Blaney, 1971; and see the summary and discussion in Blum with Kreitman, 1981).

In the hospital, although it is changing somewhat and varies with specialty, the notion of the expert professional and the passive patient still dominates. The domination of this notion is aided by the complexity of the social organization, the elaborated division of labour and the impressive and mysterious high-technology apparatus used. In the domestic domain, folk make up their own minds, guided by their understandings of illness and its treatment, and are clearly the dominant actors. In addition and in different ways both the medical profession and the state from time to time intervene to alter the mode of patient treatment or care and its locale, either bringing into hospital what was formerly handled at home or returning home cases formerly cared for in hospital. Furthermore, some modifications are taking place in the economic base (see pages 214–5). Individuals may take their troubles privately to healers who are outside biomedicine and outside the NHS, as we saw in Chapter 11. Corporate groups may establish privately financed medical facilities, either as provident or as profit-making institutions. From the beginning of the 1980s government has encouraged these private developments and is seeking to alter the public–private mix. The greatest amount of the financial cost of health care in the UK continues to be borne out of taxation; the largest amount of health labour continues to be provided, unwaged, by people in their own homes, mostly but not exclusively women. Both these workers and the state-provided health care remain dependent on the privately organized and profit-making pharmaceutical industry.

In the following three chapters we shall try to unravel some of these issues and provide evidence for the summary statements made here. In this chapter we will look at the division of paid health labour in the late twentieth century, the locale in which the work takes place and how it is organized.

THE LOCALE OF PAID HEALTH LABOUR

Celia Davies (1979) demonstrated the extent to which British health care was hospital centred in the mid-1970s. Using data derived from government health statistics she showed the division of labour in hospital and domiciliary care respectively for the period just before the 1974 reorganization. In the hospital a relatively few qualified medical practitioners and some non-medical scientists are served by a great many nurses and ancillary workers. Outside the hospital, doctors, mostly GPs but also community physicians and clinical medical officers who work for District Health Authorities, form a much larger proportion of the paid labour force in relation to nurses and other health-care professionals. The 'ancillary work' of feeding, cleaning, clothing and caring is largely done unpaid in the home (Doyal, 1985, p. 250).

More up-to-date figures are not available in quite this way because of the integration of 'community' with hospital services. However, the determination of the general practitioners to remain independent contractors means that it is possible to separate Hospital and Community Health Services (HCHS) from Family Practitioner Services (FPS), which include not only general practice but also dentists, pharmacists and opticians. While general practitioners and dentists employ nurses and other health-care professionals, the nurses, health visitors and midwives working with people in their homes and with general practitioners are more likely to be employed by the health authority and to come under the HCHS returns. Such disaggregation as it is possible to achieve suggests that the hospital remains the hub of the health service. In 1950 the family practitioner services accounted for a third of total NHS expenditure; this had dropped to a quarter by 1965 (the year of the GPs' charter) and almost to a fifth by 1980, although it rose to nearly 23 per cent by 1983 (OHE, 1984, table 4, p. 31). Taking current and capital expenditure together, in 1980–1 at then current prices about 80 per cent was spent on hospitals.

While people treated by home nurses rose by over 80 per cent between 1971 and 1981, regular day attendances at hospitals rose by over 90 per cent, hospital out-patient attendances by about 5 per cent and hospital in-patient and day cases by about 25 per cent; at the same time the number of people health visitors visited declined by about 5 per cent (DHSS, 1983a; OHE, 1984, p. 9).

These data suggest that we must be careful about how we think of the locale of treatment. Given the high and rising costs of hospital care, there have been moves to offer people hospital treatment while they remain in their own homes. The length of in-patient stay has been reduced, day surgery has been introduced, and so have day hospitals, where patients may go daily for after-care or to avoid in-patient admission (for example, in psychiatric treatment). Taking day treatment and day surgery together, the expenditure on psychiatric day patients increased by 52 per cent between 1975–6 and 1981–2 for all other kinds of patients by 84 per cent (OHE, 1984; Social Services Committee, 1983). Nurses attending people in their own homes are in many cases attending people who formerly may have been kept in hospital longer. In some of these cases patients may still be under the direct control of a hospital consultant; in many more it is likely that the general practitioner has the medical responsibility, most probably with advice from the consultant physician or surgeon. The GP's work will be included in the figures of expenditure on family practitioner services.

The way in which labour is divided between the locales of the home and the hospital has therefore changed. The GP surgery has moved away from the domestic domain, as we have seen; hostels and halfway houses have been developed for erstwhile long-term hospital residents in the areas of mental illness, mental handicap and the elderly. Hospitals are reaching into the home. It is significant that while nursing staff have increased by 100 per cent between 1960 and 1982, and hospital doctors and dentists by 130 per cent in the same period, the number of ancillary workers has remained stable (OHE, 1984, pp. 9–10, derived from DHSS, 1983a). We should bear this in mind when we discuss unpaid health labour. It is not that the UK is any less 'hospital centred' than it formerly was; it is that the division of labour between the hospital and the world outside it and within the hospitals themselves has changed. In the hospitals about half the employees are nurses; doctors, although they have increased proportionately more than other grades, remain a small minority in terms of numbers.

So far we have looked only at those who provide professional, technical, caring and manual services. Hospitals also require managerial, administrative and clerical staffs. Notwithstanding (or perhaps because of) the reorganization of 1974, which integrated all the services except for the FPS, their numbers increased about 50 per cent between 1971 and 1981 (OHE, 1984, p. 9), that is, twice as much as the average increase in that period and higher than any other grade except the professional and technical staffs (non-medical); medical and dental staff rose about 38 per cent in the same period.

THE ORGANIZATION OF THE NHS

The successive changes in the organizational structure of the NHS itself have largely resulted from efforts on the part of government to contain rising costs and to achieve value for money. The NHS takes about 6 per cent of the gross national product, which is modest in comparison with most European countries, which run at about 8 per cent. The initial modification in structure in 1974, discussed on pages 127–8, integrated hospital and local health authority services under regional and area boards with effective management at the district level. The domiciliary services were loosely attached to this structure, the general practitioners retaining their independent contractor status. The 1982 reorganization abolished the area level, and in 1984 the Griffiths Report heralded a further stage in the application of managerialism in the health service, a managerialism which had its origins, as we have seen, in moves made way back in the 1960s.

Hierarchies of Paid Labour
All of these changes have altered the relations between categories of workers, especially those in the hospital service. At the outset of the NHS it was possible to think of a hospital as being composed of three hierarchies: medical, nursing and administrative. Of these the doctors were predominant, the nurses being there to carry out their instructions as to the patients' treatment. The admin-

istration was theoretically there to facilitate the services which these two main groups were undertaking. In practice both nurses and administrators had areas over which they had some control or at least in the latter case regulatory function. The doctors were the least trammelled in that they had the right to order whatever treatments they thought the most appropriate for their patients. The situation tended to pertain in any hospital, however financed.

Part of this arrangement was that doctors had their own beds in the hospital, to which they could admit patients, and the nursing staff was organized in wards with a sister in charge. The hospital matron, in large hospitals with a number of deputies or assistants, was in charge of the nursing service overall. The ward sister was responsible for everything which happened in her ward in terms of patient care, from the cleanliness of the ward to the medication and creature comforts of the patients. Gradually this arrangement was modified. The introduction of 'functional management' was an early change. Domestic supervisors became responsible for cleaning, laundry services were provided on an area basis, and nurses became conscious that they should not undertake 'non-nursing duties' (Central Health Services Council, 1968). The Salmon Report (Ministry of Health, 1966) led, as we have seen (page 129), to a managerial nursing structure, developing a series of managerial grades above the ward sister and replacing the hospital matron as she had been known. These grades of nursing officers extended beyond the hospitals themselves into the structure of the health authority, where nursing officers were also responsible for the control of nurses working in residential localities. The work structure of those nurses was also reorganized on lines not dissimilar to the Salmon reforms following the Mayston Committee Report (DHSS, 1969). We have already discussed (pages 129–31) the criticisms which these rearrangements attracted and some of the difficulties that were encountered.

In the same period increasing efforts had been made to involve consultants in hospital management, emerging in the Cogwheel Reports of 1966 and 1972 (DHSS, 1972a; Ministry of Health, 1966). Already the increasing complexity of modern medicine had led to many *de facto* team arrangements.

The Consensus Team

From 1974 health authorities at the level of management and planning had been run by the consensus of a team of managers. Decisions for action could be made only by agreement of the whole team. It is true that three out of six members were doctors, but the consensus mode meant that nurses were their equals at least at this level of decision-making, as were the district administrator and the treasurer. The clinically subservient role of the nurse on the ward might remain, but at least the ward nurses' bosses could dispute as equals with doctors about resource allocation and other organizational issues. The 1982 reorganization, which abolished the area level, while causing as much disruption, disarray and loss of morale among all health service workers as had the 1974 organization, did not seriously alter this pattern.

The Griffiths Reorganization

The reorganization proposed by Roy Griffiths, managing director of J. Sainsbury p.l.c., in his report of 1983 (DHSS, 1983b), on the other hand, is again altering the division of power and authority among health-care professionals, administrators and managers. The 'capitalist rationality' (Carpenter, 1977) which had inspired all health service reorganization from the 1960s, whether the government was Labour or Conservative, was now openly taken forward. There was now no disguise; the principles of business management were to be applied to the health service.

At the national level a Health Services Supervisory Board and an NHS Management Board were established, the chairman of the Management Board to be a member of the Supervisory Board, itself chaired by the Secretary of State for Health and Social Services. Secondly, accountability was increased by the 'identification' of general managers at regional, district and unit level; that is, the principle of consensus management was abolished. All professionals, including doctors, were to be accountable to these managers. It appeared that doctors were now being treated as all other health-care professionals had been treated in 1974. Furthermore, clinicians were now to be much more heavily involved in management at the unit level, i.e. the smallest units of management in a district, usually responsible for one type of service. Nurses, as a profession lost their hard-won managerial authority. They had more to lose than the doctors, for they lacked the embedded foothold in health service administration at all levels which the doctors had secured for themselves from the outset of state-provided medical care. Griffiths, in his report, made no mention at all of nurses, numerically the single largest component of the health-care labour force. A few have subsequently been appointed as district general managers. (For accounts of the effect of the Griffiths reorganization on nursing see Nursing Policy Studies Centre, 1987.)

The Griffiths reorganization implied that a health service which had been administered would now be managed. Was that really possible in the face of (1) the nature of health care (for, as I have said elsewhere, producing the elusive good health is not at all like producing a tangible industrial product: Stacey, 1976; nor can offering health services be likened to purveying goods in a supermarket) and (2) the entrenched professionalism of many health-care workers? (The situation of unionized workers is somewhat different.)

ORGANIZATIONS AND PROFESSIONS

The problems about the overall nature of the delivery of health care in so far as it involves unpaid workers will be discussed later. Here our concern must be with the division of paid labour. I have argued throughout that the organization of occupations into professions was historically specific, and that their present form and the relations between them were established in the nineteenth century and pertain to its social and economic organization and to the state of medical knowledge of the period. State intervention was also initiated to meet those conditions, particularly illness associated with poverty and with widespread infectious diseases. Is the Griffiths Report finally telling the professions that they are an outmoded form of occupational organization?

Certainly mass medicine requires organization, planning and management. It is no longer a person-to-person service. The inappropriateness of that medical credo was pointed out earlier (page 127). The rhetorics of responsibility only to the individual patient and the associated doctrine of clinical autonomy have been used to enhance and maintain the power of the medical profession.

In the 1960s and 1970s the debate was one about bureaucratic versus professional power (Davies, 1972). Then the professions were not challenged as such. Now the debate has moved to one between professions and management. To understand the latter, perhaps we should first summarize the former. Formerly, professionals everywhere where mass medicine was developing, and perhaps particularly in the NHS, were complaining about bureaucratic control of their activities. Yet the evidence was that professionals, and especially doctors, could be, and were, quite powerful in health organizations.

Concerning private US health care, Freidson (1970a and 1970b) drew attention to professional dominance and advocated administrative control to curb this (1970b, pp. 181–3 and 211). Rue Bucher and Joan Stelling (1969) identified the role creativity which is possible for hospital doctors and suggested that hospitals were 'professional organizations' rather than bureaucracies. Celia Davies (1971) argued that the notion that professionals were stifled by bureaucracy was credible only because researchers had not paid attention to the power exercised by professions in organizations. Stephen Green (1974) examined empirically the alleged conflict between bureaucracy and professionals in three Scottish hospitals. He concluded that where there was conflict it was generated by differences among medical professionals (for example, university doctors versus NHS doctors, surgeons versus physicians) rather than by bureaucrats seeking to impose their views. Given a conflict among professionals, the administrators had to come down on one side or the other.

In many ways the professional-versus-bureaucrat debates of the 1970s distracted sociologists from underlying issues. It is important to see what may underlie the profession-versus-management debates of the 1980s. These have to do with issues in the health-care division of labour.

CHALLENGES TO THE ESTABLISHED DIVISION OF LABOUR

Developments in medical knowledge, advances in technology and the conditions which pertain in advanced capitalist societies have all been involved in the increased number of divisions in health labour. Specialisms and sub-specialisms have burgeoned in the last forty years, as have the number and range of non-medical workers, scientists and technicians – workers in the paramedical professions (the professions supplementary to medicine) upon all of whom doctors rely. None of these developments is peculiar to the NHS, but the form they take may be affected by it and its political and economic context.

To suggest that sociologists may have been decoyed into an inter-occupational debate is not to say there was no challenge to doctors' freedom and status from administration and now from management or from other occupations and professions in the NHS. This was inevitably the case from the moment doctors went into partnership with the state and third parties were involved in the doctor–patient relationship (see also Gill and Horobin, 1972). As Larkin (1983, p. 184) reminds us, 'The medical profession has never controlled the evolution of the division of labour independently of the state, or attained an authority which has not been delegated to it.' Furthermore, latterly the state has helped to enhance the status of paramedical and non-medical occupations associated with health care. This represents a considerable change of tack from 1946, when Aneurin Bevan said: 'It is obvious that the [health] auxiliaries must remain under the supervision and tutelage of the general medical profession. Only in that way can we ensure that the craft is kept in proper order' (quoted in Armstrong, 1976, p. 157).

However, by 1960 all the paramedical professions had achieved state registration (the opticians through the 1958 Act, and the remainder through the Professions Supplementary to Medicine Act 1960). The Seebohm reorganization, following the report of 1968, had already established Social Services Departments in local authorities with considerable budgets and power. Social work had become a profession clearly distinct from medicine and, nominally at least, equal to it. The equality of nurses at the managerial and planning level in health authorities was added to that from 1974. It would seem there was government encouragement to challenge or reduce, if not to end, the dominance of medicine and that the discontents of the subservient professions were being used to this end. In 1973 the ancillary workers had defiantly struck, ceasing to obey doctors' orders.

THE END OF MEDICAL HEGEMONY?

These events led some to suppose that an 'end to medical hegemony' was on the way. David Armstrong (1976) was one such, but see also Alaszewski (1977) and Baer (1981).

Armstrong came to his conclusion after examining a whole series of reports. They include those dealing with medical auxiliaries (HMSO, 1951a), social workers (HMSO, 1951b and 1959a), opticians (HMSO, 1952), district nurses (HMSO, 1955), health visitors (HMSO, 1956), midwives (HMSO, 1949, 1959b and 1970a), technicians and scientists (HMSO, 1968a), pharmacists (HMSO, 1970b), nurses (HMSO, 1968b and 1972) and physiotherapists (HMSO, 1973). He shows how throughout this period these professions became more self-conscious, extended their knowledge base and attempted to extend their control of their work situation. He concludes that 'state intervention in ensuring the provision of a "comprehensive health service" has also served to sponsor "professional mobility" among the paramedical groups' (1976, p. 162).

Those who foresee the end of medical hegemony appear not to have taken account of all the evidence, nor have they, as both Larkin (1983) and Øvretveit (1985) point out, sufficiently disaggregated concepts such as medical domination and professional autonomy. Armstrong, for example, fails to point out that not all the changes have gone against the doctors. He refers to midwives, but he does not discuss the way in which developments in obstetric practice and the associated changes in the locus of childbirth from home to hospital have effectively demoted the midwife from an independent professional to an obstetric nurse. The outcome of this struggle also demoted the general practitioner, who formerly did a good deal of obstetric work, as we will see (pages 239–40), in favour of the specialist obstetrician.

Gerald Larkin's (1983) careful historical analysis of the relations between medicine and the four occupations of ophthalmic optician, radiographer, physiotherapist and chiropodist from their origins until 1960 when all had state registration led him to modify the notion of medical dominance or medical hegemony. Pointing out that power and immediate responsibility must be distinguished, he argues persuasively that the recognition of paramedical skills does not necessarily imply that medical hegemony is changing. Boundaries may be redrawn without equalizing all the parties. Distinguishing occupations whose power is constructed around a few tasks from those who are agents of the division of work itself, he agrees with Freidson's (1970a) description of medicine as belonging to the latter category. Paramedical occupations, on the other hand, are of the former sort; they consequently can negotiate about, but cannot define, the boundaries of their competence.

The Nature of Medical Domination

So far from any boundary redrawing consequent upon negotiation challenging the whole system of medical domination, 'Collective upward mobility for one or several groups does not in itself alter but rather exemplifies the organizing principles of the division of labour' (Larkin, 1983, p. 184). That the state has supported these paramedical occupations to the extent of agreeing to their registration does not necessarily mean that medical hegemony is ceasing, for medical dominance may still continue. Furthermore, 'a medically imposed division of labour may survive an apparent diminution of the direct powers of doctors over it' (p. 184). To understand whether medicine will continue to dominate we need to pay attention to the nature of that domination and the challenges to it.

Gerald Larkin is in disagreement with Eliot Freidson (1977) about the nature of medical dominance. He does not dispute the continued dominance itself. He argues that Freidson is *describing dominance* rather than *analysing control*. The distinction is important to an understanding of the nature of dominance and the relations between medical and paramedical workers. While paramedical workers have wrested some control from doctors in the division of labour, they have not been able to challenge their dominance (Larkin, 1983, p. 190). Indeed, they did not intend to do that. They, like the doctors, were seeking for an occupational monopoly in their sphere of competence. In this sense medics and paramedics are similar in their tactics. What the paramedics did was set out 'to negotiate role boundaries with a senior and more powerful partner' (p. 191). They were not seeking domination in Freidson's terms, whose analysis is liable to demean paramedical strategies.

The Nature of Autonomy

Øvretveit (1985) also has disagreements with Freidson (1970b). In Øvretveit's case the grounds are that Freidson's structural analysis 'gives rise to an all-or-none conception of autonomy where other health occupations can never achieve the "true autonomy" of medicine' (p. 77). Øvretveit points out, following work at Brunel University (Rowbottom, 1978; Tolliday, 1978), that different amounts of autonomy in different aspects of work may be achieved by occupations at different times and in various circumstances. Looking at physiotherapy, he concludes that

a number of aspects of professional autonomy have been gained which correspond to a decline in complementary forms of medical dominance.

However, there is no evidence that [this] ... is either associated with, or a result of, an overall decline in medical dominance.

(p. 90)

In this context we can perhaps see more clearly the dilemma facing proponents of alternative healing systems and modalities which we discussed in Chapter 11. Are they to go for a defined and protected place within the medical division of labour or should they maintain the total separateness of knowledge and therapy systems? The answer may be different for each, depending on their goals.

Healers who wished to be accepted as complementary to biomedicine were mentioned in Chapters 11 and 12. They appear to be an example of an occupational group which wants a place in the biomedical division of labour; they do not propose to challenge that order. This can be seen from the willingness to accept trials within the biomedical epistemology, although some at least of them would appear to have healing 'powers' more like those reported for the sixteenth and seventeenth centuries.

INCREASING THE DIVISION OF LABOUR IN GENERAL PRACTICE

It is not only in the hospital that the division of biomedical labour has increased. We noted in Chapter 12 the moves made by general practitioners to claim specialist status, a specialism based on their very generality (page 166). As Jefferys and Sachs (1983) show, this development went along with an elaboration of the division of labour in general practice and changes in general practitioner's working arrangements. Evidence nationally shows that in this period, led by the Royal College of General Practitioners, GPs moved away from single-handed practice to two-person partnerships and then into group practices (see Figure 13.1).

The Jefferys–Sachs analysis relates to a particular group of practices in the London area which moved into a health centre during their study. Their description and analysis of the increasing division of labour in which the GPs were involved is of particular interest. The study carefully documents GPs' relationships with nurses, health visitors, geriatric visitors, social workers, receptionists and administrative and clerical staff. In these practices the days when the GP's wife acted as receptionist, chaperon, nurse, accountant and general surgery factotum (in addition to her role as wife, housekeeper, houseworker and mother) have gone. However, the majority of the supportive people working with the GPs are women. Nurses, health visitors, receptionists, all clearly employees and not partners, tend to be women, playing a typically 'handmaiden' role, whatever their personal marital status may be.

Other evidence shows that there are still few women principals in general practice. It seems that many partnerships carefully control their number to one woman in a partnership of five or six men; others employ women doctors, often part-time, rather than taking them into partnership.

THE HEALTH-CARE TEAM

In general practice, in acute hospital work, in the care of the mentally handicapped, indeed throughout contemporary medicine, the concept of the

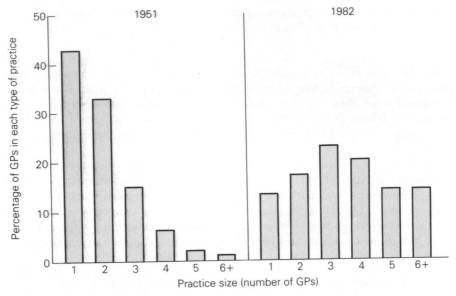

Source: Office of Health Economics (OHE), 1984, p. 31.

Figure 13.1   *Proportions of family doctors working in practices of various sizes, 1951 and 1982.*

team has emerged. It has been evoked as a principle around which the co-operation of many occupations can be organized. When discussed in terms of the delivery of care to the patient, 'team' has a cosy connotation, rather like 'community' in another context (cf. Stacey, 1969) and, upon inspection, at least as woolly (Evers, 1981b and 1982). Having begun to understand the messages that health and ill health are multifaceted and involve areas of human life beyond the narrowly biomedical, doctors have been anxious to involve an array of experts from other disciplines in their work. They have also been anxious to pass on the 'dirty work' (Hughes, 1971) to others so that they may themselves do the more prestigious and less menial tasks. The development of team-work has not been without its difficulties for them, however.

The British Medical Association in its evidence to the Royal Commission (BMA, 1977) made it plain that it wishes to continue team-work (paras. 3.7–3.10). It is happy about teams so long as the general practitioner is in full charge, but other team members in some cases dispute what this means. Hospital teams also worry the BMA. The General Medical Council (GMC) added its authority to the BMA point of view, but perhaps with greater subtlety, taking the line of *primus inter pares*:

Doctors must be educated in the implications of their clinical decisions for members of the other professions, and the doctor must exercise his overall responsibility for the patient as a leader of the team and not as an autocrat. Nevertheless ... the leadership of the health team in general practice must continue to rest with the doctor in charge of the patient and not with other professions or administrators.   (GMC, 1977, para. 39)

Not all doctors agree with this point of view, and some are experimenting in a reordering of the division of labour. In a child assessment centre where the author has researched, the doctor does not assume he should be the team leader or chairperson of the multi-disciplinary meeting which makes the final assessment of the patients (Stacey, 1980, reports some aspects of this study). This is not an isolated case. Indeed, the BMA drew particular attention to its anxiety about the loss of medical control in paediatrics and psychiatry (BMA, 1977, para. 3.9).

PROFESSIONS WHICH CLAIM EQUALITY WITH MEDICINE

It is important to make a distinction, one which Larkin (1983) does not stress, between those professions and occupations which are happy to have a defined place in the medical division of labour (even if they would like it to be bigger or higher) and those whose claim is to work beside medicine on other aspects of the patient's well-being. Social work is one such. We noted that in addition to concepts of health as total physical and mental well-being, of health as functional fitness, there was a notion of health as welfare. Such a model stresses the importance of human beings whatever their productive capacity may be and lays emphasis on the importance of caring. Social work, while not disputing the value of biomedicine in controlling or ameliorating disease, is based upon a largely different body of knowledge and is not prepared to take a subordinate position in the biomedical division of labour.

The social work view of ill-being includes social, economic and psychological factors which not only cause suffering in themselves but may impede the healing of biologically caused ailments. Social workers therefore believe they can contribute to patient cure and care in ways which biomedics are not trained to understand. They claim parity of ability with biomedics in aiding the general welfare of human beings. They are not prepared to accept biomedicine as a senior partner in the sense that Larkin (1983) suggests paramedics are prepared to do.

However, the way in which all this works out in practice may be somewhat problematic. Dingwall, Eekelaar and Murray (1983) have shown what difficulties may arise between the health and social workers caring for children at risk of abuse. Not only different concepts of health and welfare but the different organizational structure of the health and social services may conspire to fail to protect such children.

Psychologists are another occupational group who, while respecting medicine, claim independence and parity of status. However, in practice, these claims may not be seen to be accorded. Here the distinction between group and individual autonomy which Øvretveit (1985) has made is helpful. The occupational organizations of these workers may have negotiated parity with biomedics. The space which is accorded to them as workers in the treatment situation may lack that parity. In a psychiatric NHS hospital Goldie (1977) found that at the level of the individual practitioner, social worker, or psychologist, we are more likely to see accommodation to the status quo of medical domination associated with an endeavour by social workers and psychologists to gain acceptance from particular psychiatrists (p. 158).

	Men	Women
Medical practitioners	£406	n.s.
Nursing administrators and executives	£199	£170
Registered and enrolled nurses and midwives	£148	£128
Nursing auxiliaries and assistants	n.s.	£102
Average for Non-manual III*	£221	£155
Ambulance men	£166	n.s.
Hospital porters	£124	n.s.
Hospital ward orderlies	n.s.	£104
Average for Manual X*	£130	£94

n.s. = not sampled. * Occupational class.
Source: Department of Employment, 1986, pt D, tables 86 and 87.

Figure 13.2   *Health workers in full-time employment: average gross weekly earnings, 1985–6.*

HEALTH OCCUPATIONS AND PROFESSIONS IN THE CLASS STRUCTURE

So far we have been looking at the division of health labour almost as if it existed in a vacuum. This is of course not the case. Now as hitherto the stratification system which exists in health care, both public and private, is part of and also helps to sustain the class system as a whole. There are particular questions, such as those we have explored about the boundaries between occupations and relative competences, which are specific to health care. Many of the skills involved are also specific to health care and not readily transportable. Others, however, are common to a much wider range of industries – portering, catering, cleaning, managing, administering, for example.

The differentials in pay are large. It is not easy to get a complete picture, but Figure 13.2, which is derived from the Department of Employment (1986) sample survey of earnings, illustrates the differences. Thus medical practitioners earn on average more than twice as much as nursing administrators and executives. In their turn this group earn a quarter as much again as registered and enrolled nurses and midwives, and about twice as much as nursing auxiliaries, whose earnings are similar to those of ward orderlies. The gender differences are obvious too, women earning consistently less than men even in the traditional female occupations. The continued sex segregation of many health occupations presumably accounts for the failure to include the same occupations in the male and female samples.

Figure 13.2 conceals the big differences between the top and bottom of the medical profession; these differences are justified, but not to the satisfaction of the junior hospital doctors, by the definition of the latter as being in 'training grades'. Thus in 1985–6 a consultant was earning between £21,460 and £27,700, a senior registrar between £12,380 and £15,630, a registrar from £10,760 to £13,030, while a house officer received £7,610 to £8,590, that is, about a third of a consultant's salary (*Guardian*, 23 May 1986).

Figure 13.2 shows the striking differentials between fully qualified doctors and nurses and, even more, between the former and ancillary workers. Furthermore, Figure 13.2 gives the average earnings of all workers in the relevant occupational class so that some comparison can be made with workers in other industries.

The big differentials also cumulate in terms of pay increases. For example, when the government in 1986 agreed to pay increases of effectively 5.9 per cent for nurses and 5.7 per cent for doctors and dentists, the annual improvement in the pay of the latter was much greater than in that of the former. Thus the lowest paid nursing group, nursing cadets, got an increase of £200 a year to £3,880, while staff nurses gained about £455 p.a., making their salaries £6,225. Consultants, on the other hand, had *increases* of £2,000 to £3,000 a year. Top-grade consultants with the highest merit awards will have salaries of £56,000. The health service is clearly highly stratified, as is British society as a whole.

There has been a good deal of discussion as to what if any is the relationship of the professions to the class structure. In so far as professions are occupations which make special claims about their place in the division of labour (which may or may not be recognized in whole or in part), the relationship of health-care occupations to the class structure can be analysed in similar ways to any other occupations. Some structural analysts of the professions (for example, Freidson, 1970b and 1977) who take a similar view of professions nevertheless work without a concept of the class structure. For them the problem is entirely inter-occupational. For those who, like myself, find concepts of social class critical to contemporary social analysis, health care raises problems in an acute form, as indeed does the entire tertiary sector. The central feature of 'people work', which is so characteristic of health-care work, means that what is produced is unclear, as are what the means of production are and also what might be the relations of all those involved.

The alliance which the medical profession made with the bourgeoisie in the nineteenth century was discussed in Chapter 6. There I suggested further that medical practitioners could probably not be considered to be all of one class. Not only are they divided between entrepreneurs and salaried, but the salaried also undertake entrepreneurial activities. It is perhaps not surprising that Navarro (1978) is somewhat contradictory in the class alignment he allocates to doctors, seeing them sometimes as upper class and sometimes as middle class, even at times allied with proletarian workers.

Some things are fairly clear, however. No part of the medical profession, despite the variation in its power, remuneration and life-style, could be called proletarian in any strict sense. On the other hand, ancillary workers – porters, cleaners and other manual workers – by virtue of their terms and conditions of work, their remuneration and their place in the division of labour are undoubtedly proletarian. There is evidence, referred to in Chapter 8, that nurses are divided between those who are members of the proletariat, for whom advancement to senior or managerial grades is not a realistic possibility, and those in managerial grades, with vastly greater remuneration, who could be definitely called middle class on account also of their working situations.

In so far as those with high skills can command high remuneration, the more economically powerful of the health-care occupations not only reflect but also help to reproduce the values of a class-divided capitalist society. Their high level of remuneration permits them to invest, to become property owners or shareholders. These opportunities are denied in any more than very modest ways to the great majority of health-care professionals. While there is upward social mobility of individuals, it is also the case that the medical profession and the higher ranks of nursing are more likely to be recruited from offspring of upper- and middle-class parents (HMSO, 1968c)

The consciousness of the lower paid, the ancillary workers in particular but also the nurses, has been raised as to their relative disadvantage over the past fifteen years, as we have seen. Their more recent attempts to improve their position have been rejected, as witness the unsuccessful strike of 1982 when ancillary workers were protesting a pay award which was only something like a third of other pay awards then current. When ancillary workers strike, their importance to health care becomes clear; the whole enterprise is seen to be reliant on them. They are not rewarded for this contribution, nevertheless. Ancillary workers, like other health-care workers, have problems in making a strike 'bite' because of their wish not to damage patients. Grigg (1979) shows in relation to their 1973 strike, and the junior hospital doctors' 1975 strike, that they share this with doctors. He suggests that their concern not to hurt fellow human beings inhibits them, as does their wish to maintain their service image. This is a further example of the way in which the values and actions, rewards and sanctions of health care are intermediary between those of the domestic and of the public domain.

In a situation in which public expenditure cuts have been applied to the NHS as to other sectors, it may be that alignments will change. However, the greater opportunity of the more powerful to do better out of the system will restrict the extent to which this is possible.

If health care is still as closely associated with the class system in the late twentieth century as it was in the nineteenth, albeit now in different ways, what of the gender order? What effect have the removal of professional barriers in 1919 and the later sex discrimination Acts had? The short answer is, not a lot.

GENDER DIVISION IN PAID LABOUR

As Doyal (1985, pp. 250–5) points out, NHS work is predominantly women's work but generally speaking it is controlled by men. About 75 per cent of NHS workers are women, but they are more often to be found in the lower occupations and in the less favoured posts within each occupation (see also Elston, 1977). Three-quarters of the ancillary workers are women; the men mostly do portering and maintenance, while women do catering and cleaning. What it is to be a maid in a hospital kitchen has been graphically described by Elizabeth Patterson (1981) including the not always hygienic solutions to the problems of the boredom and difficulty of the work which are found. Doyal's evidence indicates that not only are many of the most disadvantaged workers women, many are also foreign and many black (Doyal, Hunt and Mellor, 1981). The dominating occupations, on the other hand, remain largely male, notably the senior administration of NHS hospitals and the higher echelons of medicine.

In 1985 about 23 per cent of registered medical practitioners were women (125,390 men to 38,318 women in September 1985: Towers, 1985), but currently about half the medical students are women. Women are found disproportion-ately in the 'opportunity specialties' such as psychiatry and geriatrics where they find it easier to get appointments and promotion (as do overseas doctors, black or Asian). Women, further, tend to select specialties which they, encouraged by their male partners, feel women can combine with their domestic duties, including child rearing. We have noted their few numbers in general practice (page 185). We saw earlier how women were put into the less prestigious posts under mostly male Medical Officers of Health in the child health services (pages 111–12). It seems likely that, if, as is possible, general practitioners take over child care and surveillance from the salaried health authority service, clinical medical officers may be employed on a salary or fee basis to work for principals in general practice.

As the number of women doctors increases, it may become increasingly difficult to sustain the male domination. However, if the notion remains in society at large that there are some sorts of doctoring which are more appropriate for women because women's is the prime household and child-rearing responsibility, it seems likely that women doctors will continue to be found more often in some medical occupations than in others. They are already more likely to move into general practice than surgery. (For a woman doctor's view of medical education see Young, 1981.)

Gerald Larkin (1983), in his study of the relations between medicine and other health-care professions, does not make a particular point about the gender order in his theoretical conclusions, but he does make the sex differences plain in the cases he discusses. Historically, the problems faced by opticians and ophthalmo-logists were not those of mainly women versus mainly men; that was a case of the increasingly dominant medical profession as such seeking to contain a rival and the older occupation's counter-attack. In the case of radiographers versus radiologists, it was largely a case of the women's occupation becoming subord-inated to the male medical practitioners. Physiotherapy was from the outset largely a female occupation; the number of men remains small. In the 1920s chiropodists, who were descended from the itinerant corn cutters, were trying to refurbish their image and find a respectable place in the biomedical division of labour. Chiropodists then used an argument that theirs was a suitable occu-pation for women, since its training costs were low and the work could be done part-time. The pattern which we have found throughout of both medical domination and male domination clearly applies to the paramedical professions.

The male domination of administration remains. In 1981 the DHSS and SSRC commissioned studies to research the possibility of sex discrimination in both administration and nursing. The detailed case study undertaken by Celia Davies and Jane Rosser (1985) of a rural and a city health authority district to establish what were the processes leading to this are interesting. In both authorities, taking clerical and administrative staff together, they found a bottom-heavy structure, with men dominating the senior posts and women monopolizing the large base of junior administrative, clerical and secretarial grades (as they put it, a submarine with the women at the bottom and the men in the periscope, for there is a tall thin hierarchy of senior administrators). Upon investigation they found that although there was no widespread feeling of discrimination among the women in the lower grades, it was also not true that the women were in those grades because that was where they wanted to be. While they did not feel discriminated against, the women were more dissatisfied than the men about promotion and training prospects.

Davies and Rosser (1985) concluded that there were two hierarchies, the one numerically dominated by women and the other by men, with movement across the hierarchies very difficult to achieve. Furthermore, at the top of the lower hierarchy women classified as clerical/secretarial were doing management functions, although this was not recognized. Finally, what they call the 'golden pathway', the route taken by both women and men to the periscope, makes demands and has requirements which are based on the conventional male career which men thus find it easier to comply with than women (p. 17). What amounts to a 'hostile climate' towards women's employment and advancement exists, although not derived from prejudice or overt discrimination: 'rather the whole way of thinking and way of organizing work assumed that it was men who would fill the senior posts and that women were seen as women first and workers second' (Davies and Rosser, 1985, p. 18). This situation is essentially similar to that in the medical division of labour, at least until the present (see also Davies and Rosser, 1986; Rosser and Davies, 1984a and 1984b).

We noted in Chapter 8 that a consequence of the Salmon Report and the introduction of managerialism into nursing had led to a disproportionate increase in the number of men nurse managers. About a quarter of all posts above staff nurse are now occupied by men, while about 90 per cent of nurses are women. This had generally been thought to be associated with the image of management as men's work (Carpenter, 1977; Stacey, 1985a). However, Davies and Rosser's detailed study found *'no support at all for the notion that men were career-minded and women were not ...* Neither sex expressed great interest in the conventional nurse management career', being more interested in nursing work, patient contact and professional development (1985, p. 23, original emphasis). Some support for the 'management is men's work' hypothesis was found in that men put themselves forward for management because they felt confident to do so or because they were formally encouraged, which women were not (p. 23). As for the SEN grade, made up almost entirely of women, there was much discontent because of the almost complete lack of chances for advancement and the lack of recognition for the amount of work and responsibility they carry (Davies and Rosser, 1985, pp. 24–5).

All in all, Davies and Rosser (1985) found that there was little if any active discrimination in the health districts they studied to account for the heavy weighting of the more prestigious and better paid jobs to men. However, normative assumptions about the gender order led to an absence of policies consciously directed to equal opportunities, leading in turn to a situation in which women were systematically disadvantaged so far as upward occupational mobility was concerned. Many women wished for opportunities to move upward.

CONCLUSION

What we see, then, in the contemporary organization of health care in the public domain, is a division of paid labour which both mirrors and reproduces the class structure of society as a whole. At the same time the nature of people work, of professional–client relations, suggests that modifications are necessary in the way in which sociologists have conventionally seen the class structure. However, class analysis itself is inadequate, for the stratification of health labour also reflects and reinforces the male-dominated gender order.

The two systems, the latter deriving originally from the domestic domain and the former established in its present manner in the public domain as a consequence of the rise of industrial capitalism, are interwoven throughout the service. Both women and men are found in subservient positions; both are also found in superordinate ones. However, far more women are subordinate than men.

14 Unpaid Workers in the Division of Health Labour (1): the Patients

The theoretical and empirical grounds for thinking of potential patients, patients and their unpaid carers as health workers were laid out in Chapter 1, pages 4–7. This chapter will look at the roles which each of these categories of health workers plays, is expected or is permitted to play. It will also look at the relations between them and the paid health workers. We noted in Chapter 11 a small but not insignificant minority of people who have consulted non-biomedical healers of various kinds, either as well as or instead of practitioners on the Medical Register. In the same period there have been two other developments: first, a great deal of official encouragement to people to look after their own health and, in the case of minor acute illness, to treat themselves in the first instance at least; second, reliance on unpaid carers has increased. Policies of decarceration, i.e. the return of long-stay patients to the 'community', and of shorter hospital stays for acute episodes have led to a greater reliance on unpaid carers; so has the increasing use of volunteers both in hospitals and to help care for the ailing in their own homes.

In this chapter we will examine some of the issues involved, looking first at the potential patient and her/his work in keeping well; second at the sick who do not adopt the sick role (Parsons, 1951; and see pages 196–7) but care for themselves in a morbid episode with or without the help of others, making mention also of self-help groups in this context; third, we will look at patients who have adopted the sick role and are being treated within the biomedical division of labour. In the following chapter we will turn to the unpaid carers.

POTENTIAL PATIENTS

As we saw (pages 4–6), everybody every day undertakes (more or less well) work to maintain their health. Generally speaking this is something which everyone does (and mothers do for children) without thinking much about it. It is routine, although as we saw in Chapter 10 people are aware that there are some things they 'ought' to do to keep fit, ward off damp, colds and draughts, for example. They also believe that some things 'just happen' and cannot be prevented. The 'health cult' has increased the amount of work Chicagoans feel they should put in (see pages 148–9).

Prevention and Health, Everybody's Business (DHSS, 1976a), was published in 1976 by a Labour government (DHSS, 1976a). Its publication was associated with another document, *Priorities for Health and Personal Social Services* (DHSS, 1976b), which talked about 'reallocation of resource priorities' rather than 'public expenditure cuts' because it 'sounds much nicer' (BBC commentator, 1977, quoted Radical Statistics Health Group, 1978, p. 367). *Prevention and*

Health sought to show that specific preventive measures have been the most important causes of disease reduction. In a sense it follows the arguments of Thomas McKeown, discussed in Chapter 9, in so far as the argument is that prevention is better than cure and that the health of the people has been improved more by the preventive measures taken than by the curative activities of clinical biomedicine. While acknowledging the importance of personal hygiene and family limitation, McKeown judged that most of the reasons for the nineteenth-century fall in death rates were associated with collective action of some sort: improved food supply, clean air, water and proper sewerage disposal. *Prevention and Health*, on the other hand, stresses that 'the prime responsibility for his [*sic*] own health falls on the individual' (DHSS, 1976b, pp. 62–3).

In Chapter 9, pages 134–7, we saw how the evidence which the DHSS produced to demonstrate how important immunization programmes have been in the prevention of such infections is disputed by the Radical Statistics Health Group (1976 and 1978). The Group argues that using the log scale rather than the linear scale exaggerates the importance of the immunization programmes. There is a consequent lack of attention to the collective preventive measures which led to the decline, and heavy stress is placed on individual responsibility.

Individuals not only have to take up immunization, they must adopt healthier life-styles, stop smoking, eat healthily but not too much, nor drink too much, not drive carelessly, but take exercise and keep fit. Attention is not paid to those factors which prevent people from living a healthy life-style, as the Radical Statistics Health Group (1976 and 1978) points out. It has to be said that the conclusion to which government came is consistent with a major conclusion of Thomas McKeown himself, who feels that preventive measures are of a different nature in the late twentieth century compared with the nineteenth century. Having reviewed the causes of disease as reported in Chapter 9, he says:

> the requirements for health can be stated simply. Those fortunate enough to be born free of significant congenital disease or disability will remain well if three basic needs are met: they must be adequately fed; they must be protected from a wide range of hazards in the environment; and they must not depart radically from the pattern of personal behaviour under which man evolved, for example by smoking, overeating or sedentary living.
>
> (McKeown, 1976, p. 100)

The Radical Statistics Group complains that insufficient attention was paid in the *Priorities for Health* document to the first two and perhaps especially the second. The Group is not alone in this. It is, as we saw in Chapter 9, also the view which the Black Committee (DHSS, 1980) took (Townsend and Davidson, 1982). Drawing attention to continuing inequalities between social classes, the Committee concluded that these derived from differential material conditions which individuals alone were powerless to redress.

The Black Committee therefore recommended a radical programme to reduce these health inequalities which included measures inside as well as outside the health service (such as measures to eradicate child poverty). The Committee had been appointed by a Labour government (the same that was responsible for the 1976 *Prevention* and *Priorities* documents) but by the time it reported the government had fallen. The Conservative administration was not prepared to undertake the public expenditure which would have been involved in implementing the Black recommendations. The tendency to concentrate on 'life-styles' and health education as ways of improving the national health, to blame the victim (Crawford, 1977), has continued.

The implication is that ordinary people are health workers, indeed that they have a moral responsibility to look after their own health. Governments have increasingly encouraged and cajoled the population to this end. However, ordinary people are not referred to as health workers and are rarely praised for their efforts. There is dispute as to how free people are to do good health work because of constraints on their income (perhaps they have fallen into the 'poverty trap' as increasing numbers now do because of mass and long-term unemployment); constraints too are imposed by the built environment – houses, roads, vehicles, factories. Women as unpaid health workers have particular difficulty in guarding their own health, as we shall see (pages 206–8).

ILLNESS BEHAVIOUR

We may use the term 'health behaviour' for those activities which people undertake to try to maintain their health. 'Illness behaviour', on the other hand, is what people do when they feel unwell; in Parsons's view, except in cases of transitory ailments, they should then adopt the 'sick role'. For Parsons (1951, pp. 436–7) the sick role involves the following four characteristics:

(1)   exemption from normal social responsibilities;
(2)   the sick person cannot be expected to get well by an act of decision or will;
(3)   s/he must want to get well;
(4)   s/he must seek technically competent help.

In effect this is a typology of behaviour which might be accepted by the medical profession and the sick person in a society where a system of professional healing is available and not under strain and which the sufferer accepts and can gain access to. Specifically, while put forward as universally applicable, it relates best to mid-century US medicine as practised among the white middle class. It also relates specifically to acute illness. Freidson (1970a, ch. 11) has discussed the limitations of the notion when applied to illnesses of other kinds (see also Gallagher, 1976; Gerhardt, 1979). David Robinson (1971) has indicated some of the circumstances in which professional help may or may not be sought, showing that surrounding social circumstances may determine the outcome. Irving Zola (1966) has also shown that it is not so much the onset of an illness which leads a person to seek treatment, but some change in social circumstances which precipitates the consultation.

In practice there are a variety of choices open to people when they feel unwell. They may attempt to ignore the sensations and do nothing, aiming perhaps to 'work it off' (see, for example, Cornwell, 1984). They may consult close relatives or friends, what Freidson (1961) called the 'lay referral system'. They may approach a biomedical practitioner, in the UK most likely their general practitioner, or they may go to one of a range of alternative healers.

How people conceive of health and illness affects their illness behaviour.

Herzlich (1973) suggested from her interviews with middle-class Parisians and Normans that there were three main ways in which people thought of illness: as a liberator; as an occupation; as destructive. This conceptualization has recurred in recent work (see, for example, Pollock, 1984). Those who saw illness as destructive were active people who thought of themselves as indispensable. Such people experienced illness as intolerable and destructive. Initially denying their illness and continuing to work, when they finally had to accept that they were ill they swung to a position of total impotence.

Those who saw illness as a liberator also saw it as desocializing. But in their case they found it a pleasant and valuable experience which took them out of their normal responsibilities; they could withdraw and find themselves. However, this is possible only if others will co-operate.

The third category of illness as occupation comes up frequently in the field studies. It fits the Parsonian model in so far as the ill person must admit the illness, seek professional advice and actively co-operate in achieving the goal of recovery. The patient does not see her/himself as desocialized as both the other two categories do; many others are in similar situations. What may be the implications of this model for relationships with professionals is something we shall refer to later.

PATIENT SELF-CARE

At the outset of the NHS there was a widespread feeling that many people (perhaps deriving in part at least from the evidence in Margery Spring Rice's *Working Class Wives*, 1939) were suffering from illnesses that could be 'nipped in the bud' if they were 'caught soon enough'. This was not just a lay view but shared by many, especially general practitioners, appalled when they were not called in until a disease was far advanced. Initially when health care became free at the point of delivery people were encouraged to take any illness to the doctor in good time. All too soon general practitioners found themselves overwhelmed with consultations and rapidly began to label a great many of the conditions they were presented with as 'trivia' (Cartwright, 1967). Encouragement to 'come early' seemed to be replaced by the message 'don't bother your doctor unless it's serious'. (What's serious? Who can tell but the doctor?) The confusion about viruses and bacteria referred to earlier led people to consult in flu epidemics, resulting in broadcast messages on behalf of overworked doctors to 'go to bed, take aspirin and nurse yourself'. Nevertheless, doctors' complaints about people who do not come soon enough, 'the problem of patient delay' (Murcott, 1981 pp. 130–3), continue. These seem more often to come from hospital consultants than GPs. Murcott sees these complaints as a way of handling day-to-day treatment problems, removing the problem from doctor to patient.

Alongside the alleged excess consultation by patients with 'trivia' there also exists the 'symptom iceberg' (Hannay, 1979). Studies for many years have shown that the population that does not consult is in medical terms and in terms of its own reported symptoms not much different from the population that does consult (e.g. Last, 1963; Wadsworth, Butterfield and Blaney, 1971). David Hannay's (1979) study of a population in Glasgow found that 86 per cent of all the respondents had physical symptoms; of those about a third consulted a professional and 10 per cent a lay person. Of all the adults who consulted professionally, 9 per cent thought their symptoms were not serious, i.e. could be called 'trivia'. Hannay called cases where professional or lay advice was sought, although the respondents did not think the syptoms severe or serious, 'incongruous'. Again using a system of symptom grading he found that 'twenty-three per cent of all subjects had at least one physical, mental or behavioural symptom for which they did not seek professional advice, although they said the pain or disability was severe, or they thought the symptom was serious' (p. 57). Proportionately most of these were physical symptoms. He calculated that the 'iceberg', i.e. symptoms which he judged should have been taken to a professional, was more than twice as large as the number of incongruous referrals (p. 58).

We do not know from Hannay's study what action those with symptoms who did not go to a professional took. Some will have treated themselves, on their own advice or that of the lay people they consulted, with medications bought over the counter from the chemist's shop. Karen Dunnell and Ann Cartwright (1972) found that self-prescribed medicines outnumbered prescribed ones by two to one (p. 22). Nearly half (and the most common) self-prescribed medicines were analgesics and antipyretics (designed to reduce fever) and ones for the digestive system; less than a fifth of prescribed medicines fell in this category (p. 27 and table 15, p. 28). As Dunnell and Cartwright point out, prescribed and non-prescribed drugs are neither mutually exclusive nor independent of each other. Buying self-prescribed drugs is an indication of self-care, however, and indicates the extent to which people experiencing symptoms do attempt to look after their own health.

In this discussion I am distinguishing self-care from self-help groups. The former are individual acts, although lay people may be consulted and, in the case of over-the-counter drugs, perhaps also the pharmacist. Fifty-seven per cent of Dunnell and Cartwright's respondents thought the chemist was a good person to ask for advice when they were not feeling well (p. 96; and also see Stimson and Webb, 1975, pp. 129–31).

SELF-HELP GROUPS

In the self-help group we can also see the patient as an active health worker. No doubt folk suffering from the same sorts of complaint have always got together to help each other (Henry and Robinson, 1979). There is, however, a good deal of attention paid to this today, and it can be seen as another example of encouragement to the patient to do more work, which has been associated both with the attempt to control costs in mass medical systems, with the increase in high-technology medicine and the associated prolongation of life and with feelings of loss of autonomy on the part of patients.

It would be incorrect, as Stuart Henry and David Robinson (1979) point out, to imagine that these are entirely lay developments divorced from biomedicine. Many are encouraged, some even started, by biomedical professionals. The Ileostomy Association, the Society for Skin Camouflage, the Possum Users' Association, for example, themselves acknowledge that their origin lay in some professional initiative. Other groups exist because off biomedical failure to handle their problem. Perhaps Alcoholics Anonymous is the best known example, but that association, while running itself and providing therapy for its members on a mutual help basis, works with and has the blessing of doctors. Indeed, there are AA groups specifically for alcoholic doctors. Self-help, in the opinion of Henry and Robinson (1979, p. 196),

> works for people whose problems are unsolvable by conventional means of transcending short-term solutions ... In self-help helping the problem is integrated with life. Rather than living everyday life and having problems, self-help group members live their everyday life through their problems, which requires them to change their everyday lives.

THE PATIENT IN THE SICK ROLE

Generally speaking patients adopt the sick role, or at least go and consult the doctor, of their own volition. However, at the outset it is well to remember that this is not always so. Young children have no choice but are taken by parent or guardian. (In the NHS young women and men at the age of 16 may consult in their own right. In practice some may consult on their own before that age.) Sometimes the elderly also are presented rather than presenting themselves; the line between encouragement to consult and coercion by concerned carers is a fine one. The mentally ill may be committed to care under the Mental Health Act. Some illnesses of sudden and severe onset, and some accidents, when the patient is unconscious for example, are also circumstances in which others will have to act on the patient's behalf. The issue of resuscitating suicides is a complex ethical one which cannot be dealt with here.

The great majority of decisions by adults to consult are taken by themselves. The consultation process itself is a rather special kind of social interaction which Gerry Stimson and Barbara Webb (1975) studied in two general practices in South Wales. They show how patients rehearse beforehand what it is they have to say, what happens in the face-to-face consultation and what the patients make of it afterwards.

They find that patients have expectations of what will happen, which include background expectations, based on general knowledge about what usually happens in GP consultations; expectations of this particular interaction, given what it is they are consulting about and what they know about the doctor; and finally they have expectations of what the doctor's actions will be, two-thirds expecting a prescription although not all necessarily wanting one. Patients who have to attend repeatedly with a chronic condition, and patients with an acute illness experienced before, know quite clearly what to expect and what they want from the doctor. Sally Macintyre and David Oldman (1977) explain this phenomenon well so far as migraine sufferers are concerned.

Stimson and Webb (1975) argue that in the actual consultation both patients and doctors pursue strategies in which each tries to influence the other in terms of their preferred outcome which is achieved through a series of negotiations, although a number of features constrain what is possible. The patient is not entirely powerless or passive, however, for s/he can decide what to tell the doctor out of all the things s/he knows about her/himself, although often experiencing difficulty in finding the appropriate language in which to do so. The patient is at somewhat of a social disadvantage being on the doctors' territory, perceiving the doctor to be much more competent both in the matter of illness and in social matters. The patient is also constrained by time, as is the doctor, but in a different sense.

The patient's health work does not end, however, when the doctor has decided what action to take. There is reappraisal and there are decisions for action which the patient must now make. Patients evaluate the consultation and its outcome. The latter may have been what they expected and hoped for, or they may feel that it is appropriate even though they had not known what to expect. This may be reinforced by talking to others. On the other hand, expectations may be thwarted; the prescription may turn out to be one that has been found to be inappropriate for this condition on another occasion: 'As soon as I saw the pills I knew they were no good. I said to Terry ... "I've had them before and they were no good" ' (Stimson and Webb, 1975, p. 71). Or perhaps the patient had hoped for antibiotics for a cough and sore throat and had just been given a gargle and cough linctus, neither of which s/he believed would be efficacious. Patients' decisions whether to take the treatment are not arrived at lightly; it is not possible to say they are 'satisfied' or 'dissatisfied'. They weigh up the pros and cons and decide whether to 'obey doctor's orders'. 'In the consultation, the doctor makes the treatment decisions; after the consultation, decision-making lies with the patient' (p. 87). Gerry Stimson (1974) has also reviewed elsewhere the many rational considerations which may lead a patient to disobey doctor's orders.

Other studies of general practice consultations have been undertaken from various points of view and using different methodologies (Byrne and Long, 1976; Cartwright, 1967; Cartwright and Anderson, 1981; Fitton and Acheson, 1979). All make plain how much health work patients have to do and the sorts of constraint they experience.

It is also the case that how patients conceive of illness modifies what they expect from the professional. Thus Williams (1981a, 1981b and 1983) has shown that those who conceive of illness as occupation in Herzlich's terms (1973; and see pages 142–4) require information on which to base their health work, demands not forthcoming from the accepting or fatalistic position of those who conceive of illness as liberating or destructive.

Mick Bloor (1976a and 1976b) studied the consultation process at the specialist level when he looked at what consultants decided in particular cases, i.e. the disposal decisions made. The ENT consultants were examining child patients who had been brought to them as possibly requiring their tonsils and/or adenoids out. It became clear from the many consultations Bloor observed that the surgeons had a number of different routines, each of which was likely to lead to a different disposal decision: to operate for Ts and As or to wait and see if the condition would clear up, for example. The question here is less the action which the child can take than the action taken on behalf of the child by the parents. Clearly the parents had taken action before this consultation. They had presented the child to the GP and either had persuaded her/him to refer them onwards to a specialist or had not objected, indeed had complied, when the GP made this proposal. However, in the course of the specialist consultation Bloor noted that the parents were able to influence the outcome only if the routine of the consultant gave them space so to do.

Elsewhere I have argued that, rather than being considered a consumer of health care, the patient should be considered a partner in the health-care team and a producer as much as a consumer of health care, if one is to use the producer–consumer analogy which, I have argued, is not altogether appropriate (Stacey, 1976). More recently (Stacey, 1984) I have attempted to sort out a misunderstanding on the part of some who suggest that to think of patients as partners in the health-care process implies that they are equal partners. This is not the case. There are two points here; one is that, theoretically and empirically, as we have seen, the patient is indubitably a health worker; the second is the empirical question of what at any given time and place may be the nature of the power relations between professionals and patients.

THE PATIENT IN THE IN-HOSPITAL DIVISION OF LABOUR

As soon as we begin to think about this question we can see that where the patient comes in the division of labour in the hospital much depends upon what kind of social order we understand there to be in the hospital. It is also necessary to distinguish between the social order in the hospital ward and the social order of the hospital as a whole. A modern hospital is a highly complex set of social arrangements. What it seems to be must to some extent depend on the stance one is taking and the reasons for the description.

Managerial authorities are likely to see the hospital in terms of units which are accountable upwards to manager or administrator. We have already seen that the division of labour between the paid professionals, as delineated in agreements reached between them as to their mutual relations and their respective areas of autonomy, differs from the division of labour in practice in the clinical situation.

An Imposed or Negotiated Order?
Celia Davies and Arthur Francis (1976) asked senior and junior members of NHS hospitals, both nurses and doctors, how they *perceived* the hospital. They all said they saw it as highly hierarchically structured, contrary to the way in which Anselm Strauss and his colleagues (1963) had seen it. In studying a psychiatric hospital they found that the rules were ignored as much as they were followed, and new ones were invented when a rule was called into question. They characterized the social order as 'negotiated'.

In response to the Davies–Francis inquiry both doctors and nurses denied role creativity, something which, as we saw earlier (page 182), Rue Bucher and Joan Stelling (1969) report they observed in US hospitals. British evidence suggests that consultants are free to alter the way in which they perform their tasks in comparison with the way in which the last incumbent performed it. Their ability to do this and to alter resource allocation in the process by the introduction of new procedures or expensive new techniques has been explored by the Council for Science and Society (1982).

We have seen that the patient was accorded a passive role in biomedical treatment and that hospitals were developed initially for teaching and research as much as for patient care. The role consequently allotted to patients in NHS hospitals caused them distress, which was articulated in the 1950s and 1960s. Gerda Cohen (1964), for example, exclaimed that under the system exemplified by a hospital of considerable repute her experience was that 'patients had no rights, no dignity, no status' (p. 7). What Strauss *et al.* (1982b) call the 'sentimental work' of the hospital staff was not being done or not well done. So Cohen set to and wrote a popular Penguin, *What's Wrong with Hospitals?* (1964). Even passive patients, however, have to be reckoned with. Nurses say that in their experience the character of a ward can change with a change of patients.

Technology and the Status of the Patient

Writing in 1969, Rosengren and Lefton sought to compensate for the failure of many previous studies of the hospital as an organization to pay attention to the patient as an actor who affects the organization. They introduce the notion of the patient's biographical career and stress the technological skills available for various conditions. Where there is a clear technology available, they argue, patients are seen in the light of that – for example, the short-term quick repair in an acute hospital. Where there is no clear technology, then the hospital sees the patient differently – for example, the long-term psychiatric hospital. Further-more, they argue, the kind of compliance or co-operation needed is variable, again depending on the technology.

Thus they argue that, depending on the technology available, the hospital will want a longer or shorter amount of the patient's time and will invade more or less of the patient's social space:

> the *longitudinal* patient career extends in social time, but the *lateral* dimension extends in social space. A patient treated for an acute condition in an acute general hospital may not experience any extensive lateral or longitudinal extension, while a patient treated in a long stay psychiatric hospital will experience extensive involvements on both dimensions. However the lateral and longitudinal extensions may vary independently of each other. Thus a patient in, for example, a rehabilitation hospital may not suffer much invasion of social space but a good deal of social time. In a short stay psychiatric hospital the reverse would be the case.
>
> (Rosengren and Lefton, 1969 pp. 124–5, original emphasis)

Further evidence for the way in which the treatment a patient is to receive may affect the social order of the ward comes from Rose Coser's (1972) comparative study of authority and decision-making in medical and surgical wards. She noticed a marked difference which she concluded derived from the need in surgery for decisions to be made quickly and carried out unquestioningly and instantly, compared with the careful consultation and deliberation required for the solution of medical problems, essentially those of diagnosis and choice of treatment. The surgical chief (cf. consultant in charge in British terms) made the decisions, and in this sense the war was run 'despotically'; below that level there was a good deal of camaraderie, chattering, laughter and swearing. In the medical ward the tasks were approached through team-work, reflection and deliberation rather than through a single authority. In the medical ward nurses were quieter, more polite and stuck to rules and routines more.

Coser was focusing on the relations between doctors and nurses rather than on the activities of the patients, or the impact of the social order on them. She is however making a similar point to Rosengren and Lefton, namely, that the condition of the patient and the way physicians and surgeons believe it should be treated have important consequences for the social order of the ward. However, in these studies it is the attributes rather than the actions of the patients which are seen to have significant impact. In the case of Rosengren and Lefton (1969), the social relations between staff and patients appear to be technologically determined.

The Patient as Active Initiator
It is undoubtedly invaluable to draw attention to the ways in which the patient's condition or the application of particular medical procedures modifies the social order. It would, however, be inappropriate to see technology as the only influence or to imagine that it is only through technology that patients may influence their paid carers. Julius Roth (1963), in a classic study, showed how patients in a long-stay TB hospital negotiated with their doctors to move them on to a further stage of treatment. Patients had learned what they might expect and how to argue for it from the experience of other patients. Treatment for TB was long drawn out, and there was time to learn. The ultimate sanction that could be used was to leave the hospital before treatment ended, something which the physicians would not want on a number of grounds and especially not if the patient were actively infective.

Goffman (1961) in *Asylums*, another classic, also demonstrates the patient as actor, notwithstanding the stripping and humiliation to which mental patients were submitted on admission and the repressive and routinized regime to which they were subjected. Within the constraints imposed upon them patients developed their own 'underlife' which might take a number of forms. More recently Strauss and his colleagues (1982a) have demonstrated in empirical studies how much work patients have to do in high-technology hospitals and in cases of chronic illness. That study also suggests that these features have important implications also for the trained staff.

The Nature of the Organization
In a useful review of the nature of social order in the hospital, David Hall (1977) suggests that studies have been based on two fundamentally opposed views which derive from the way in which organizations have been seen. The first puts the emphasis on common goals, and the second on co-ordination towards those goals. The first, he argues, leads to the organization being treated as a series of interrelated parts oriented around a system of goals or sets of goals. In the second the organization is seen as the outcome of the actions of members in which co-operation is achieved rather than assumed. Following from Silverman (1970) he argues that the first does not take into account purposive human action because it emphasizes system and the self-regulatory qualities of the system. The second treats even the taken for granted as problematical and something which has to be worked out.

Rosengren and Lefton's (1969) work constitutes an example of the former, for having identified the way in which patients' and the relevant medical procedures have varied consequences, they then go on to argue that certain authority patterns go along with the implications of these procedures. Apart from the observation that there is insufficient evidence for the conclusions they reach, which certainly do not apply to NHS hospitals, at a theoretical level their view is one which sees the hospital much as an organism, rather than composed of numbers of people with problems to solve and wills to solve them. How this approach works out at a more theoretical level may be seen in a work such as Croog and Ver Steeg (1972), who write of the hospital as a social system.

Problem-Solving Patients

In his work on children in a hospital ward, Hall (1977) did not deny the existence of a structured social order, of a series of hierarchies which in one sense constitute the hospital, but he did not feel that the ward any more than the hospital itself could be said to be rigidly rule governed. Undoubtedly the outside world impinged on the hospital in various ways, just as other facets of the hospital itself impinged on any one ward. Hall's approach is thus much nearer to that of Anselm Strauss and his colleagues (1963), to which we referred earlier. In their view, the hospital *is* the combination of rules and policies, agreements, understandings, pacts and contracts and so forth which currently obtain. When changes are made in any one of those things negotiation and renegotiation are called for. This results, not in a return to some previous equilibrium, but in the establishment of a new order. What Hall observed was that the social order of the hospital ward was a constant matter of all members in the division of labour, including in this case the child patients and their parents, seeking to solve the day-to-day problems which they found themselves faced with. Only at a very abstract level could there be said to be a goal shared by everybody in the ward; each category of worker might have different goals from another. A child might want attention just now while the nurse had to make a report to sister or answer a doctor's inquiry.

The studies of which Hall's was one (Hall and Stacey, 1979) make it plain that even children on traction in an orthopaedic ward are not without ability to influence the social order. Children on traction are bedfast and dependent on the staff for their every need. Being bored, from time to time they would demand a bedpan. Nurses knew that this might be a ruse to achieve, temporarily at least, a different position from the permanently horizontal. On the other hand, the child might really have a bursting bladder. What should they do? Assume they were being put on and ignore the call for help, thus risking a wet bed and all the attendant work of changing it, or answer the call and be taken for a ride?

The children in this and other ways were relatively, but not utterly, powerless. How much unintended suffering they experienced is documented in those studies, some of it simply because the nurses lacked adequate psychosocial training at that time and did not realize what they were doing or what was the nature of the children's distress. Some of the unintended suffering arose because it was easier for the staff to pursue their own goals at the expense of the children's goals, which, being in the more powerful position, staff were able to do. In such circumstances how patients use the little power available to them can be important.

In a study of geriatric wards, Helen Evers (1981a) has described the differences she observed in the treatment received by elderly women in long-stay care. Of women who still had their wits about them Evers characterized three types: 'Dear old Gran', 'Poor old Nellie' and 'Awkward Alice'. The 'Dear old Grans' were smiling, pleasant and conforming, praising the nurses. The 'Awkward Alices' had a good idea of what they wanted and were entitled to and said so. The former received a good deal more attention than the latter, who came in for quite a rough time. To this extent the work 'Alice' put in regularly went amiss.

The Locale of Care

An important issue which the children in hospital studies (Hall, 1977; Hall and Stacey, 1979; Stacey, *et al.*, 1970) addressed was the implications for the child patients of the change in the locale of care from home to hospital and of having their carers changed from primarily unpaid carers, i.e. their mothers, to primarily paid carers, i.e. the ward staff. The children's status changed markedly in this transition from being one of a son or daughter in a small face-to-face group to being one of many in the category 'child patient' and perhaps in the case of T-and-A patients one of a 'batch' of children in hospital at the same time for precisely the same procedure (Pill, 1970). The sort of work that the children could do to improve their own well-being changed along with these changes. They did not understand their new situation; they were faced with constantly changing personnel; their mothers knew their foibles, whereas these people did not. For a few children the experience was apparently liberating; they rode it well, and their mental health was subsequently apparently improved. But they were the minority. The majority of children were greatly distressed by the experience, a distress which continued for some weeks or months after they returned home. An unhappy minority apparently suffered damage to their mental health which lasted beyond six months. Most had recovered by that time (B. Brown, 1979). Fred Clough (1979) was able to show, using semantic differential tests, that even much older children perceived the two locales of home and hospital quite differently, the former being seen much more positively than the latter.

The meaning of the labour which parturient women have to undertake is also much changed by their removal from the locale of home to hospital. In this case, from being the central focus around which the household, including the paid and unpaid carers, revolves, they again, like the children, become one of a category of many others in a similar situation. Labouring women are of course a category of patient where it has always been recognized that the patient is a health worker; she labours. This issue is more fully discussed in Chapter 17. For the present we will turn to unpaid carers.

15 *Unpaid Workers in the Division of Health Labour (2): the Unpaid Carers*

Jane Taylor (1979) has referred to the unpaid carers as the 'hidden labour of the NHS'. Unpaid carers are involved in health promotion, health maintenance, health restoration and caring for the disabled. Most of them are women. We have already seen (Chapter 7) the way in which the state recruited the mothers of the nation as unpaid helpers in the bid to improve the quality of the nation's health. The process of teaching and encouraging mothers continues through the work of health visitors. It was also backed by government resources in the form of grants to the Health Education Council (now succeeded by the Health Education Authority). There is no doubt that many mothers are appreciative of the help and advice that they are given, but some still find the entry of health visitors into the home an affront to their privacy. Others are frankly ambiguous (Buswell, 1980a and 1981).

THE RESPONSIBILITY OF WOMEN FOR CHILDREN, PARTNERS AND PARENTS

Around the time when *Prevention and Health, Everybody's Business* (DHSS, 1976a) was published, Hilary Graham (1979) wrote an article which she perceptively titled 'Prevention and Health: Every Mother's Business'. She demonstrated that mothers already felt remarkably responsible for their children's health; so far from neglecting them the majority in her sample played their role traditionally and put their husbands and children first. The mothers, however, were in some difficulties to know how to fulfil these obligations. As between the care of the baby at home who was due to go to the child health clinic and the child in school who needed meeting when school came out, what should she do? If she felt that violent sex might damage the foetus *in utero* and her husband wished her to join in violent sex, what should she do? Which obligations should she fulfil?

Each woman is made responsible for her husband's health also. In order to help him avoid heart disease she should encourage him by stopping smoking herself, replan his diet to make it more healthy, encourage him to take exercise (and join him in it), listen to his worries and take over some of his work, like paying the bills, and getting the plumber – according to one advice pamphlet Graham quoted. As she says, such advice presumes a woman wants to shape her life-style, and that of her family, around her husband; but, perhaps more important, it also assumes that she is able to do so, which research suggests she may not be (Graham, 1984, p. 72).

These conflicting role obligations may have deleterious consequences for the women's own health. Devices to help women cope with the labour of caring may bring solace without damage, such as listening to the radio. On the other hand, 'Cigarettes, psychotropic drugs, and alcohol offer women this contradictory kind of support, helping and hurting them at the same time' (Graham,

1985b, p. 39). Furthermore, she then feels guilty at providing a bad role model for her family. Mothers are often reluctant to visit the doctor about their own health problems, both physical and emotional. Research evidence indicates that there is a considerable iceberg of suffering in women who are mothers of young children (Boulton, 1983; Brown and Harris, 1978; Buswell, 1980b; Graham, 1984; Graham and McKee, 1980; Pill and Stott, 1982).

If women have the primary responsibility for maintaining and promoting the health of their family, it is upon them that the burden of care for the ill and handicapped falls. This development has undoubtedly accelerated since the recent recession and government policies to contain, and now to cut, public expenditure on health (Graham, 1985a and 1985b; Taylor, 1979). The return of long-stay patients to the 'community' and demands that mothers stay at home with their children or go to hospital with their children have been around since the 1950s.

Many of these movements have been initiated by people whose intentions are essentially humane. How could I say otherwise having been involved in the movement for the admission of mothers to hospital with their young children? There is no doubt also that many psychiatrists, paediatricians, other health-care professionals and policy-makers also have the most humane of intentions. At the same time I am only too well aware that the same arguments which support requests for the opening of hospital wards to parents can be, and have been, used to limit the freedom of choice of women as to how we should rear our children, to confine women to the home and to make us feel guilty if we are not able to go to hospital with our children. The moral pressure upon women, and indeed upon both parents, is strong. Any parent having read *Better Services for the Mentally Handicapped* (DHSS, 1971) who then decided that she or they could not cope with home care (perhaps because of the sacrifice they judged the other children would have to make) would be made to feel guilty.

Furthermore, inadequate services have been provided to support the hidden carers who are sustaining chronically ill or handicapped relatives, as Taylor (1979) argues. Phillipson (1981), for example, discussed the large amount of women's work which is involved in caring for the elderly. As he says:

> The caring role which is allocated to women moves from caring for her own children to caring for her parents (or her husband's parents) and back to her grandchildren. Even in her 60s and 70s, a woman may find her life predominantly shaped by the image of her as a caring and mothering figure.
>
> (Phillipson, 1981, p. 187)

His research shows that three times as many old people live with married daughters as with married sons. Even those daughters who are not in the same house as their elderly parents are more often called on for help than sons. Hundreds of thousands of single women look after an elderly parent, spending more than eight hours a day on it and at any time of day or night. Such carers frequently have to give up their jobs and also have their own personal and social lives severely curtailed; their situation is much like that of the captive wife at the beginning of the family cycle. It is similarly affected by expenditure cuts which remove both nursery facilities and relief care for the elderly (Equal Opportunities Commission, 1979; National Council for Single Women and their Dependants, 1979).

It would be untrue to say that such sacrifices never fall upon men. Having a handicapped child in the home has consequences for the father as well as the mother, even if they both follow fairly conventionally sex-segregated domestic roles. Where elderly women become dependent some men take over full responsibility not only for running the house but for looking after their wives as well. Such men have probably often started undertaking the caring in the way in which they have always 'filled in for the wife' when she has been ill, but this illness did not end, and the obligation continued and deepened. Helen Evers (1985, p. 96) has shown that this is often the way daughters slip into responsibility for the care of their ageing parents or parents-in-law. It is not so much that a rational decision has been reached but that the arrangement has developed from small assumptions about helping out among kin.

State Assumptions about Women as 'Natural' Carers
The assumption in state health and welfare policy has been that women do the caring (Finch and Groves, 1980; Land, 1978). In 1982 the Equal Opportunities Commission (EOC) heeded their message and that of others and analysed the implications for women of the 'return to the community' policies and also the increasing calls for volunteers to help with day care. These movements made heavy demands on women; the EOC concludes: 'The Government's "community care" policy is revealed as a euphemism for an under-resourced system which places heavy burdens on *individual* members of the community, most of them women. It represents "care on the cheap"' (1982, p. 3, original emphasis). What is more, as the EOC points out, the costs also 'are borne individually and do not figure in any public expenditure account. The price is paid in restrictions on women's opportunities' (p. 40).

At the same time that these implicit assumptions are made about the 'naturalness' of the health work which is done in the home, there are ways in which there is a blurring of the domestic and public domains. We have already seen how, from early in the century, public officials entered the private domestic domain for health and welfare reasons. Essential differences remain.

> In the public domain the prime reward is monetary, a wage, salary, fees or profits. Sanctions are loss of pay or profits, ultimately in the case of the employed, the sack, for others loss of clientele or collapse of the firm. Honour, standing, worth are also involved but flow from the prime rewards. In the private domain rewards are more diffuse, as are sanctions: the smile, the gift, the loving hug, or their absence or opposites (see also Bell and Newby, 1976). The ultimate sanction of separation or divorce loses the life partner, for the man a houseworker and child rearer, for the woman her daily occupation and possibly her children as well as her life partner.
> (Stacey, 1984, p. 167)

Allowances for Caring
Although health and welfare policies assume that health work is women's work, the extra cost has been to some extent recognized of recent years. Allowances may now be paid for 'attendance' upon a handicapped member of the household, and in some cases where the attendance allowance is paid an invalid care

allowance may also be payable. The conditions for receiving attendance allowance are stringent, and exhaustive medical inquiries are made as to the amount of care involved. The invalid care allowance is even more restrictive; only those in receipt of attendance allowance are eligible, and it is available only to men and to certain categories of unmarried women who have given up work to care for the handicapped relative (or in some cases have never worked for that reason). Married women and women who are cohabiting are not eligible. This is a most blatant case of the assumption that a woman's domestic health work is a duty which flows from the attachment to the man she is living with (Groves and Finch, 1983). It remains to be seen how the 1986 judgement of the European Court against this practice as discriminatory will work out.

The allowances are small when looked at in terms of wages people might get for doing the same work as paid health employment and they appear even smaller when compared with the cost of institutional care. There is little enough evidence about how much these allowances are taken up and what effect they have. A small survey by the EOC (quoted in Ungerson, 1983) indicates that of 111 households looking after a member only 15 per cent received an attendance allowance. The interventions in the domestic economy are obviously not great. Much larger allowances are paid in some other countries. They are, furthermore, often too little and too late (see the suffering caused in the examples described by Oliver, 1983). Nevertheless they represent a further development of the intermediate zone, between domestic and public domains, in which so much health care takes place and in which the unthinking (and unrecorded) consequences of male-dominated health and welfare policy disadvantage the unpaid carers, be they male or female.

THE INTERFACE BETWEEN THE PAID AND THE UNPAID CARERS

A number of features make the relationship between paid and unpaid carers less than easy. In the light of the totally different system of rewards and punishments to which we have referred, this is perhaps not surprising. There are further problems. As I have pointed out elsewhere (Stacey, 1984), one of the problems which health workers face is that in providing a service they are in some sense carrying into the public domain mores which are valued more highly in the domestic domain. We saw in the section about paid carers how these values inhibit all-out strike action on the part of doctors as well as of ancillary workers. The problems, I believe, are felt most acutely in the conventionally female health-care occupations such as nursing. Indeed, I have suggested that the expectation that nurses should offer love and care for pay has underlain many of the problems which they have encountered in developing effective strategies for occupational enhancement.

In addition, so many of the tasks which are done as paid work in the health service can be also, and indeed are also, done for love or duty in the domestic domain, as we have seen. This has had the consequence that members of paid occupations like nursing have learned to draw the boundaries between themselves and the untrained and unpaid very sharply. We saw how health visitors were from the outset instructed to withdraw from their clients and set themselves apart. We saw also (page 130) that the same insistence on training-derived status led to discontent among SENs, who were neither remunerated nor recognized for the work they did, so much of which was the 'same as' that of SRNs. The health-care occupations where women predominate consequently have two problems to contend with: one, that in part of their work at least they are expected to do work and behave in a way similar to that of women in the domestic domain. (A similar phenomenon pertained with those high-powered medical secretaries still in the clerical grade which Davies and Rosser, 1985, reported on: see page 192.) The second problem of the professionally trained is that unpaid workers constitute a threat to them in so far as the unpaid and untrained are doing similar work. The extent of the overlap is limited, of course; there are many highly sophisticated and technical tasks which require a great deal of skill and experience. The trained may feel threatened nevertheless.

Mothers in the Wards

The problems can be seen acutely in the case of the hospitalization of children where the parents and mostly the mother had been caring for the child day and night before admission. Roisin Pill's (1970) early work showed how in 1964 there was no role 'mother in the ward'. Mothers were not staff, and they were not visitors (visitors came for defined and limited periods only; the mothers were there all day). Staff were exposed to view, watched at their work, and they found it most uncomfortable. Nurses are now more experienced in and understanding of how to cope with parents in the ward. Experiments are in hand to see if 'care by parent' will work in NHS hospitals (Cardiff Care by Parent scheme). The research shows just how carefully such arrangements have to be worked out, not only because of the possible hazards to the children of untrained carers where the children have a serious illness, but also because of manifold problems in the division of labour. Some lack of conviction on the part of the nurses has resulted in a relapse to the parent-visitor from the parent-carer role (Cleary *et al.*, 1986).

Mothers as Mediators

Graham (1985b) has drawn attention to the important role which unpaid carers – mothers, wives and daughters – play at the interface between paid and unpaid care. They serve as mediators of services from outside the home:

> Their responsibilities within the domestic health services unavoidably bring them into contact with professional welfare workers: the doctor and health visitor, the social worker and the district nurse. Their caring role places them at the interface between the family and the state, as the go-betweens linking the informal health care system with the formal apparatus of the welfare state.
> (p. 26)

In playing this role women all too often find that our knowledge and understanding is devalued. Obviously lay women do not have the technical language but know and understand more than many professionals imagine. Nick Spencer (1984) has shown that mothers recognize serious illness in their children (although they could not name it biomedically) just about as well as trained professionals. This makes a strong case for suggesting that professionals should pay more attention to these lay health workers. There is some evidence that some medical tragedies could have been avoided if more attention had been paid to anxious parental statements such as, 'I don't think the drug is agreeing with her, Doctor,' when repeated more than once, or, 'He's really not at all himself.' The mother's knowledge is in a different form but it is about the same thing as the doctor is concerned with. The tragedy is the professional's 'trained incapacity' (Merton, 1957, pp. 197–8) to hear what is being said.

Sentimental Work by Lay and Professional

Strauss *et al.* (1982b) have discussed an interesting interface between paid and unpaid carers in hospital wards in the Bay area of California. They are analysing the 'sentimental work' which professional staff do for and with patients, which they contrast with the instrumental medical work of servicing their bodies. What has often been referred to as 'psycho-social support' they divide into interactional work and moral rules, trust work, composure work, identity work, awareness context work and rectification work. All are facets of work which is done to sustain the patient as a person through suffering, physical or mental. Much of this work is not part of the formal activities of the staff, is neither prescribed nor recorded. In my terms it comes under the heading of all those activities which are part of domestic-domain social relations rather than of vocational training or the market-place. Interestingly, in a number of case accounts which Strauss *et al.* report, kin members work alongside staff; the mother of a very ill child helps her with 'composure work' while the nurse undertakes various procedures, but the nurse is gentle and does not infringe the moral rules associated with interaction. She minimizes the necessary assaults. Strauss *et al.* discuss the division of labour in sentimental work in the ward which most often (but not invariably) appears to be undertaken by the nurses and kin members. Strauss *et al.* do not give any examples of where co-operation in sentimental work (or psycho-social support) between paid and unpaid carers broke down, but this can also happen.

Members of a kin group are not the only people who get involved in unpaid health care. There are also very many volunteers, some individual, others organized in groups such as Leagues of Hospital Friends. Their number has grown, and increasing reliance is being placed on them.

THE VOLUNTEERS

One of the triumphs about the establishment of the NHS in the eyes of Labour supporters and those to their left was that the days when hospitals and other parts of the health service would have to rely on volunteer workers were over. They rejoiced that, now the service was state funded, health care would be provided properly and professionally by paid workers. It would also be properly financed: no more rattling the money-box in collections for necessary but unfunded developments or just to keep the hospital open. The days of volunteering were over. However, those days did not last long, any more than the days of 'free' prescriptions did. It was a difficult decision for Nye Bevan to make to call for volunteers, but so he did. From that time on, the NHS has actively recruited volunteers to do all manner of things from washing-up to driving patients to and from hospital, providing tea kiosks and visiting people in their homes. In the 1970s, and even more in the 1980s, the need for volunteers has increased as cash limits have bitten harder, real cuts have been made, and the numbers in need, especially the elderly, have increased.

The relationship between volunteers and paid health workers has never been easy. There are questions of accountability, of reliability and also of skill involved. While I have stressed the extent of overlap of skills between paid and unpaid health-care workers, it is also the case that volunteers may feel that they lack competence and training. This was something which Philip Abrams and his colleagues found when studying neighbourhood care schemes. People whose formal training had taught them how to care, such as nurses, fitted in readily to such schemes; so did mothers who, as Abrams *et al.* (1986) point out, received their training informally. However, some volunteers dropped out 'because they did not know *how* to be useful'. The extent to which the untrained were frightened, deterred by their own incompetence emerged strongly (Bulmer, 1986, p. 114).

Abrams and his colleagues did not discuss the problems of the interface between the paid and unpaid in terms of the quite different systems of reward and punishment which apply among kin and in the market-place. They were well aware of the problems which arise from those differences, however: for example, when volunteers are paid, as many, especially working-class women, need to be if they are to be able to sustain their caring role; and in particular the problems of undercutting paid carers. They do not find that paying diminishes caring, however, a point which Diana Leat has stressed (Abrams *et al.*, 1986, pp. 73–4). In their studies they found, as is repeatedly recorded, that most caring for the dependent is undertaken by kin members, generally near kin and usually women. (Gordon Grant, 1986, has reaffirmed this finding in the case of the home care of the adult mentally handicapped in North Wales.) In round numbers it amounted to about nine-tenths of all care given in the home. However, there are between 5 and 10 per cent of people who need help who do not have available relatives. Their care if they are not to be institutionalized requires the 'provision of surrogate kin'. Abrams (Bulmer, 1986, pp. 232, ff.) is much exercised as to how one can build functional equivalents to the commitments of close relations among non-kin. He speaks of the importance of developing competence and reciprocity and of researching further why it is that the religious are more inclined to undertake volunteer work. The absence of any analysis of the domestic economy and of the motives which lead to the acceptance of caring within that framework, especially on the part of the women, sets limits to his analysis of the relationship between the formal and the informal. Albeit that Abrams is fully aware that while such an acceptance appears to be 'natural' it is socially constructed (see, for example, Bulmer, 1986, p. 233), he quite frequently uses 'naturally' occurring social relations as a concept when contrasting them with the contractual arrangements. At the same time, it is not altogether correct to refer to these kinship arrangements and the norms and sanctions that back them as 'informal'; they are part of an elaborate and formal set of social arrangements of ancient origin, even if those in question here may not have legal sanction.

It is clear that the NHS would be unable to provide the health care which it does without the help of the unpaid carers, both kin and volunteers in hospital and community. Problems which arise between the unpaid and the paid carers derive in large measure from the different origins and allegiances of the carers in domestic and public domains. However, these problems and others in the division of labour in health care which we discussed in Chapter 13 among the paid carers do not entirely derive from within the health-care system itself. They also derive from the situation of health care in a capitalist society. We have referred to the way in which the stratification system is related to the social class structure of the society at large. In employing female labour in lowly and less well-paid positions health authorities are behaving as capitalist employers also behave.

We have seen, however, that there are particular facets of health care, namely, the nature of 'people work', which mark it off from other forms of industrial production. While some health care is undertaken for profit, its extent in the UK is less great than for example in the USA. In the NHS in particular there are no profits to be made, although there are lucrative positions to be gained.

Nevertheless all health workers within the NHS, as in all other health-care systems except those of the Soviet-bloc countries, are directly dependent upon capitalist industry for the work they do, be they paid or unpaid carers. Hospital supplies and pharmaceuticals are all manufactured and sold for profit by industries not bound by professional service ethics. It is to these that we now turn.

16 Health Care and Late Twentieth-Century Capitalism

The development of the National Health Service, as we saw in Chapter 8, removed the delivery of health care in Britain from any direct involvement with the profit motive. Even those physicians and surgeons who had been unconvinced about the NHS quickly came to appreciate the advantages of being able to treat the condition presented with the best available mode rather than having to consider who the patient was and what treatment they might be able to afford. They appreciated, also, the advantages of state capital to back expensive establishments such as hospitals and their equipment.

In this chapter we will look at the extent to which, and some of the ways in which, capitalism impinges upon health care: first, in terms of the profit motive and health-care delivery; second, in the provision of pharmaceuticals; and finally in relation to hospital supplies and especially the installation of expensive medical techniques. Two considerations will be borne in mind; one is in terms of intrusions into the doctor–patient relationship itself; the second relates to the triangular set of relationships between the health-care provision, the state and capital.

FOR-PROFIT HEALTH CARE

In the United States the capitalist mode of production has infused health care more directly from the outset than in Britain. Although health-care delivery in many parts of Europe is more capitalistic when compared with the NHS, the USA stands out in contrast to most European countries in this regard. While there are many not-for-profit or provident hospitals and also public hospitals in the USA, there have been fewer inhibitions there than in the UK about providing health care in a directly capitalist mode, i.e. investors providing the capital, controlling the facility and employing the health-care workers with the precise and overt aim of making a profit. 'For-profit hospital systems presently own fifteen per cent of non-government acute general hospital beds in the United States (but more than fifty per cent of non-government psychiatric beds)' (Salmon, 1984b, p. 144). Self-sponsorship by groups of physicians may also take the capitalist mode, although income may be derived from fees (Derber, 1984, p. 230).

The comparison of the USA with the UK is instructive. It helps us to recognize more clearly what the relationships have been between health care in the UK and the capitalist society of which it is a part. It also helps us to understand how the new involvement of corporate capitalism in health-care provision is changing the British scene.

Until these developments, which have taken place only in the last ten to fifteen years, the influences of the capitalist mode of production have been indirect rather than direct. They have been important nevertheless. The influences have been indirect because facilities such as hospitals have for the most part been provided in the provident, not-for-profit mode or by the state, although some private nursing homes have followed the for-profit mode. Major facilities have not generally been provided by profit-making companies or corporations. This is a new development. At the same time, the NHS, along with all other health-care providers, has been dependent upon the capitalist pharmaceutical and hospital-supplies industries. Hitherto this has been the most direct economic influence which capitalism has had on British health care.

MEDICINES AND THEIR USE

In Chapter 7 we saw the development of the pharmaceutical industry had transformed the division of labour in health care from early roots in the late eighteenth century, through the bench-mark provided by the discovery of the sulpha drugs and accelerating from the Second World War. No longer did housewives brew their own medicines; no longer did physicians rely on well-tried formulae or pharmacists dispense the mixtures by themselves. By the 1960s medical practitioners were faced with an ever-increasing array of pharmaceutical products. Unpaid health workers seeking to maintain or restore their own or their family members' health were similarly bombarded with many over-the-counter products to choose from: vitamin pills to help maintain fitness, analgesics to calm pain, cough mixtures, skin creams, balms and digestive aids. By that time granddaughters had lost the knowledge of their foremothers about how to make up many of these pills and potions; others now available were derived from the new biochemistry and most from synthetic materials, rather than herb gardens and hedgerows.

Slick judgements as to whether these developments have on balance been advantageous or otherwise would be inappropriate. No simple divisions into medicines which are 'good' or 'bad', 'safe' or 'dangerous', 'effective' or 'ineffective' may be made. Many preparations, both herbal and synthetic, are poisons, possibly lethal poisons if taken in large doses, although they may be life-saving if taken in small quantities. Digitalis, an ancient remedy still in use and derived from the common foxglove, is one well-known example. It can stimulate the heart and thus save life, but it can also kill. All medicines are likely to have certain specific uses, to be dangerous in overdose, or to have undesirable side-effects even when used in appropriate doses for the appropriate conditions. The more serious a patient's condition the more appropriate it may be to risk the side-effects, a risk not worth taking for minor or self-limiting ailments.

Commonly most of us think of medicines as 'curing' illnesses; one may even say, 'I took an aspirin, and it cured my headache.' Biomedically what it did was reduce the pain. With luck the (probably unknown) cause of the headache will have disappeared before the analgesic effect of the aspirin has worn off. Andrew Herxheimer and Gerry Stimson (1981, pp. 36–44) categorize the biomedical uses of medicines as follows: prevention of disease (prophylaxis); diagnosis; cure; maintenance therapy; and symptomatic treatment. They point out that 'medicines cure illness much less commonly than most people believe, if cure is defined as the restoration of health' (p. 39). In the terms we have been using in this book, I think they mean diseases rather than illnesses; i.e. they are referring to biomedically recognizable pathological conditions. The main medicines which cure in the sense they have defined are anti-microbial and anti-parasitic drugs, anti-cancer drugs and antidotes to poisons (p. 39).

The best known example of the other biomedical uses is the preventive use of medicines in infectious diseases (immunization or inoculation), although there are others. 'The essential feature of prophylactic medication is that it is given to people who are judged to be at risk of developing a disease or condition that they may be protected against' (Herxheimer and Stimson, 1981, p. 37). Most methods involve some risks. The judgement is made that the risks of the prophylactic are less than of the disease or condition. Contraception is a special case because here a normal condition is being impeded. The risk of contraceptive use has to be balanced against the risks, physical, social and emotional, of repeated child bearing and the feasibility of heterosexual abstinence.

The use of contrast dyes in X-ray examination is an example of the diagnostic use of medicines. Maintenance therapy may be divided into replacment therapy – as for example in nutritional or hormonal deficiency; the take-over of homoeostatic control, for example, to reduce hypertension or excess body fluids; and finally the suppression of a disease process, so that its manifestations are removed or reduced, as for example in the reduction of inflammation from rheumatic conditions, although the rheumatic condition itself is not overcome.

The overwhelming majority of medicines in everyday use in the late twentieth century are provided by the pharmaceutical industry, to which we shall now turn. It must be noted at the outset that any review of the literature is made less than easy because of the way much of it is divided between the bland analyses of apologists for that industry and the violent polemics of those who oppose its present structure and practices. We shall look at the relationship of the industry with each of a number of categories of workers in the health-care division of labour.

THE PHARMACEUTICAL INDUSTRY AND THE UNPAID HEALTH WORKERS

When Karen Dunnell and Ann Cartwright (1972) asked a representative sample about the medicines they had in their homes, 94 per cent had some self-prescribed medicines bought over the counter (p. 82). Respondents had twice as many non-prescribed as prescribed medicines available at home (p. 96). Most were medicines the respondents already knew about; only a tenth had recently been bought for the first time (p. 97). Of the medicines people kept, the four most important categories were preparations acting on the skin (27 per cent); analgesics and anti-pyretics, i.e. pain-killers and fever-reducers (18.5 per cent); digestives (nearly 16 per cent); and preparations acting on the ear, nose and throat (10.5 per cent). Self-prescribed medicine tended to be kept for general use and not for a particular person, and this was especially true for households with children (p. 90). Furthermore, self-prescribed medicines were kept longer than prescribed medicines (p. 90) although generally they were taken less often (p. 38). We can see how in this way the houseworker continues her long-established role of guardian of the household health. She no longer makes up the formula; her task now is to have the basic mass-produced remedies available and to know how and when to use them. The health-maintenance responsibilities are reflected in the report that tonics and vitamins were the types of self-prescribed medicine which had been taken every day in the last fortnight (p. 120).

The evidence is less clear as to how unpaid health workers came to buy self-prescribed medicines in these categories or in the particular brands they chose. Over a fifth of Dunnell and Cartwright's (1972) respondents could not remember where they had first heard about the medicine they bought; 18 per cent said it was from parents or grandparents, 7 per cent from their spouse, 10 per cent from friends (the unpaid workers still fulfilling their traditional role), 10 per cent from doctors and 4 per cent from other paid health workers, and 6 per cent from chemists. Only 8 per cent admitted to advertisements as their source. Advertising may well have been more important than this, perhaps being the source for some of the 22 per cent of those who could not remember. And how did parents, grandparents, spouses and friends hear about the preparations in the first place? Clearly the pharmaceutical industry thinks advertising its over-the-counter (OTC) preparations is important since it spends a good deal of money and effort on it.

THE DOCTORS AND THE PHARMACEUTICAL INDUSTRY

A great many drugs, however, are available only on prescription; these are known as the 'ethicals', which it is thought ought not to be freely available to those who do not understand their pharmacological content or their mode of action on body and mind. There is a further category of even more tightly controlled drugs, those which have major mood-changing properties, which are drugs of addiction and liable to be used (or misused) in ways that are damaging to people's bodies, minds and social relations. Medical practitioners, within wide limits, are themselves responsible for the ethicals; as to the latter, the state in the form of the Home Office also maintains an oversight.

In Dunnell and Cartwright's (1972) study half of the prescribed medicines were for drugs acting on the cardiovascular, genito-urinary and central nervous systems, those taken internally for infections (antibiotics) and those affecting metabolism and allergic reactions. Most of these drugs are available only on prescription (p. 27). Of the prescriptions dispensed by chemists in 1968 a fifth were those which act on the central nervous system (p. 29). Of the prescribed medicines which people had in their homes, the single largest group (13.9 per cent) were also preparations of this kind. They were followed by preparations acting on the skin (12.8 per cent), those affecting metabolism (11 per cent) and analgesics and anti-pyretics (10.3 per cent) (p. 85). The mood-changing drugs were also among those taken the most frequently (p. 40).

At the time in the late 1960s when Dunnell and Cartwright were funded to survey the use of drugs in the population, there was a good deal of anxiety about inappropriate prescribing, especially with regard to the mood-changing drugs. This arose from the addictable nature of some of them; from the thin line between use and abuse, a line not to be drawn simply by the legality of the method of obtaining the drug; from their being a major cause of accidental poisonings and suicides; and from beliefs that they were masking social and economic problems. Added to cost, these thoughts led to campaigns against the use of 'tranquillizers'. It would be interesting to know how the holdings of medicines in people's medicine cupboards may have changed in the seventeen years since Dunnell and Cartwright (1972) collected their data. Their evidence, which is backed by other data, does suggest that Blum *et al.* (1981, p. 18) are correct when they say that what people 'are mostly medicating is something in their heads' (see also Blum with Kreitman, 1981).

PRACTITIONERS' SOURCES OF KNOWLEDGE

There is now a vast array of drugs available. According to Lall (1981, p. 195), 'Some 700–1,000 drugs are sold under thousands of brand names in almost every country.' He calculates that 35,000 or more product specialities were available in the USA in the 1970s; in the UK, 10,000; in West Germany, 12,000 to 15,000. However, those 700 to 1,000 different kinds of drugs appear under a variety of brand names depending on which company has marketed them. There may be ten brand names for what is essentially the same chemical compound. How the nature of the pharmaceutical industry makes this possible we will discuss shortly. At present let us think about the implications for the physician faced with a suffering patient. How is s/he to decide what to prescribe?

Initially after the pharmacological revolution broke upon them medical practitioners had little training in how to select and prescribe. Many had been educated in medical schools before the new pharmacology developed; those educated later were taught in medical schools where therapeutics and toxicology were insufficiently stressed. Since the new products were being promoted by for-profit industry the main source of information which the practitioners had was that which the industry itself provided.

The promotional activities of the industry are intense; a great deal is spent on advertising, on promotional gimmicks of various kinds. The level of these activities upset many physicians.

> Practicing physicians are inundated with gifts, patient educational materials, and free samples, all promoting the latest brand name products. A practicing physician myself, I am actually writing this manuscript [critically analysing the industry] with an Eli Lilly pen, on a Pfizer scratch pad, with a SmithKline calendar reminding me of my deadline, and a Squibb paperweight perched on top of the Parke-Davis paperclip holder.

So writes Bodenheimer (1984, p. 202) of the advertising bombardment to which US physicians are subjected. He goes on to refer to the *Physicians' Desk Reference* as the book he reads more than any other and from which he can most easily get information about prescription drugs. In Britain the equivalent is *MIMS* (*Monthly Index of Medical Specialities*), which is used more than any other listing. Both these books are produced by the drug companies. The *Lancet* comments that

> wiser prescribing would surely ensue if doctors stuck resolutely to the *British National Formulary [BNF]* and eschewed the list of proprietary preparations entitled *Monthly Index of Medical Specialities*, the undiluted use of which by prescribers does not favour economy in the NHS drug bill and deprives them of the pharmacological guidance supplied by the *BNF*.

(2 March 1985, p. 497)

The *BNF* is produced by the British Medical Association and the Pharmaceutical Association, both organizations of professionals. There is, in addition, the *Drugs and Therapeutics Bulletin*, produced by the Consumers Association. According to Arabella Melville and Colin Johnson (1982, p. 215), most copies are bought by the DHSS for distribution to doctors.

In the UK, as in the USA, indeed anywhere outside the socialist societies, all professional medical journals include a large number of drug advertisements, often at the rate of every other page. The journals could not survive without this advertising revenue. Furthermore, medical practitioners regularly receive professional journals which are delivered free as part of the pharmaceutical industry's promotion efforts. Medical meetings are subsidized by drug companies, which may provide the participants with food and drink as well as advertising their wares. Doctors receive many free gifts to encourage them to prescribe particular branded products. Increasingly the ethicality of accepting these encouragements is questioned. Some doctors systematically throw all drugs advertisements into the wastepaper basket without looking at them; others refuse to see the representatives of the industry who so constantly call on them; some postgraduate medical centres may accept a company's financial support for seminars but will not permit anything more than a discrete acknowledgement of the company's name. Others do not have such scruples; they find they learn a great deal from the reps and the advertising material; they find the free gifts and samples helpful. I have personally been invited to dine with doctors' organizations where the hall in which the preprandial drinks (kindly provided by one of the pharmaceutical firms) were taken bore a greater resemblance to a trade fair than to the annual dinner of a professional medical association.

In 1983 a scandal developed which was exposed on the BBC *Panorama* programme with regard to the drug Opren which was later withdrawn (Mangold, 1983). Opren is alleged to have been associated with sixty avoidable deaths and a great deal of suffering from photosensitivity dermatitis. The drug, which was used to treat rheumatic conditions, was anti-inflammatory and not a steroid. The film included exposés of the ways in which the manufacturer, Eli Lilly, had involved doctors with, for example, a lavishly hosted seminar in Paris (Marigold, 1983, p. 3). Perhaps the most blatant piece of advertising was undertaken by Farmitalia when they decided to launch another anti-arthritic pill, a successor to Opren (*Lancet*, 1983, p. 219), with a free trip for rheumatologists on the Orient Express to dine in Venice at the firm's expense. The BBC programme also exposed the setting up and publication of dubious research in support of particular drugs.

PROFESSIONAL RESPONSIBILITY

This experience gave the medical profession pause for thought. The *Lancet* in an editorial expressed considerable disquiet, including about the revelation that 'doctors were either unwilling to admit the powerful influence of commercial pressures or unconscious of it' (1983, p. 219). The *Lancet* concluded that 'Doctors should be more careful about the invitations they accept: the drug firms' own guidelines ... are too easily bypassed' (1983, pp. 219–20). The General Medical Council's response was to refer the problem to its ethical committee, which held a private symposium about how the various codes of practice which exist, in the profession itself as well as in industry, can so easily be bypassed (GMC Minutes of Council 25–26 May 1983, para. 16, pp. 7–8). The matter was raised in open Council by the Chief Medical Officer for England.

Medical attention is frequently paid to general practitioners when control of prescribing is concerned, because they write so many scripts for so many conditions. However, the role played by hospital consultants should not be forgotten. They are responsible for hospital prescribing and may start patients off on a drug regime which general practitioners then follow. The doctors on the train to Venice were apparently rheumatologists, i.e. specialists, not GPs (*Lancet*, op. cit.).

THE INDUSTRY, THE DOCTORS AND THE RESEARCH

According to Jasper Woodcock (1981, p. 30), director of the Institute for the Study of Drug Dependence, most new drug discoveries occur in the pharmaceutical industry's own research laboratories. Much of this research is concerned with variations in existing products to overcome competition or avoid patent problems (see page 221). According to this account, university and hospital laboratories are then recruited to test clinical safety and efficacy. Others (for example, Bodenheimer, 1984, p. 200) have claimed that the major innovative work has been done in universities. It is in any case increasingly difficult to disentangle this issue. Industry has always funded academic research; with the reduction in public expenditure in the 1980s this tendency is increasing. Indeed, a new pattern is being developed, not only in biochemistry, but in scientific research more generally, whereby university research teams are set up in industrial establishments.

The same BBC programme which attacked the Venice trip funded by Eli Lilly also challenged the scientific validity of published research articles purporting to have rigorously assessed drugs. The *Lancet* (29 January 1985) felt that the attack upon drug-firm-funded research raised the most important questions of all. Not altogether opposed to such funding, the editor nevertheless felt that there was a danger of university departments becoming too dependent on industrial funds.

HOW THE INDUSTRY IS ORGANIZED

The pharmaceutical industry is not only big business, it is transnational in its scope and dominated by a small number of firms, mainly based in the United States, Switzerland, Great Britain and Japan (Bodenheimer, 1984; Lall, 1981; Melville and Johnson, 1982). Many approach the size of the large oil and finance-house transnational corporations. The majority rate among the most profitable of the giant corporations. The English Beecham Group and Glaxo are among the world's top ten pharmaceuticals (*Fortune*, 1982, quoted in Bodenheimer, 1984), the sales of which constituted nearly 28 per cent of total world sales in 1974 (Lall, 1981, p. 189). Some indication of the scale of operations is given by ICI's annual report. With a turnover of £2,984 million in 1985, pharmaceuticals constituted about a third of the total turnover of the company and its subsidiaries. They made a trading profit of £27 million, nearly three-quarters of ICI's total trading profit. Their products sell world-wide.

Patents

The system of patents greatly aids the profitability of the industry. This system provides a legal monopoly for the manufacturers of a new drug for a defined period of time which varies from country to country. Manufacturers give brand names to their drugs which are easier for doctors to remember than the generic name. The latter is derived directly from the chemical constituents of the drug. Some brand names are invented from these, e.g. Brufen for ibuprofen, Nystan for nystatin. Others link with the intended therapy. 'Pfizer called its antidiabetic, chlorpropamide, Diabinese. And Glaxo's branded combination of iron and folic acid for use during pregnancy is called Pregaday' (Melville and Johnson, 1982, p. 68).

Brand names in association with the patent system have a marked effect on pricing, for where the patent laws prevail the industry can charge what the market will stand for as long as the life of the patent. This can be shown by the case of Italy, which is unusual among highly industrialized nations in not having patent laws. Italian prices for the same drugs are much lower than they are elsewhere, showing what an important part the patent laws play in the profitability of the pharmaceutical industry. Brian Abel-Smith (1976, p. 81) has pointed out that this pricing policy has induced Italian firms to undertake raw material production. Some Eastern European countries have done the same thing. This has resulted in 'two world markets of the main pharmaceuticals – the patent market with prices set by the multinational companies and the non-patent market where prices are much more competitive' (Abel-Smith, 1976, p. 81).

There is no real competition among the for-profit transnationals. Rather, there is a structured coexistence whereby corporations develop lines where there seems to be a chance of exploiting the market. The game has become more sophisticated than it was in the days when 'molecular roulette' was commonly played to avoid patent rights; that is, small molecular changes were made in what was essentially the same product. There is, however, still some tendency to the 'me-too' type of activity whereby companies develop similar products where a market seems worth further exploitation.

Sales Promotion

This form of controlled capitalist competition has led to more of the industry's research potential going on modifications and developments of existing products than upon real innovation. However, even more has gone on sales promotion. Mention has already been made of the pressures exerted upon doctors by sales representatives. In the late 1970s sales promotion as a proportion of sales amounted in the USA to 22 per cent and in the UK to 15 per cent, the lowest of seven nations quoted by Lall (1981, p. 195). It is claimed that expenditure on sales promotion includes expenditure on continuing education for doctors faced with massive changes since the days they were trained (Abel-Smith, 1976, p. 83). However, there is considerable dissatisfaction about the data which are provided. Thus Peters (1981) shares with others such as Herxheimer and Lionel (1978) a conviction that prescribers are insufficiently well informed about the properties of the drugs they prescribe.

THE STATE AND THE SAFETY OF MEDICINES

Everywhere the state has found itself inevitably involved with the safety of medicines. Involvement or increased involvement has generally followed disaster. The Food and Drug Administration (FDA) in the USA was early faced with a difficulty. In 1937 the Tennessee Massengill Company produced a form of sulphanilamide for children called Elixir Sulfanilamide-Massengill. It was made by dissolving the sulphanilamide in diethylene glycol (a principal constituent of antifreeze). Over a hundred child and adult deaths resulted; there was no known antidote. Subsequently the FDA, whose powers have been progressively extended, has been called 'the most onerous regulation in the world' (Lumbroso, 1981, p. 72), on the one hand, and, on the other, a body whose only interest appears to be the avoidance of the worst scandals of pharmaceutical abuse, scandals which undercut people's faith in "private enterprise" and which can lead to extremely expensive lawsuits for drug companies' (Bodenheimer, 1984, p. 210).

British government involvement with medicines began because of its responsibility for purchasing drugs for the NHS. In 1949, only a year after the NHS was inaugurated, the Joint Committee on the Classification of Proprietary preparations was set up to advise ministers on the status of proprietary preparations and to indicate where less expensive forms existed. After the thalidomide disaster the Committee on Safety of Drugs was established in 1963 to monitor the way the industry tested drugs before they were put on the market. Thalidomide, prescribed to pregnant women, turned out to be a teratogene; that is, it changed the body shape of those children whose mothers had taken it during pregnancy. About 8,000 children survived with absent or shortened limbs (*Sunday Times* Insight Team, 1979, quoted in Melville and Johnson, 1982, p. 20).

The Committee on Safety of Drugs continued after the Joint Committee was dissolved in 1964. The Sainsbury Committee of 1965 was followed by the Medicines Act of 1968 which established the Committee on Safety of Medicines (CSM) as the successor to the Committee on Safety of Drugs. The CSM's responsibilities lie in licensing new drugs and removing drugs from the market. Under the 1968 Act no drug can be put on the market until a product licence has been applied for and received. The criteria used are safety, efficiency and pharmaceutical quality. The need for the drug and its comparative efficacy in relation to other drugs on the market are not criteria which are used (*British Medical Journal*, 5 January 1985, p. 58). The Committee receives a great deal of information about the new drug which includes clinical trials on 1,000 patients, 100 of whom have been treated for a year, several hundred for six months and the remainder for less than that. This means that long-term effects have not been thoroughly studied, and post-marketing surveillance is therefore important. The Committee runs the 'yellow card' system, whereby doctors are issued with yellow cards on which they are asked to report suspected adverse drug reactions. The CSM does have what has been called 'the draconian power of immediate suspension' (*British Medical Journal*, 5 January 1985, p. 58), which is rarely used although it was used for benoxaprofen (Opren; see page 219) and indoprofen (Flosint) because the alleged damage being caused by these drugs was so great.

The Industry and the State

The British government has two further interests in the pharmaceutical industry. As a major purchaser it is concerned to keep the price of drugs as low as possible; at the same time its responsibilities for the promotion of exports from British pharmaceutical companies lead it to encourage high profitability in those companies. There is some evidence that the NHS bulk purchase of drugs does mean that they are available at cheaper rates to the NHS than they are elsewhere. The case of Librium in 1964 is an interesting example. The basic cost was four shillings for 1,000 tablets. La Roche sold it to the NHS at £10 per 1,000, a profit of 5,000 per cent. In the summer of 1973 the DHSS refused to continue paying these inflated prices. Hoffman La Roche retaliated by taking the case to the House of Lords. Ultimately the company paid back £1.6 million to the British government in compensation for excess profits (Lang, 1974; Melville and Johnson, 1982). In its role as promoter of British pharmaceuticals the Industries and Exports Division of the DHSS was formed in the mid-1970s with resultant sharp increases in medical exports. The loans made by Ministry of Overseas Development for health aid projects involved the purchase of British medical equipment (Doyal with Pennell, 1979, pp. 270–3).

The Limited Drugs List

The DHSS is concerned not only with the price it pays for drugs but also with the number of NHS prescriptions that are written and filled out. These constitute about 10 per cent of the total NHS bill (OHE, 1986, table 11, p. 25). There has for many years been a medical lobby which suggested that doctors should prescribe using only generic names, rather than brand names, since this would reduce the pharmaceutical bill. At one time doctors could not prescribe by brand name on the NHS where there was a BNF equivalent. Thus soluble aspirin was to be prescribed rather than Disprin, for example. Then the powerful pharmaceutical lobby in Whitehall persuaded the DHSS that there were real differences in the brand-name products.

Some hospitals, encouraged by the DHSS, have instituted restricted drug lists to their hospital pharmacies. Wandsworth group are one such; Joe Collier and John Foster (1985, p. 333) have reported the experiment:

> A restricted drugs list has now been used in the hospitals of the Wandsworth district for five years. The list has reduced costs to the district and risks to the patients. It has also saved time in the pharmacy which now has to handle fewer drugs, it has probably improved prescribing by junior staff who have fewer drugs with which to become familiar, and it is likely to have improved the welfare of patients since such a system can direct those conducting 'unofficial trials' to the ethical committee.

The 1985 edition of the list contained 'about 2,000 of the possible 18,000 dosage forms available in the UK and just over one quarter of the items listed in the *BNF*' (Collier and Foster, 1985, p. 331). And there are possibilities for consultants to prescribe outside the list. Modes exist for admitting new drugs and deleting existing ones; the latter has turned out to be quite difficult to do.

Controlling prescribing in hospital practice is a different kind of exercise from control in general practice, however.

For many years some medical practitioners have favoured the use of a restricted drug list in general practice, similar to the hospital list described. Others have argued for voluntary restrictions on the part of GPs. The DHSS has exhorted them over many years to prescribe responsibly with an eye to the cost. The Regional Medical Officers have from the outset of the NHS visited GPs whose prescribing bill is considerably higher than the average in their neighbourhood to encourage them to reduce their prescription costs. The World Health Organization has drawn up a list of about 200 drugs which it feels are adequate for all basic needs, whereas probably about 15,000 are in use in the UK (Woodcock, 1981).

In 1984 the government moved and indicated that it would impose a limited drug list upon all GPs (*Lancet*, 17 November 1984, 8412, p. 1166). Around the turn of the year it announced the members of the panel who were to draw up the list (*Lancet*, 5 January 1985, 8419, p. 62), and by the end of February the list was published and due to come into operation on 1 April 1985. The original proposal created a great deal of opposition from practitioners who felt that their clinical autonomy was being infringed. The BMA was extremely heated, as the pages of the *British Medical Journal* make plain. There was even more opposition from the pharmaceutical industry itself. One of the latter's ploys seriously misfired. La Roche had sent letters to doctors to sign and send on to their MPs in protest against the limited list proposals. The MPs' sympathies for the company were not evoked; they thought they were being got at by La Roche. The prescribable list of drugs was published along with a second black list of drugs and preparations which are not to be available through the NHS. These include certain antacids, laxatives, analgesics for mild to moderate pain, cough and cold remedies, bitters and tonics, vitamins, sedatives and tranquillizers. In each of these categories, however, there is a prescribable limited list. This list the DHSS advisers say includes examples of all drugs which might be needed in general practice. The *Lancet* and the *Drugs and Therapeutics Bulletin*, the latter published by the Consumers Association, concur with this view.

Undoubtedly the whole exercise has made the profession more conscious of its prescribing responsibilities. Already the Royal College of General Practitioners had a responsible prescribing campaign afoot. In 1985 also the *British Medical Journal* started a regular column on the Committee on Safety of Medicines. It can be seen from this debate that the medical profession is divided in its attitude to prescribing. Those who have supported the notion of the limited list clearly have defined their professional responsibilities and the interests of the pharmaceutical industry in a different way from those represented in the pages of the *BMJ*.

PHARMACEUTICALS AND THE THIRD WORLD

The marketing and testing of drugs in the Third World have long been of concern to responsible medical practitioners, administrators and others (see, for example, Abel-Smith, 1976; Bodenheimer, 1984; Doyal with Pennell, 1979; Melville and Johnson, 1982; Silverman, 1977; Silverman and Lee, 1974; Silverman and Lydecker, 1981; Vass, 1985).

The charges are that the industry is more concerned to seek its profits than to improve health; that it adopts different standards in advertising and promotion in countries where there are strong governmental controls and a well-educated and informed medical profession from those which it adopts elsewhere. Silverman and Lydecker (1981) report a 1974 study which showed what they call 'unbelievable' and 'sickening' differences between the way multinationals were promoting identical drugs to medical practitioners in the USA and ten Latin American countries. Thus, for example, doctors in the USA were warned of the possible serious or fatal side-effects of chloramphenicol, but doctors in Central America were not warned. This proved also to be true for other antibiotics and for drugs in the following range: oral contraceptives, non-steroid anti-arthritics, steroid hormones, anti-psychotic tranquillizers, antidepressants, and anticonvulsants. The authors report the tragic toll not only from direct adverse side-effects but also from the development of drug-resistant strains of organisms consequent upon the excessive and inappropriate use of antibiotics (Silverman and Lydecker, 1981).

When an inquiry was held in the USA following the publication of these data, some improvements in practice were noted. Bodenheimer claims, however, that since that time the FDA has not been sufficiently firm with the industry. The latter claims that the FDA controls limit its chances of competitiveness in world markets because it has to wait for clearance while extensive tests are made (Bodenheimer, 1984, pp. 198 and 110–11).

British as well as US-based multinationals are implicated. *MIMS* (see page 218) is produced in a number of editions. The editions for Third World consumption contain information which is different from that in the British edition, being less explicit than that available to physicians in the home market.

The representatives of the pharmaceutical industry seek to influence governments as well as physicians. Allegations of bribery are made. There are also problems about lack of control by government and profession (Vass, 1985, p. 12).

The heavy promotion of 'a pill for every ill' philosophy includes vitamins for senility (for which there is no known specific) and, perhaps most emotively cruel, of appetite stimulants as a cure for childhood malnutrition and steroids to promote growth.

The pattern of drug-taking which has developed and is promoted in the Third World has two serious consequences, one which is serious for inhabitants of the Third World themselves, the second which is serious not only for them but for all the world. The problem which specifically assails the Third World is that vast sums are spent on expensive branded products, some useless or dangerous and many inappropriately used, and too little spent on essential drugs. Health workers find they lack the essentials, such as penicillin, when many branded but irrelevant products are widely available.

The second problem is the development of antibiotic-resistant strains because of the misuse of antibiotics. The problem has been known for over a decade but persists. Resistant strains of typhoid have already led to uncontrollable epidemics in Latin America and the Far East; a visitor may contract and bring home strains of VD which are resistant. Perhaps now overshadowed in the public mind by the risks of AIDS, these hazards are nevertheless real.

EXPENSIVE MEDICAL TECHNIQUES (EMTs)

The bill for high-technology equipment may be smaller than that for hospital labour, but it is not unimportant. (Excluding doctors, dentists and pharmacists, over half the cost of the NHS went on wages and salaries in 1984: OHE, 1986, p. 13; while probably three-quarters of the cost overall derives from labour costs: Butler and Vaile, 1984, p. 54.) Expensive medical techniques (EMTs) not only involve the cost of the high technology itself but also have knock-on labour and other costs. An example may suffice. On account of the reluctance of health authorities to invest in whole-body computed tomography (CT) scanners in the 1970s, there were many public collections of money to buy the equipment. This in itself was expensive, but its staffing and maintenance were even more so. The equipment could cost as much as a small hospital to run. Thus there are two economic facets to the purchase of expensive medical technological equipment; the first is the capital cost, and the second the running costs in terms of labour and maintenance. There may also be social costs, as in the widespread introduction of induction, to which we shall turn later (see page 240).

The NHS has always been dependent upon private industry for the provision of hospital supplies as it has been dependent on it for the provision of drugs. It is only more recently when increasingly expensive techniques are being introduced that serious attention has been paid to the problem. The attention has been directed mostly to the control mechanisms, or their lack, whereby expensive new techniques are introduced. The issue of expenditure on technology has not become an emotive popular issue as pharmaceuticals have. The anxiety has expressed itself in various ways; the Royal Commission on the NHS in 1979 discussed the introduction of technology into medicine and recommended an independent health service research unit to evaluate EMTs, (HMSO, 1979, S.17.39). In 1982 the Council for Science and Society (CSS) was concerned that things were going wrong and set up a working party on EMTs. An earlier working party on aspects of new reproductive technology had raised a number of doubts about the way those procedures had been introduced and the problems involved, a matter to which we shall turn in Chapter 17 (CSS, 1980). Among the EMTs the example of CT scanners, already mentioned, was one instance where the effect was an unplanned change of direction in the allocation of health resources and thus of health care. A disaster revealed by the paediatrician William Silverman (1980) was the serious damage to the eyes of infants by retrolineal fibroplasia when units for the new-born were first supplied with piped oxygen. The concentrations were too strong. Inadequate testing had taken place. The damage was distressing.

The Case of CT Scanning

An early careful analysis was the study by Barbara Stocking and Stuart Morrison (1978) of the introduction of computed tomography (CT scanning). They chose this as one example; there could have been others – for example, the introduction of renal dialysis machines, implantable cardiac pacemakers, or automatic analysers (Stocking and Morrison, 1978, p. 1). The interplay of ideas developing in industry, guidance in the shape of encouragement or discouragement from the DHSS to invest in development and the demands of doctors for the new technology all emerge. A scientist in EMI's central research laboratory in Britain recognized the implications of his work on imaging for radiology. Advised by a panel of experts, the DHSS decided to fund a prototype brain scanner and later two others. It also subsidized the staffing and running costs of a further two prototypes (p. 9). The brain scanners proved to be clinically valuable in diagnosis, and by mid-1977 there were about thirty brain scanners already installed.

· While the DHSS had a high degree of control over the initiation and introduction of brain scanners, 'with the body scanner, events overtook evaluation and the same orderly procedure was not followed' (Stocking and Morrison, 1978, p. 11). The DHSS no longer had funds to buy enough scanners for a thorough evaluation, and furthermore philanthropists had already donated a number to private and NHS hospitals. The result was that the body scanners were diffused rapidly throughout the service, without adequate evaluation and at great cost. Brain and body scanners each cost about a quarter of a million pounds and about £50,000 per annum to run at mid-1970s prices. This may be compared with the cost of a renal dialysis machine at that time of £3,500 (Stocking and Morrison, 1978, pp. 12 and 15).

The technology having been made possible by industry, Stocking and Morrison (1978, p. 14) suggest that the prime movers for the new body scanners were the consultant radiologists, who could see their potential. The clinical uses and safety of CT scanners were not properly evaluated before their wide diffusion. Their uses were not set against other medical imagining techniques such as ultrasound and the use of radio-isotopes and the isotope scanner. When Stocking and Morrison were writing, nuclear magnetic resonance was not much more than a gleam in the eye. It was 'probably a number of years away'. That technique, also expensive, is becoming increasingly widespread. It is the view of Stocking and Morrison that medical technology 'can be pushed in socially desirable directions which may not be the same as the route industry would take if left to itself. But to achieve such movement, a better mechanism of interaction between the NHS and industry is needed' (1978, pp. 45–6). The interplay between industry, DHSS and NHS is complicated.

The State and EMTs

As in the case of pharmaceuticals, the DHSS has an interest in encouraging developments in British industry just as much as it has in controlling NHS expenditure. As the Council for Science and Society point out:

> EMTs do not emerge from out of the blue and then oblige the NHS to make up its mind to devote funds to them or reject them. On the contrary, encouragement given to technologists and manufacturers by individuals and groups in the NHS influences what new techniques are developed. NHS policies create more or less favourable conditions for a manufacturer to develop and produce new equipment. DHSS, with the encouragement of the British Technology Group (formerly the National Enterprise Board), may give some assistance to produce equipment to meet a known need, especially when there is a good prospect of export sales. The manufacturer then promotes it with the interested clinicians or even charities.
>
> (Council for Science and Society, 1982, p. 15)

Individual clinicians, while knowing what they would like to improve their practice, have no, or little, sense of the overall demands on the health service and do not, unencouraged, balance their claims against those of others. In this way they may play into the hands of industry rather than forwarding overall health needs of patients.

Within the DHSS is the Supplies Division, which has a Technical and Scientific Branch. This keeps in touch with services divisions. Within the service divisions there are advisory groups relevant to most types of equipment, laboratory, radiological and so on. Clinical evaluations are mounted to test whether equipment does what it says it will do, but such evaluations on behalf of the Supplies Division do not usually question clinical needs and whether the equipment meets them (CSS, 1982, p. 14).

In terms of health policy, like Stocking and Morrison (1978) the Council for Science and Society (1982) argues strongly for a better evaluation of EMTs before they are put into service use. This evaluation should take account of the technique's effectiveness and efficiency; it should furthermore take account of patient acceptability and acceptability to their lay carers, not merely of the technique's perceived appropriateness from the point of view of the consultant and the health service manager. There should also be much wider involvement of interested persons in the evaluation process than there is at present. 'That an EMT is rational in the sense that it has been shown to correct a fault in an internal bodily process is not sufficient evidence that its clinical application is efficacious, or effective, and safe' (CSS, 1982, p. 50).

As I pointed out at the start of this discussion, studying some of the consequences of the new obstetrics had already alerted the CSS to the wider implications of introducing new techniques and the problems that might arise in the process of correcting 'an internal bodily process', for there is more to healing than that. Furthermore, patients and potential patients are active participants. Had the advice of the CSS been available and taken when the new reproductive technologies were being developed, had a wide array of interested parties been involved and had account been taken of the psychological and social consequences, the story that will be told in Chapter 17 about human reproduction in the late twentieth century and its prognosis for the future might well have been different.

17 Reproduction for the Twenty-First Century

The knowledge and techniques available to us as human beings to control and manipulate conception are greater now than they have ever been; the manipulation of inherited characteristics is understood and on the agenda. The way these various techniques are applied is likely to have profound consequences for reproduction in the twenty-first century – not only for reproduction but for the social structure and social values more generally. If the framework of analysis which has been used throughout this book has any merit, it should help to guide us through the complexities which now confront us.

In previous chapters we have discussed aspects of gender and the division of health labour. We saw how biomedicine developed as an exclusively male profession until towards the end of the nineteenth century; we noted that it was not until the 1970s that women began to be admitted to medical schools in anything like equal proportions with men. Consequently men remain for the present time heavily dominant in all the positions of power and influence in medicine and health care. In the area of reproduction we saw how the 'men-midwives' (obstetricians) ousted the midwives from the control of reproduction; for many hundreds of years previously women had helped others give birth, using skills and customs passed down from generation to generation of midwives, using accumulated wisdom and personal experience. By the outset of the twentieth century, although the great majority of births were still attended by midwives, these women were now legally required to call doctors in when any abnormality was discovered. Since 1902 midwives have had a clear place in the British health-care division of labour, but one which was subservient to the doctors, still mostly men. We also saw, following Gamarnikow (1978), how in another aspect of the division of labour, that between nurses and doctors, the gender order of the Victorian bourgeois family was recreated with the doctor-father, nurse-mother and patient-child. What we have not yet discussed, which must be addressed in this chapter, are the implications for reproduction of the medical take-over of childbirth. This has particularly crucial implications for the uses to which the new reproductive techniques are being and will in the future be put, and by whom.

We have also reviewed the nature of medical knowledge and paid some attention to its mode of production and reproduction. We saw that biomedicine has fairly limited goals, being predominantly concerned with the functioning of the human body as a piece of apparatus liable to malfunction in various ways and from time to time. In principle the knowledge is based on systematic scientific study, much of it undertaken in the laboratory. In addition, it accumulates through clinical trials when the efficacy of a particular treatment is tried out on patients. In the best practice this is done systematically through techniques such as the randomized controlled trial, but some clinical practice is based more on hunch than on scientific method.

Knowledge about the female reproductive system was developed in this way. The use of the speculum to view the interior of a woman's vagina, and of surgery in childbirth and gynaecological surgery, in the case of things being amiss in the female reproductive organs, gave medical men an increasingly clear map of the female genitalia, such that not only did her doctor know more about her body than a woman did, but men came to know more about women's bodies than women did (Arney, 1982; Oakley, 1984). This led much later, in the 1960s and 1970s, to women seeking to reclaim control of our own bodies, lay women teaching each other how to use the speculum with the aid of a mirror to see themselves for themselves (Phillips and Rakusen, 1978).

Both science and its application to reproduction were developed by men. It has been argued, and with some justification, that in consequence the mode of science is a masculine mode; that the questions it has asked are those which are the primary concern to men in a sex-segregated society; and that it has sought solutions in a masculinist manner (Oakley, 1984; Rose, 1983; Wallsgrove, 1980). I have argued elsewhere (Stacey, 1986a) that the charges against Wendy Savage, the obstetrician from Tower Hamlets who was suspended from duty by her health authority, arose at least in part because of her attempts to take women's experiential knowledge into account in her practice of obstetrics (Savage, 1986).

On the question of sexuality we saw how the nineteenth-century attempts to control venereal diseases followed a mode which was quite different from the way in which the control of other infectious or contagious diseases was sought; control, exercised by men, was through women and not at all through men. We also saw the part which the medical profession played, not only in supporting those measures, but in creating the images of masculinity and femininity and their definition of any sexual activity, whether by women or men, which fell outside heterosexual intercourse as pathological.

In this chapter I propose to look at the way sexuality and reproduction are handled in the late twentieth century; at the orientation of biomedicine towards them and the interventions which are considered appropriate; the attitudes and actions of the state; the problems perceived, protests made, and alternative solutions suggested. The area is of critical importance because it has to do with the reproduction of the entire society, both its physical biological reproduction and the reproduction of its most crucial values.

FERTILITY CONTROL

Attempts to control fertility must be as old as copulation and childbirth themselves. In many societies women had shared understandings about when to admit male lovers; prolonged breast-feeding afforded some protection, it seems; withdrawal and abstinence were well known and widely used; abortion was practised anciently, as well as infanticide when unwanted children were born. What is new in the second half of the twentieth century is not the attempts at fertility control itself, but the much more successful modes available and also the form of their control.

Abortion and Infanticide
Infanticide is perhaps the oldest and the least preferred way of controlling fertility. It is wasteful of women's life and labour and of the life that has been

born. Not only is it uneconomic, it raises and has always raised manifold moral problems. While overtaken in many parts of the world by other methods, it still persists. Thus Madhu Kishwar (1985) attributes the low ratio of women to men in parts of India to continuing female infanticide.

Rather than carry to term and then destroy the infant, women always and everywhere have sought to abort an unwanted pregnancy (even when dominant religious or secular norms or rules forbid this). Abortion has raised many problems, about rights in the unborn child, rights of the unborn child and the woman's right to control her own life. For the majority of women seeking or achieving abortions, however, the question has not been so much one of rights but of being driven by social and economic necessity. A child born out of wedlock in a society with strong mores about marriage and fertility will not only bring disgrace or disaster to its mother but will itself have poor life chances. Many women have felt in these circumstances that they have no choice but to attempt abortion. Rosalind Petchesky (1985, pp. 156–60), discussing the importance of state aid for abortion in the United States, has demonstrated the social and economic imperatives which lead poor women there to seek abortions, whether legal or illegal, at considerable cost to themselves. The women are convinced that these risks are less than the consequences of carrying the child to term and of rearing it (see also Rich, 1977, pp. 266–7). Nor in cases of poor women is it necessarily that a child is not wanted; rather, that it is not going to be possible to rear this child appropriately.

Abortion nevertheless arouses a good deal of emotion and has been rendered sinful or illegal or both by many religious and state authorities. In religious terms the notion has most often been that women should experience sexual pleasure only for the intended purpose of procreation. Such rules have prevailed in patriarchal societies. According to Mernissi (1975), before Islam, Arabic women were self-determining in a way which became impossible after the establishment of the Islamic patriarchal kinship system. Previously they were able to select lovers and had greater possibility of controlling their fertility. It seems likely that the strict control of abortion has been associated with patriarchal societies, religious societies and religious systems which are male-dominated.

Socially acceptable abortion has a longer history in Britain than in the USA of which Petchesky (1985) was speaking. As long ago as 1936 a British feminist pressure group worked to extend the availability of legal abortions (Randall, 1982). Its antecedents went back more than a hundred years (Banks, 1954). The 1930s agitation followed the work of socialist and feminist women such as Stella Browne, Dora Russell and Janet Chance in the 1920s (Doyal with Pennell, 1979). It was not until 1967, however, that an Act was passed in Britain which effectively made abortion on social and health (as well as medical) grounds legal. While this did not meet the feminist goal of 'abortion on demand', justified by belief in a woman's 'right to choose', it was welcomed and has been supported by women nevertheless. The extent of its welcome by many women may in part be judged by the increase in legal abortions which followed. Alison Macfarlane and Miranda Mugford (1984) have gathered together the data derived from the notification of abortions required by the 1967 Act. Figure 17.1 reproduces their findings. The data from England and Wales and from Scotland 'both show an

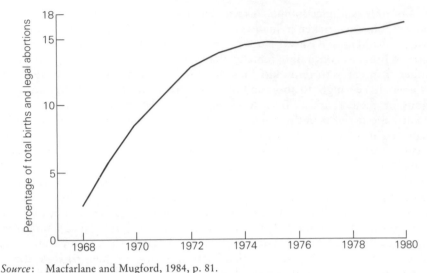

Figure 17.1   *Legal abortions as a percentage of total births and legal abortions, 1968–80.*

increase in legal abortion up to 1973 as the services developed, then a decrease in the mid-1970s, followed by another increase' (p. 81). They point out further-more that this rise in legal abortions coincided with a rise in the birth rate. Satisfactory explanations of birth-rate fluctuations are still lacking.

When there was an attempt by John Corrie MP in 1979 to amend the Abortion Act a remarkably united demonstration on the part of many women's organizations took place to retain the legality of abortions. The great majority of women's organizations, except those linked with LIFE and SPUC, the major anti-abortion agencies, demonstrated together. At that time there were still many women who remembered the tragedies of 'back-street abortions' of the pre-1967 and prewar days. In those days women who could not afford to buy a private abortion had recourse to less than hygienic or safe methods undertaken in the back streets by persons some of whom were humane while others unscrupulously exploited their 'patients'. The same could be said, of course, of the medical practitioners who 'obliged'; some did it from high moral motives (despite the illegality), others for the fat fees they could earn. In these circumstances the 1979 anti-Corrie campaign slogan, 'Keep it legal – keep it safe', can be readily understood. The opposition of medical practitioners' organizations to the Corrie Bill was crucial to its defeat. The depth of feeling and belief, however, of those who hold that any termination of pregnancy is murder has to be recognized. In a personal communication one pro-LIFE person likened the consequences of the 1967 Act to the decimation caused by the Black Death (see Simms, 1985).

Legal abortions may be performed under the National Health Service, but their availability varies from one part of the country to another. The Act includes a 'conscience clause' whereby those medical practitioners who are opposed to abortions are not required to perform them. In some regions the appointment of a rather high number of pro-LIFE obstetricians and gynaecologists has meant that NHS abortions are not easily available (Doyal, 1985, pp. 244–5). Women have either to travel to another part of the country, possibly using an accommodation address, or to 'go private'. Many of the private abortions are undertaken at cost or sometimes less by charities of which the British Pregnancy Advisory Service (BPAS) is the largest (Macfarlane and Mugford, 1984, pp. 81–2). Private, for profit, facilities with high fees are also available.

Practitioners may be selective about the women to whom they are prepared to offer antenatal care, abortions, or sterilizations. Sally Macintyre (1976a and 1976b) found that they used social typifications which are generally available to guide them in these decisions rather than any scientifically derived evidence.

> Promotion of childbirth is therefore regarded as reasonable for young married women. It is not regarded as reasonable for those who are too young or too old, have 'enough' children already, are unmarried or who wish a child by someone other than their husbands.
>
> (1976a, p. 187).

Other rules are used to typify those who may reasonably wish not to have children. Thus difficult marital circumstances might constitute a reason, but generally speaking young married women without 'too many' children cannot reasonably expect an abortion or sterilization. Unmarried women on the other hand are not expected to want to carry a baby to term, and may have trouble engaging the pro-natalist skills of the doctor. Macfarlane and Mugford (1984, p. 82) note that terminations in non-NHS premises include proportionately more operations on single women than those in NHS premises. (They also include proportionately more first trimester abortions.) Non-NHS premises are generally set up solely for fertility control and do not suffer the same contradictory pro- and anti-natalist pulls of NHS clinics.

Contraception
Thomas McKeown (1971, p. 36; and see pages 76, 136) has argued that contraception was one of the main reasons for increased longevity and health. But this was no thanks to the medical profession. The birth control movement was largely lay (see Aitken-Swan, 1977; Banks, 1954 and 1981). In the middle of the twentieth century the contraceptive modes available were those which had been available in the 1880s. In 1945 a woman wishing to be fitted with a diaphragm, or 'dutch cap' as they were called, had to find a family planning clinic or, if her income was too high to be accepted at such a place, to be referred privately to a friendly gynaecologist, possibly one working in the clinic prevented from helping her. The sheath for men was commercially and widely available, but mostly in back-street shops. Sheaths were never on obvious display in chemists' shops, nor were the various spermicides. Hurdles made up of cost and embarrassment assailed the responsible married contraceptor, who had to know what she wanted, where to find it and how to ask for it. The unmarried had more to dare.

In a useful review of the history of contraceptive technology Vivien Walsh (1980) discusses why it was that the pharmaceutical industry was so slow to develop a contraceptive pill. The scientific knowledge was available, but despite the vast potential market of fertile women wishing to control their fertility, the industry did not invest in it. The industry's contribution to the profitable but largely clandestine contraceptives which did exist was kept quiet. The failure to develop the technology from available understanding partly arose from the fragmented arenas in which the scientific work was done, the lack of interaction between biological, chemical and clinical studies. The opposition or indifference of doctors meant there was little or no pressure from them for clinical applications. The industry was afraid of coming out publicly in support of contraception, fearing that it might lead to losses of support and trade from Roman Catholic and other sections of the public opposed on principled grounds to contraception.

It was not until 1960 that Searle, the US pharmaceutical company, introduced the first contraceptive pill ('*the* pill'); it came to the UK about two years later. Throughout the 1960s the manufacture and development of the pill expanded, greatly to the profit of the pharmaceutical industry. Its distribution was controlled by doctors, who were, it appeared, more prepared to handle this form of contraception and began to withdraw their opposition from birth control (Walsh, 1980, pp. 186–7). Although opposed to its general use, medical professionals had themselves used contraception extensively in their private lives for many years (Walsh, 1980, pp. 185–6). Initially patients wishing contraceptive advice had to pay a fee, for it was not available on the NHS until 1974. Under the 1974 arrangements general practitioners get an extra fee for their contraceptive services, now paid for by the NHS and not the patient. It seems strange that, when contraception has improved the health of women and their children by the avoidance of repeated child bearing and of too many bodies to clothe and mouths to feed, medical men were so slow to support birth control. General practitioners still see it as an extra activity for which they should be paid, rather than as central to the health care of their patients.

The arrival of the pill was hailed as a great liberation for women. Now they could be as free sexually as men had ever been; a solution had been found, it was thought, to the problem of the 'double standard', albeit not a solution that Josephine Butler would have approved of (see pages 74–5). The solution was rapidly found not to be so liberating for women as was first thought. Two separate problems emerged; one was the unwanted side-effects of the pill experienced by many women; the second was the increased sexual exploitation of women by men.

The enthusiastic reception of the pill in the 1960s had stressed its positive advantages for women including those over and above its contraceptive properties. Women with irregular periods welcomed the regularity it induced; advertisements suggested that the pill would help them retain their youthful appearance. That every drug is a potential poison (see page 215) was perhaps for a while overlooked. It was some years before the side-effects were publicly recognized. It was established that deaths from thrombosis could be and were a side-effect, and associations with cancer emerged. Side-effects are now well recognized, although not all associations are clear. Adjustments have been made to the pills to change the proportions of oestrogens and progestin, and new forms of progestin have been synthesized. It seems that before launching the pill extensive tests had been undertaken to show it was an effective contraceptive, but insufficient tests had been made to assess any harmful effects (Walsh, 1980, p. 203; see also Phillips and Rakusen, 1978, pp. 244–59).

In addition to side-effects that to start with were not well understood, general practitioners appeared, and in some cases still appear, to be insufficiently careful, before prescribing or represcribing, in taking a woman's history and checking her physically to ascertain if she is likely to fall into an at-risk group, for thrombosis, for example. These matters have led to a good deal of space being made available in women's magazines and feminist publications for the discussion of problems associated with the contraceptive pill and to self-education in women's groups. Some women's groups advocate methods such as the diaphragm and spermicides rather than any of the pills, on the grounds that all continue to have unacceptable consequences for the woman's health.

The Depoprovera Debate

Depoprovera, the long-acting injectable contraceptive (which acts for three or six months, thus avoiding the daily ingestion of a pill), has been the cause of a great deal of controversy. For long it was licensed only on a temporary basis by the Commission on the Safety of Medicine (CSM) because of suspicions that it caused cancer, particularly of the breast, and had other side-effects. However, after an inquiry in 1983, although banned in the USA, the CSM licensed it for long-term use in Britain.

Many women were opposed to it, not only because there were doubts about its safety, but also because of the way in which it was administered in some cases. It was alleged to have been injected into women, generally of low social status, who were deemed by their doctors to be incapable of remembering to take a daily pill, without the women being given a proper choice or really understanding what was being done to them (Rakusen, 1981). However, it is also argued that for some Muslim women it is the only contraceptive they could use, for their husbands would throw away any device or pill which they found about the house. For them any risk would be less than the risks of repeated child bearing (but see Balasubrahmanyan, 1984, pp. 156–7). Its use with mentally handicapped women also reveals contradictions. In the past, sexual relations were denied to women and men categorized as mentally subnormal, on the grounds that they should not reproduce, either because their condition was hereditable, or because they were judged not to have the wit to raise children satisfactorily. With injections of depoprovera it was felt that there need be no impediment to their mating and marrying. Herein are starkly revealed all the paradoxes of liberal humane attempts at solutions to difficult problems. A better life is available but only on these paternalistic terms.

Pill as Liberator?

The second problem which began to be recognized about the use of the pill was that it was in practice more liberating for men than for women. Men tended to assume that all nubile women were on the pill and therefore available. Men thus took even less thought for the consequences of their sexual acts than heretofore. True, a woman on the pill could avoid pregnancy with a reasonably high degree of certainty. However, she had to take the pill daily for at least three out of every four weeks throughout the year. This is a chore in any case, but a bitter pill if she has no lover. These understandings began to emerge in studies of unintended teenage pregnancies. Women with steady boy-friends contracepted responsibly. When the relationship broke they ceased to take the pill and thus were all too likely to 'fall' at the start of a new relationship. Contraception turned out not to be the rational procedure that many in the birth control movement had imagined. Life is not altogether rational and especially in matters of the 'heart'.

Evidence now available of possible adverse consequences of the long-term use of the pill suggests that the young women who take the pill only when they are in a steady sexual relationships are probably behaving wisely. Many young men nevertheless continued and continue to assume that women are protected all the time and readily available to them for the 'one-night stand' or a longer affair. Not so liberating for the women after all, who may not always find themselves able to say 'no', or have that 'no' heeded.

The slowness with which the pharmaceutical industry took up the pill may now seem surprising. The major responsibility for contraception was left with the women. Little research has been done on male reproduction (Pfeffer, 1985). The industry has not developed contraceptives for men other than the condom. The AIDS epidemic has reinstated that mode, at least in the DHSS propaganda, as the best means of giving protection from AIDS. This stress on male responsibility is new and, it has to be noted, has arisen in the context of an epidemic disease, not of fertility control.

Apart from the condom, the only contraception which has more recently come into use has been vasectomy for men, a simpler and less hazardous operation than is sterilization for women. Numbers of men who do not wish for more children, or who do not wish for children at all, have had vasectomies. Many more refuse, feeling apparently that their masculinity would thereby somehow be impugned, leaving their wives to contracept or to undergo the far more serious and disruptive operation (e.g. Roberts, 1981; see also Simms and Smith, 1982).

The rhythm method of contraception is acceptable to those who believe that mechanical or chemical modes are sinful. However, unless the date of ovulation can be known with a reasonably high degree of certainty, the method is not reliable. It is reported that a simple test is now available, but is being promoted for artificial insemination and *in vitro* fertilization rather than for contraception. It has been suggested that this is associated with the threat to the contraceptive market which it might pose (*British Journal of Sexual Medicine*, December 1985, quoted in MIDIRS, 1986).

CHILDBIRTH

Doctors may have had problems in recognizing their role in controlling fertility but, as we have seen (page 234), once they had overcome their difficulties about engaging in obstetric practice at all, they became fully and increasingly involved with reproduction. These developments have led not only to the almost complete medicalization of childbirth, but also to its transfer to hospital; from the private domain of the home under the control of experienced women to the public domain of the hospital under the control mainly of men.

This process has changed the image of childbirth. Whereas at one time it was seen as a normal physiological activity which might occasionally go wrong, every pregnancy is now considered as potentially pathological (Arney, 1982; Oakley, 1984). The settlement of the dispute between midwives and obstetricians led to the 1902 Midwives Register which left midwives as independent practitioners in charge in their own right of normal births, but with a responsibility to call a medical practitioner should any abnormal circumstances present. This legal status with its attendant rights and obligations still remains in force. However, developments since 1902 and particularly in the latter part of the twentieth century have reduced midwives to the status of technical nurses working under medical direction in the majority of cases. The confidence of general practitioners in their ability to deliver a baby in the mother's home has also been destroyed. The confidence of women in our ability to deliver without a great deal of technological back-up has also been shaken.

Pregnancy Testing and Antenatal Care

A woman who suspects she is pregnant does not now wait for three months before becoming privately convinced that she is right. If she wants to be pregnant she seeks urgent confirmation which will help her feel she has some control over the matter; if she does not want to be pregnant she wishes to know quickly so that she may arrange for an abortion. The presence of a pregnancy can now be known quickly and cheaply – one end-result of the work of the 1930s on endocrinology (Oakley, 1984, pp. 95–8). Thereafter, if she is pregnant she will follow the regime laid down for her by the obstetric policy of her health district. She will report at regular intervals during her antenatal period to her GP or perhaps to a midwives' clinic; she is likely to go at least once to a consultant clinic at her local maternity hospital so that she may be checked by the obstetrician for any abnormalities which GP or midwife may have missed. Those with known or predicted difficulties will find themselves under tighter medical surveillance.

The routines which govern the work of antenatal clinics were laid down in 1930 by a Departmental Committee of the Ministry of Health (Oakley, 1984, pp. 79–80). They cover the purpose of antenatal care and include the frequency of visiting. No evidence was provided in support of these guidelines, which seem to have emerged from the practice of a number of existing clinics. The guidelines remained largely unchallenged for fifty or more years and are still followed in many clinics. Marion Hall, a consultant obstetrician, and her colleagues examined the efficacy of antenatal care and the justification for the received wisdom (Chng, Hall and MacGillivray, 1980; Hall, Chng and MacGillivray, 1980). There had been doubt in the 1930s because the increasing attendance of pregnant women at antenatal clinics did not appear to have the expected effect in reducing birth complications and maternal mortality. The evidence of Hall and her colleagues shows that while women with a potentially serious problem are diagnosed and treated, suspicion is cast upon many women whose raised blood pressure is transient. The evidence also showed that few potentially dangerous cases were picked up in early pregnancy, suggesting that antenatal visits for that purpose early on were a waste of resources for both staff and pregnant women. The study also showed that many obstetric risks remain unpredictable. Yet in that same year a working party of the Council for Science and Society (chaired by Geoffrey Chamberlain, consultant obstetrician) could say:

> Modern antenatal care has progressed to become one of the most important branches of preventive medicine ... provides opportunities for educating the mother and preparing her physically and psychologically ... screening methods are used in order to detect any condition which might endanger her or the fetus.
>
> (CSS, 1980, p. 16)

The claims made for antenatal care include the detection of rhesus-factor incompatibility, abnormality in the foetus (see also pages 254–5) and the measurement of placental function.

The Aberdeen study (Hall, Chng and MacGillivray, 1980) looked systematically at the births for an entire year and, while not denying these possibilities, came to more modest conclusions, as we have seen. Consequently in Aberdeen a revised schedule of antenatal visits, a changed division of labour between midwives and consultants and a move of some services from the hospital to the community have resulted. These researchers have had some influence elsewhere (see the discussion by Oakley, 1984, pp. 284–5).

Diverse Images of Pregnancy

The obstetrician's goal in antenatal care is to detect if possible the presence of serious disorder, especially those which may lead to maternal or infant mortality. He (most commonly but not always he; 15 per cent of obstetricians are women) is less interested in the many small discomforts of pregnancy which can make life unpleasant for a woman, heartburn for example; nor in listening to her worries about the immense changes which are taking place in her body and which she does not know how to interpret (Homans, 1985). Women have a different image of pregnancy from obstetricians, as Graham and Oakley (1981 and 1986) have demonstrated using evidence from samples of mothers in York and London. The frames of reference of obstetricians and of women differ as to both the nature of child bearing and its context. In addition, women's experiences and image vary by ethnic group (Currer, 1986; Homans, 1985). Obstetricians see pregnancy and birth as medical matters, mothers as a natural biological process. The obstetrician has a limited view of the woman as a patient through her pregnancy and until after the birth; for the woman it is not an isolated episode but an event integral with the rest of her life. Her notions of a successful outcome are far more complex than his. These differences lead to conflicts, but the differential social positions between them leave the consultant in command.

From Home to Hospital

The progress which British obstetricians made towards moving the locale of birth from home to hospital can be traced through three government reports. The Guillebaud Report of 1955, whose main task was to look into the unexpectedly high cost of the NHS, pointed to the division of responsibility for maternity care among the three branches of the NHS: local authority, GP and hospital services (Ministry of Health, 1955). This led the following year to the appointment of the Cranbrook Committee to review the maternity services (Ministry of Health, 1959); while suggesting that services for home deliveries should be continued and improved, the Committee recommended that hospital deliveries should rise to 70 per cent of all births. This had happened by 1965.

In 1967 the Peel Committee was appointed to look into the future of the domiciliary midwifery service and the provision of maternity beds in hospital (DHSS, 1970). That committee recommended 100 per cent hospital deliveries. The evidence it adduced included as a main plank a table which showed that as the proportion of hospital births had increased, so the incidence of maternal and infant mortality had decreased. In a withering attack on the lack of sound research data on which to base this major and expensive change of policy, Archie Cochrane (1972) pointed out that because two factors co-vary (i.e. move together) it does not follow that one is the cause of the other – something of which any first-year student of elementary statistics is aware. In the years from 1955 to 1968 which the Peel Committee surveyed there had been many other changes: improved housing standards and improved nutrition, for example. Although class differences remained, the all-round longevity and health of the population had improved. It is likely that some of these factors were also associated with the improvements in perinatal and maternal mortality. These possibilities were not examined.

The composition of the Cranbrook and Peel committees reflected the reliance upon the expert, the expert being defined as pre-eminently the obstetrician. They included a token midwife, but no lay women (see also CSS, 1980, pp. 32–3). In its commentary the Council for Science and Society stresses the importance of the increasing demand for hospital services which came from the public. Public opinion is used as a reason for the transfer. The normative expectations of women, their assumptions about what the proper thing to do in childbirth is, had of course been strongly led by the medical, and particularly the obstetric, profession. It is not an independent variable. Thus, while in 1955 a woman would consider not only that she had a choice between home and hospital but that it was a decision to be thought about and discussed with her midwife and her doctor, by 1970 there was a strong normative expectation that first babies at least should be born in hospital. From this one cannot infer that women were happy to have their babies in hospital or happy when they did. Evidence mounted that there were a number of problems with hospital deliveries. It had not, however, been a part of the work of the Peel Committee to collect data from women who were having or had just had babies in home or hospital.

In the case of the Peel Committee it seems likely that the hospitalization policy had been formulated before it was publicly articulated. British obstetricians had already decided that births should be transferred from home to hospital; it was the logical consequence of developments from early in the century. The task of the Committee was really to secure resource reallocation for a policy the obstetric profession already agreed about.

An Inter-Professional Struggle
This history can be seen as an inter-professional struggle between obstetricians, general practitioners and midwives in which the first won at the expense of the

other two and in which parturient women had their minds made up for them, their choice taken from them. It was not the only way to run the maternity services, as many protesters were quick to suggest. The Dutch maternity services were pointed to, with their great stress on home deliveries and their excellent record with regard to maternal and perinatal mortality.

Childbirth had at one time been the facet of a GP's work which some most enjoyed, at least so far as those who opted for it were concerned. (From the inception of the NHS not all GPs involved themselves with maternity work.) They became convinced by the obstetricians' arguments that 'no delivery can be regarded as safe until it is over' (CSS, 1980, p. 17), that is, that one could not tell in advance what might be a 'normal' delivery and therefore that all deliveries must be regarded as potentially abnormal. They had been 'softened up' from the time of Cranbrook onwards. The general practitioners suffered a loss of only part of their work; they had plenty of primary-care activity left.

Domiciliary midwives on the other hand lost the core of their work. It is not the same looking after a woman who has been discharged from hospital forty-eight hours or more after delivery as it is being responsible for that delivery. That was only one aspect of what the midwives lost, however. The application of high technology in the active management of labour has reduced the majority of midwives to nurse technicians and has taken from them *de facto* the autonomy which *de jure* they still have.

The Active Management of Labour

Along with the dawning notion that all births are potentially abnormal came the idea that consequently one should monitor the birth to ensure that a 'normal' delivery is taking place. This may be by foetal heart monitoring, for example, so that intervention can promptly follow any indications of foetal heart failure. Another concomitant has been that one should intervene to ensure a normal delivery. Routine acceleration of labour is an example of the latter. The observation that prolonged labour is associated with distress for both mother and child, and possible fatality, led to the proposition that there was a 'normal' delivery time which could be achieved by active intervention. The artificial rupture of the membrane (ARM) has become routine in many hospitals. The use of oxytocin and prostaglandines for the induction and acceleration of labour was facilitated by the commercial production of the Cardiff pump. The commercial spread of this apparatus was associated with a rapid increase in the rates of induction. It was installed throughout the NHS without its effectiveness, efficiency and acceptability to the patient having been established (CSS, 1980). In the event, many women found the procedures and the changed style of childbirth distressing; medical evidence also suggested that the outcome of these interventions was less unequivocally desirable than had at first been thought (Chard and Richards, 1977).

Midwives

The upshot in terms of the midwives' role has been a further demotion and a situation in which many have left the profession. Midwives had already lost their independent status in the 1930s, having found it impossible to work except as an employee (Palmer, 1987). In some other countries, notably the Netherlands, they remain self-employed and can compete with medical practitioners for maternity work.

In Britain midwives work as salaried members of a multi-disciplinary team. They rarely have full clinical responsibility for a birth (Robinson, Golden and Bradley, 1983), although this is more likely to happen in a GP unit than an obstetric unit. Forty-five per cent of them have never done a home delivery (98 per cent of births are now in hospital); less than 10 per cent have done ten or more. Many midwives felt that they were under-used and that they should be able to take charge of more of the procedures associated with the new style of childbirth: apply scalp electrodes, suture the perineum, set up intravenous infusions, for example; smaller proportions were in favour of being able to deliver breech births, insert intra-uterine catheters, apply and use low forceps.

Midwives Protest

It was not until the 1970s that midwives began to protest about both their diminished status and the more unsatisfactory aspects of the new childbirth. The midwifery leadership had not protested the new developments as they took place. The Association of Radical Midwives which was formed in 1976 has a programme which would change the division of labour radically. The Association argues that midwives should be responsible for the 80 per cent of normal births; that midwives should be independent practitioners contracting with the NHS as GPs do; that 60 per cent of deliveries should take place at home attended by midwives; that women should have choice of place and manner of delivery (Flint, 1986).

Susanne Houd and Ann Oakley (1983) have looked at the alternative birthing arrangements (for example, home births and births without high-tech) which are available in ten countries in Europe and North America. Perhaps only 2 per cent or so of births are covered by these alternative arrangements, but clearly methods with an underlying philosophy and birth practices different from biomedicine exist widely. The theory and philosophy generally combine high levels of continuous social support for the birthing woman, low levels of intervention, birth at home (or sometimes in a birthing centre) and an holistic approach to the whole event, which is seen as physiological. Midwives in some of these traditions claim that high-risk births in particular benefit from this approach; that the methods used (laying on of hands, and massage, for example) can help the high-risk woman through in cases where the high-tech and the clinical and impersonal hospital atmosphere exacerbate the woman's problems and eventuate in forceps or a caesarian section.

It is easier in some countries than others for women to avail themselves of these alternative arrangements. The existence of independent midwives is a help; so is it if insurance companies will cover the alternative birth in the insurance-based health services of Europe; in limited areas in the UK the practice is possible within the NHS. The grip of biomedical obstetrics is in many places so strong that women may have to go private to achieve an alternative; this restricts the service to those with money to spare. This alternative birth movement, like the Radical Midwives in the UK, can be seen as part of a revolt against the new obstetrics, which has a number of facets.

Women Protest
The active management of labour (see page 240) aroused a good deal of unrest
among women. Perhaps no facet of biomedical practice has had such lay
scrutiny. The protest was expressed through pressure groups such as the
Association for the Improvement of Maternity Services (AIMS), although this
body had originally demanded increased beds for parturient women in hospital.
It moved on to campaign for improved hospital facilities and now also defends
the right of women to home births. The National Childbirth Trust, whose work
focuses on training women for childbirth to encourage satisfactory birth
experiences, also ultimately expressed concern. Individuals, such as Sheila
Kitzinger (see, for example, her publications 1962 and 1971; Kitzinger and
Davis, 1978) and Jean Robinson, one-time chairperson of the Patients' Association, were active. Women objected to the early foetal heart monitors because
they restricted movement in labour. Induction, however, earned the greatest
adverse attention. In *The Dignity of Labour?* (1979) Ann Cartwright showed
that generally speaking women would prefer to have similar arrangements for
the next birth as they had for the present one. She also showed that there were
variations in the treatment that women received according to their class and also
in their wishes. However, the one thing which was steady at about 80 per cent
across all classes was the women's wish to be asked whether they wanted an
induction or not (Cartwright, 1979, table 59, p. 114).

It was characteristic of the feminist movement of the late 1960s and early
1970s that some women began for the first time to criticize the way in which
they were treated by the medical profession; they began to develop the
hypothesis that medicine was an active agent of their continued oppression.
Reactions of many women, not themselves feminists, to the increasingly passive
and subordinate role which the new obstetrics thrust upon them fuelled these
arguments. It is in this context that an association like the Radical Midwives
deviates from the paternalistic pattern of male-dominated obstetrics and has as
the first statement in its programme, 'The parturient woman is the central
person in the process of care' (Flint, 1986, p. 14).

A Vessel or a Person?
This is a radical statement because, as the histories of maternal care have made
plain, the object of obstetric practice has been the safe extraction of a healthy
baby. The mother has not been regarded as a person in her own right, but rather
as a vessel for the production of the baby (Arney, 1982; J. Lewis, 1980; Oakley,
1984). The implications of this emerge in a number of ways. One is in the
question of risk-taking and who is to take the risks. Around the time of the Peel
Report the obstetric profession decided that women were not to be permitted to
take the risk of having a child at home. They further decided that they should
intervene to reduce risks; that women had 'placed themselves in their hands',
and therefore the decisions should be professional ones.

The suspension of Wendy Savage, consultant obstetrician, in April 1985
appears in part at least to stem from disapproval of her practice by her male
colleagues because she was prepared to let women take some risks. She would let
them try in labour even though there were indications that they might not be
able to labour successfully. One of the women whose child died, one of the five

cases arraigned against Wendy Savage, was upset that her case had been used by the prosecution and has said publicly that she would go to Mrs Savage for care in a subsequent pregnancy. It has been argued that the cases which have been produced against Mrs Savage would have their equivalents in any practitioner's obstetric history, unfortunate though they may be. It has also been argued that her perinatal mortality rates are better than those in the same hospital group. Medical practitioners rarely arraign each other; it is hard to believe that Wendy Savage's avowed socialism and feminism, which she tried to practise in the deprived Tower Hamlets area, are totally unconnected with the problems she has experienced (Savage, 1986).

Societal Implications

What these developments in obstetric practice signal is the emergence of a new form of patriarchy: benevolent, but not the less repressive for that. It has been emerging in an intermediate zone somewhere between the public and the domestic spheres. It is perhaps epitomized by the scene enacted in the privacy of the labour ward.

In the 1960s AIMS was not alone in requesting that the loneliness of women in labour should be overcome. Its request that a companion be permitted to accompany the labouring women entering hospital was resolved by an agreement to permit her male partner to accompany her. This had not been AIMS's original request and it cut out mothers, sisters, female lovers, women friends, among others. However, it was male partners (presumably legal husbands) who were permitted. Brown (1981), Richman (1982) and Richman and Goldthorp (1978) have interestingly discussed what happens in this intermediate zone between the public and the domestic which is constituted by the labour ward. Their accounts shed light on the new patriarchy, the modified paternalism, which is being created within the health service.

OVERCOMING INFERTILITY

In a society where a dominant norm is that couples should conceive and be fruitful, infertility is a great sorrow. Its impact upon men and upon women is probably different (see, for example, Owens, 1982). For a man it seems important that 'his' woman should bear the fruit of his loins. Men have found the blood tests indicative of paternity important. Not to conceive seems a denial of her womanhood to a woman who has internalized the dominant values. There have always been women who have refused to accept the wife-mother role as their destiny; more of us have been prepared to take this stand since the latest upsurge of the women's movement. Many more accept the dominant mores of heterosexuality, child bearing and child rearing. The wish to become a mother is not, however, confined to married or to heterosexual women; it is shared by single and lesbian women. While some women may wish to have children to establish long-term solidary ties with offspring, others see it as the means to achieve a satisfying identity; married, single and lesbian women share this view (Lewin, 1985, pp. 126–9). From wherever they come, whether derived from the values of patriarchal society, from personal experiences, or from other cultural influences, the feelings of distress of the infertile are real (Pfeffer and Woolett, 1983).

The infertile of all societies consult experts for help with their infertility. Una MacLean (1969), for example, has discussed this important facet of healing in traditional Nigeria. Biomedicine has offered infertility services which, until *in vitro* fertilization, had, apart from attempts with fertility drugs, remained static for nearly fifty years. Little attention has been paid to the causes of infertility or to its prevention (Doyal, 1985). The infertile have found the facilities and attention they have experienced in clinics and consultations distressing (Pfeffer and Woollett, 1983). More resources appear to have been put into developing alternatives to sexual intercourse as the mode of conception. This is where the focus of infertility research has been placed; it has brought fame and fortune to the practitioners involved as well as to the supplying industries (Pfeffer, 1987; Stanworth, 1987b). There are implications in these new modes of conception which are likely to have consequences far beyond the clinician's straightforward and doubtless honest intention of relieving a couple of the suffering which their infertility has created. The new reproductive technologies (NRT) have many facets, of which we will start here with AID. (This entire chapter has been about reproductive technologies; for a definition of NRT, see Klein, 1985; Standworth, 1987b.)

Separating Sex from Conception
Artificial insemination by donor (AID) is not new. According to Snowden and Mitchell (1983), it was first practised in the USA in the 1880s secretly and without the women initially being told. When the matter came to light controversy raged around issues of morality and legality of a similar kind to the arguments which still continue. Seriously discussed in Britain in the 1930s, it has been regularly practised since the Second World War (see also Lewin, 1985, pp. 129–31; Pfeffer, 1987, pp. 81–97).

Of the roughly 10 per cent of infertile couples, the husband's sterility is thought to be responsible in about a third of the cases. The introduction of the semen of a fertile man into the vagina of the wife can lead to conception and birth of a child. The legal status of the child is in some doubt.

> As the law stands, an AID child is illegitimate and the birth registration entry for such a child should either have the name of the donor, the words 'Father not known', or a blank space left where the father's name should be recorded. But almost invariably a husband enters his own name as the father of the child and in doing so he is in contravention of the Registration Act of 1965, unless he is under the impression (rightly or wrongly) that there is a genuine possibility that he may be the father.
>
> (Snowden and Mitchell, 1983, p. 17)

Men prepared to accept their wife's child gotten by another man have of course done this sort of thing for many years.

The technology involved in AID is simple; all it requires is a surgical syringe with the needle removed, or, as American lesbians discovered, a turkey baster will do well (Hornstein, 1984).[1] Knowing the time of ovulation is more problematic. Major problems come from the social assumptions about what are the proper ways to make babies.

Thus the research which Snowden and Mitchell (1983) report shows that AID children and their parents suffer from problems with which adopted children and their adoptive parents are familiar. In the latter case there are two 'real' parents whom the children may well wish to know about; in the former case there is one who is unknown. (Of course in the case of AIH, where the husband is the donor and the only problem is getting the sperm to the right place at the right time, these issues do not arise.) It seems that AID parents consider the child to be 'theirs' in a way they would not have felt an adopted child to be (Snowden and Mitchell, 1983, pp. 36–7).

It is clear that problems with AID, like problems with adoption, stem from the strong norms of a patriarchal society in which biological inheritance is seen as paramount. The very use of the term 'artificial' family suggests that there is a 'natural' family. Copulation and birth may in some sense be natural; they are part of the biological base, but all family forms are socially constructed. There is no one 'natural' family, as evidence of the variation around the world and over time should convince us. Those medical practitioners and social workers who control the processes of adoption and AID could have acted in ways which would have tended to weaken the normative expectations that there is one right kind of family to have, but that is not what they have done. Rather than stressing the 'naturalness' of building a family in a wide variety of ways, such as by adoption or fostering, collective child care and so on, the conventional nuclear family has been stressed. In the UK, AID has been offered only to those in stable heterosexual relationships who could demonstrate their wish to have children, their ability to rear them and the 'maturity' to handle parenthood – very similar rules to those applied to parents seeking to adopt children before the scarcity of children available for adoption developed.

There is no reason in practice why AID should be restricted in this way, and since the 1970s lesbians, particularly lesbian couples, have used this low-tech route to motherhood without heterosexuality. Klein (1984) records the activities of the London-based Feminist Self-Insemination Group (and see also Lewin, 1985). While Snowden and Mitchell (1983) refuse to comment on the appropriateness of this, or on the practice of single women becoming pregnant by AID, it is clear that they feel this increase in its use is a factor which complicates the solution of the legal and other problems they discuss. There are medical practitioners willing to help lesbian couples and single women; the view of the medical profession is not undivided on this or any other aspect of NRT. But the view of the lay and medical establishment appears to be. These issues become clearer when we turn to the question of more high-tech modes, which will first of all be described and later discussed.

In Vitro Fertilization

In vivo fertilization, where the sperm is inserted into the woman and fertilizes the egg there, is the procedure of long standing which has just been discussed. *In vitro* fertilization occurs where the egg is removed from a woman, fertilized outside the womb and then returned to the womb (either that of the egg donor or of another). The outcomes of this procedure are commonly referred to as 'test-tube babies'. The first such child, Louise Brown, was born in 1978, under private auspices. Not long after, the NHS took up the technique. This technique, which is appropriate for perhaps 5–10 per cent, or perhaps 18 per cent at most, of infertile couples (Doyal, 1987, *BMJ* (1987), 295, 6591, 18 July p. 155), has led to the surrogate mother, who carries to term the child of other parents. This she may do simply as a service, or it may be commercially arranged and done for profit, although this is illegal in the UK. Problems arise if, when the child comes to term, she does not want to part with it, as has already happened.

Embryos Become a Problem

Both sperm and eggs may be frozen and kept in banks, and this already happens. Now that eggs can be fertilized in a dish, there is the question of embryos which can be kept alive for some time outside the womb. Ordinarily when *in vitro* fertilization is to take place more than one embryo is created, some but not all of which may be implanted. None of the first implants may 'take'; and, if embryos have been saved, a second attempt may be made without the further operation, tiresome for the woman, of further egg extraction. (Numbers implanted vary depending on the practitioner; often it is three embryos, rarely only one, and perhaps as many as nine. The large numbers used explain multiple births from *in vitro* fertilization, but, in general, overall success rates are low.) A number of questions arise about embryos which have been frozen; as to whether they may be used for research purposes, as to whom they belong and by and for whom they may be used and under what circumstances. Geneticists and other scientists are anxious that embryos should be available for research. Others deem this completely inappropriate.

CONTROLLING THE PRODUCTS OF CONCEPTION

Genetic Manipulation: Therapy or Engineering?

The intention of gene therapy or genetic engineering (which term is used reveals something of the bias of the author) is to modify the DNA to reduce the incidence of hereditable diseases such as haemophilia. This is now scientifically possible by detecting, removing and replacing the inappropriate piece of DNA. The use of recombinant DNA in agriculture is already established; DNA is recombined in plants, for example, to alter the genetic inheritance to preferred characteristics. Its medical application is thought by some to be 'just around the corner' and much more distant by others. Medical practitioners appear more convinced of immediate possibilities than some molecular biologists (for a realistic assessment of probabilities, see Rose, 1987).

The already practised mode of controlling the products of conception is the detection of abnormalities *in utero* and the subsequent abortion of the 'impaired' foetus. Certain abnormalities, such as skeletal deformities, anencephaly and spina bifida, may be detected by the use of ultrasound. Others are detectable by amniocentesis whereby a needle is passed through the wall of the abdomen to withdraw some of the amniotic fluid which surrounds the baby. An alternative method which is currently being systematically tested is chorionic villus sampling, whereby a small amount of chorionic frondosum is removed from the uterus either across the cervix or by entering the abdomen with an aspirating needle. The techniques require to be associated with ultrasound to locate the placenta and avoid damaging the foetus. While amniocentesis cannot be undertaken until the second trimester, chorionic villus sampling is done from weeks eight to eleven. Amniocentesis results take some weeks to be known; those of chorionic villus sampling are available much more quickly. The latter will detect the presence of Down's syndrome and can also be used for gene probes to detect haemophilia, muscular dystrophy and Huntingdon's chorea, for example, but not for neural tube defects (MIDIRS, 1986). Both these procedures also inevitably reveal the sex of the foetus.

THINKING ABOUT THE IMPLICATIONS OF NRT

It was in 1973 that Amitai Etzioni published *Genetic Fix* after attending a Paris conference called by the Council for International Organizations of Medical Sciences (CIOMS) which was concerned with the social and ethical implications of 'recent progress in biology and medicine', by which was meant the discovery of DNA. It was in 1976 that Hilary Rose and Jalna Hanmer sketched out to a British Sociological Association annual conference concerned with sexual division in society what might be the consequences for women of the application of these discoveries. It was not until 1982 that the British government set up the Warnock Committee to investigate human reproduction and embryology. It was also in the early 1980s that women biological and social scientists first joined together to form FINNRET (Feminist International Network on New Reproductive Technologies) and then changed their name to FINRRAGE (Feminist International Network of Resistance to Reproductive and Genetic Engineering), so anxious had they become about the implications of these newest developments in reproductive technology. (For a useful critical review see Berer, 1986.) It apparently took a decade of gestation, the successful birth of a test-tube baby and renewed agitation about the termination of pregnancy before public discussion could take place and codes of practice begin to be enunciated.

Men as well as women feel threatened by the potential which science and medicine have created. While writers in books like those of Arditti, Klein and Minten, (1984) and Corea *et al.* (1985) see the techniques being used for the greater subordination of women, John Harris (1985), the ethicist, suggests that the technologies make possible a revolution in which women will take over, keeping alive only the few men they need. The magnitude of the possibilities, and some impossibilities, revealed by the enhanced control over biological processes which the new technologies give inclines, as Michelle Stanworth has pointed out, to a polarization:

These technologies claim to offer, on the one hand, a range of possibilities for extending the pleasures of parenthood to people who have been unable ... to have a child. They offer a chance for would-be parents to know, before a birth, about chromosomal abnormalities in their offspring, and even ... eventually to eliminate some of these ... before conception ... Viewed from the vantage-point of these potential benefits, reproductive technologies validate the image of science as a realm of boundless progress, bringing triumph over natural obstacles for the satisfaction of human needs.

On the other hand, the new reproductive technologies extend the possibility of a medical and scientific practice that outreaches human understanding and public control. They bring dangers of new, unknown (and in the short term unknowable) risks to patients ... and to babies ... They allow greater scope for the application of eugenic policies that would place a higher value on some human lives than others. They appear to turn the 'precious gift' of a baby into something that money can buy ... [and] invoke the spectre of science gone mad, of a Frankenstein world in which scientists manipulate – with unforeseeable consequences – the very foundation of life itself.

(Stanworth, 1987a, p. 1)

This polarization occurs, as Stanworth correctly argues, because the new techniques alter the boundaries between the biological and the social. Areas which were previously taken for granted, where the norms appeared to have a biological base, are opened up to political debate.

Situations are presented which are difficult to think about, which many feel uncover the mysteries of procreation, making the sacred profane. Deeply held views are challenged; hitherto unquestioned assumptions are destroyed. For those who believe that nothing should ever be permitted to come between sex and the possibility of conception, who steadfastly oppose any methods of contraception on these grounds, necessarily the 'interference' with 'nature' which is involved in separating sex and conception is likely to be anathema. This is the position adopted by the Roman Catholic Church, for example, which embraces a large number of the world's population.

For those who feel that the very nature of womanhood, and whatever power women may have, is vested in their unique ability to bear children, the possibilities which the new modes of conception give to scientists to usurp that power are frightening. This prospect has led some radical feminists to fear that the techniques will result in femicide and to take a rather Luddite position in opposition to the new technologies.

Radical feminists' beliefs are rooted in claims about women's autonomy; their present anxieties rest on an understanding of how that autonomy has already been limited by obstetric and gynaecological practice over many decades. However, although based on women's rights and interests, radical feminists appear to be arguing on the same side as Catholic women. The beliefs of the latter lie in the conventional model of the mother whose highest destiny is to serve the family. Yet in practice not all Catholics may adhere to a narrow interpretation of official church policy on this issue, any more than in practice they do on the use of contraception. Nor do all women, and not even all feminists, interpret motherhood in the same way; it has different meanings for different women. In practice the values that Catholics and feminists place on motherhood may lead many of both persuasions to accept the technologies, particularly perhaps in both cases out of compassion for the infertile. Feminists, however, would want to be assured of an input into the conditions placed upon the use and control of the techniques.

The inquiries which feminists associated with FINRRAGE and others have made have revealed problems about the way NRT is already being used which merit attention.

The Use of NRT: Powerful Influences
Restraints in every society are put on a woman's ability to choose whether to bear a child or not; nowhere does she have an untrammelled right to choose. The

constraints may lead women to support a society which disadvantages us.

There are reports from India (Kishwar, 1985; Roggencamp, 1984; and for some of the background, see Sangari, 1984) that clinics run for profit offer amniocentesis to sex the foetus and abort it should it be female, notwithstanding that this is legally banned (Balasubrahmanyan, 1984, p. 160; Roggencamp, 1984, pp. 268–9). Madhu Kishwar (1985) describes the dilemma of women who find themselves in a patriarchal system where they are not valued for themselves but only as the mothers of sons. Demographic studies suggest that female infanticide has continued to be used in parts of India despite its illegality. This new mode of control will continue the deficit of women. It will also continue their subservient position in that society.

Using amniocentesis (or chorionic villus sampling) for sex typing may take a less dramatic turn in other societies, but research shows that preferences are often, but not always, expressed for male children (Holmes and Hoskins, 1985, pp. 22–3; Hoskins and Holmes, 1984, p. 237; Owens, 1982; Rowland, 1984, p. 361, and 1985, p. 81; Williamson, 1976). Feminists fear that sex typing in private US clinics is being used to ensure male first-borns. Here there is not so much a prejudice against girl babies as a wish to have one of each sex, but starting with a boy. The more that girl children are second children the more the second-class status of women will be reinforced. In these ways the normative assumptions about the higher value of men engendered initially in patriarchal kinship systems and sustained in male-dominated industrial societies may be reinforced.

While most anxiety is raised by commercial clinics where practitioners appear to be concerned with gain, paying scant attention to professional ethics, many others act responsibly. They nevertheless feel that they must act within the norms of 'society' without disaggregating what that might mean. 'Society' then becomes an abstract, but a powerful one, which renders them helpless and behind which they seem to hide.

Choice and Social Class in the Use of NRT

Lesley Doyal (1987) has pointed out that in the UK the new technology services are being introduced *despite* the lack of basic gynaecological and infertility care for all (p. 177, original emphasis). She shows that the services are more readily available to the well-to-do, although it is likely that some of the known causes of infertility are more commonly found among the poorest groups. She details, using survey data, the patchy nature of the services among the various health authorities. Even in those health districts where artificial insemination is available, only three out of twenty-eight are completely free (p. 179). Furthermore, '25 out of the 53 clinics providing this service in England and Wales are actually outside the NHS – 17 of them commercial undertakings and 8 of them charities' (pp. 179–80). Consequently, more than nine out of ten AI patients end up in the private sector. Not only, as Doyal says, does this reflect 'a basic lack of commitment within the NHS to a woman's right to choose to have ... a child' (p. 180), it also means that only the well-to-do can exercise the choice.

IVF facilities present a similar but starker picture. Only one clinic in an NHS region is entirely NHS funded, so most IVF treatments are carried out in private clinics. Since BUPA has removed IVF from its list of available benefits, 'only the

rich and those single-minded enough and solvent enough to borrow a considerable sum will be able to try the possible benefits of IVF' (Doyal, 1987, p. 181),
which she suggests has a 10 to 15 per cent chance of success; the *British Medical
Journal* (17 July 1987), reviewing the present state of infertility treatments,
suggests less than an 18 per cent success rate.

Such unevenness in the availability of services is another example of how the
health-care system – and in the case of the NHS we are talking of state allocation
of resources as influenced by practitioners and managers – not only reflects but
re-creates the class structure; in this case re-creating it by making new
inequalities, by making reproduction possible for those in higher classes rather
than in lower and attempting to alleviate the suffering of the higher rather than
the lower. More than this, by concentrating resources in this way, the health-
care system diverts them from the prevention of infertility. To do that would
benefit all classes.

Evidence of this kind about the differential use, and indeed misuse, of NRT
has led FINRRAGE to their uncompromising position, a position which has
served an important purpose in forcing on to the agenda problems which those
in power either had not noticed or wished not to take account of. Attention has
been sharply drawn to the need for careful analyses of the manifold implications
of the new technologies for academic understanding and for action; the concept
of motherhood appears to be a good place to begin.

Who Is the Mother?

Husbands have (until the recent technologies) had difficulty in knowing
whether the child their wife has borne was really theirs, i.e. whether they were
the genitor. Paternity has always been an important issue psychologically,
socially and legally, and particularly so where inheritance is involved (see Smart,
1987). The question of who is the mother formerly raised far fewer difficulties.
Until now it has been taken as obvious that she who is delivered of a child is the
mother of that child, or as the law had it *mater semper certa est* (Zipper and
Sevenhuijsen, 1987). A mother might cede her legal rights to another woman
through adoption, but the issue of who was the original mother was unproble-
matic. Does, or should, *mater semper certa est* apply to surrogate mothers who
have entered into a contract with another woman? In the UK such contracts are
not recognized; in some states of the USA they are. The consequent disputes
have led to a great deal of press and popular attention being paid to 'womb
leasing' or 'surrogate motherhood', as it has been called (or 'carrymother', as the
Dutch have it: Zipper and Sevenhuijsen, 1987 – a term I find useful.)

A number of factors require to be disaggregated. To start with, it is not
surrogacy *per se* which is new. Women have borne children for other women in
the historic past; Sara and Hagar are cited from the Bible (Zipper and
Sevenhuijsen, 1987); sisters are said to have helped each other, the fertile sister
being inseminated by her brother-in-law and bearing the child for her sister and
her brother-in-law to raise as their own.

A feature that is really new occurs when the embryo the surrogate mother is
carrying has been conceived in a petri dish in the laboratory from genetic
material derived from the infertile couple. This occurs when the couple's
infertility is not just that they are unable to conceive by sexual intercourse, but

that the wife cannot carry a baby to term. In the former case the embryo, having been fertilized *in vitro* can be replaced in the womb of the woman whose egg was used; no carrymother is needed.

A second new feature raises questions of control and derives directly from the technology, although it is not determined by it. The intervention of a third party is necessary for surrogacy following *in vitro* conception; medical practitioners, medical scientists and technicians have to be involved. Former surrogacy arrangements were done privately and without public discussion (although no doubt with some gossip and speculation), the wife accepting as hers a child another had borne, the carrymother giving up her legal rights to her offspring. Technically illegitimate, such children will presumably, from the days when birth registration was instituted, have been entered as the legitimate offspring of the hitherto childless couple. In the case of IVF, not only is a third party involved, but a third party who for professional reasons has responsibility to the state. Immediately questions of control are raised: control of the activities of the medical professionals and control of the relationship of the commissioning parents to the carrymother.

There is also the question of payment. Should a carrymother be paid for the work she does? A problem about this is that it smacks of the commercialization of health care. In Britain we have in the past adhered to a strong sense of the commonweal, of the importance of mutual support in times of suffering, the inappropriateness of exploiting suffering for profit and of buying and selling human beings; in this context we have rejected the buying and selling of body parts. The British blood transfusion service is the best known example. Richard Titmuss's classic work (1973), comparing experience in the USA and the UK, showed that giving blood on the British pattern, rather than buying and selling it as in the USA, was not only ethically desirable but technically more efficient. These arguments have been used powerfully against the buying and selling of gametes, foetuses, embryos and children and also against womb leasing (Rothman, 1985, pp. 191–2, and Stacey, 1985b, pp. 193–5).

Most people would probably accept that a carrymother should be recompensed for all the extra expenses which go with carrying and delivering a child; also that she should be recompensed for any loss of earnings she might suffer. But should she be paid for being a surrogate as she should for any other work she had contracted to undertake? Should surrogacy be an enforceable contract? Or should she carry the child from a sense of service, out of a generalized love? If she is paid, does this not smack of prostitution? Is she not in some sense prostituting not only herself but the whole idea of motherhood, as some have suggested? On the other hand, if she is not paid, is she not being exploited? If carrymothers are paid, may not poor women be exploited and forced into this way of relieving their poverty? But is not a woman's body hers to use as she will? Restrictions on prostitution and abortion suggest that that right has never been recognized, but now the question arises again in another guise.[2]

All the problems about unpaid carers, the difficult relationships between paid and unpaid, the issues of service and duty, which were discussed with regard to unpaid health work in Chapters 14 and 15, are raised in this case. They have an even heavier loading here, however, because of the emotions that are involved in issues to do with conception and birth: the feelings to do with sacredness or mystery; questions of property in the child; questions of the rights of the child; questions about the dignity of women; strong notions about the importance of genetic inheritance. When rights and property are involved, the state in its legislative and judicial aspects is also implicated.

The State and NRT

Hitherto it has been possible to recognize two sorts of parenthood: what one might call biological parenthood, where the child has genetic inheritance from the parent, and social parenthood, where the tasks of rearing the child are undertaken by a parent other than the genetic parent. The law has recognized these differences, as well as whether the child is legitimate or illegitimate. As we have seen, the legal rights of biological parents may be transferred to social parents in the case of adoption. Persons may also act as social parents temporarily, as in the case of fostering.

Step-parents are a particular category of social parents, having a legal, marital relationship to one of the child's biological parents. The number of step-parents has increased considerably with the rise in the rates of divorce and remarriage; many more children nowadays live in households with a step-parent, more often a stepmother than a stepfather (cf. Stanworth, 1987b, p. 22). AID, and even more the institution of the carrymother, has complicated matters further.

There remain two kinds of father: biological and social. There are now three kinds of mother: genetic, the social and the carrymother. It was in part to recommend how to sort out the rights and responsibilities among these five kinds of parents, and among the combinations of them that technology has made possible, that the Warnock Committee was set up.

The Warnock Committee (HMSO, 1984) when it reported in 1984 effectively followed the conservative line which has been taken about the nuclear family by adoption agencies and most AID practitioners. NRT, it argues, should be used only to overcome infertility in couples who are in a stable heterosexual relationship. Furthermore, AID should be undertaken only under licence. If this proposal is adopted, the informal use of AID by single women and lesbians wishing to become mothers would be prevented for those wishing or needing to use medical facilities rather than the low-tech self-help method.

There are no scientific grounds for this recommendation of the Warnock Committee. It can be understood only in terms of the perpetuation of the patriarchal family and an unquestioning assumption of its merits. Golombok and Rust (1986) have shown that there is little sound evidence for this decision of the Warnock Committee. Indeed, the evidence about the effects of children growing up in fatherless heterosexual or lesbian families suggests that the children suffer no more than in fathered families (see also Golombok, Spencer and Rutter, 1983). Warnock appears to have followed the received wisdom and the reticence of the Royal College of Obstetricians and Gynaecologists in this matter (RCOG, 1983). What is happening is that the new techniques, which could be used imaginatively to extend the available forms of the family, are being used restrictively to reinforce a particular set of relationships between men and women and a particular child-bearing and child-rearing role for the women.[3]

The Problem of Control

In terms of control there are questions as to who will make the decisions about how NRT is to be used; as to who is to control the sperm, egg and embryo banks; as to whether those who are likely to have the control and make the decisions appreciate the sort of scientific understanding that they need to have available to them.

As to who will make the decisions about how NRT is to be used we know that, although women are now to be found in the structures of state and in the professions, we remain very much in a minority at least in the higher echelons where critical decisions and actions are taken. A majority of women in those positions have achieved them on men's terms. At those levels there are few challenges, although they are increasing, to the values of the male-dominated gender order or to patriliny. While this is of little consequence to most people, who probably bequeath what little material wealth they have reasonably equally among their offspring of both sexes, patrilineal inheritance remains of great importance to the Lords. We all too often forget just how important the court and the aristocracy remain in setting values and behaviour. Reservations are still entered about illegitimate but subsequently legitimated children being able to inherit titles. The views of women and of 'average' men are not likely to get a strong hearing in the councils of state as things stand.

Many decisions have been, and still are being, made by professionals. Undoubtedly medical scientists and medical practitioners have at present the greatest influence upon decisions, simply because they are there doing it; they are in charge of the technology; they are on the grant-giving committees; they have the products. Increasingly they, and others in senior places, are aware of the need for legal advice, as to rights in, rights of and obligations to children born by these new techniques. There is recognition of the problems the children may face (which Snowden and Mitchell, 1983, demonstrate). The need for counselling is understood, although less is known about how it should properly be done. A powerful case can be made for the argument that 'plain women and men' should be present on all scientific bodies which in any way control the use of NRT or the storage and use of its products.

There remains the question of the range of scientific knowledge which is available to those who make decisions about and control the use of NRT and its products. Psychological inputs may sometimes be available, but mostly only so far as the problems of counselling the infertile and those who are carrying, or may carry, a damaged foetus. Medical practitioners generally lack the socio-logical understanding which is necessary to add a societal dimension to debate and decision. While much money is spent on genetic research, there is no comparable recognition of the need to research the social consequences of the new reproductive technology.

Of course, those whose business it is to reduce suffering and disease must in each individual case do what they can. The problem is that the individual decisions may aggregate into unintended social consequences. The difficulty is that those who are not trained to think in societal terms, whose focus is the individual or the individual couple, appear to have difficulty in appreciating what the larger social consequences of their actions may be. Geneticists, for example, readily recognize the need for counselling of a couple at risk of a child who will have Tay Sachs disease (a rare but inevitably fatal condition), muscular dystrophy, or Down's syndrome; and of counselling couples who are known to be carrying such a child. They have much greater difficulty, given their professional attention to individuals, in grasping wider social consequences. None of us can know definitively what may be the outcomes of these developments, but it is clear that our individual decisions, lay and professional, about NRT are actively creating and re-creating our society.

It is possible, however, to use sociological concepts to put these developments into a wider context, as has been attempted here. It is also crucial to collect and analyse data as to how these technologies are at present being used. FINRRAGE are already attempting to do this in a voluntary way. Already social scientists have made contributions which indicate some of the unintended consequences which are arising, or may arise, from the use of NRTs. Let us look at the question of gene therapy.

Trying to Remove Handicap

Obviously every woman hopes she will not bear a handicapped child. What can be wrong about any attempts to prevent that sad happening? The very real problem is that by making it possible to detect handicap, and terminate the pregnancy or remove the offending genes, further problems may be created which should be taken into account in decision-making. Three aspects may be mentioned: first, the paradox that increasing choice can increase restrictions; second, the question of the consequences of changing normative expectations; third, the implications for the non-congenitally handicapped.

Increased choices have removed other choices, as Barbara Katz Rothman (1985) argues. It is harder now that family limitation is possible to have a large family without public censure, especially for a poor family. The choice to avoid bearing a handicapped child can also become a forced choice. 'In gaining the choice to control the quality of our children, we may rapidly lose the choice not to control the quality, the choice of simply accepting them as they are' (Rothman, 1985, p. 191; see also Farrant, 1985, p. 120; Stacey, 1985b). It is already reported that some women are permitted amniocentesis only if they agree in advance to an abortion if the foetus is abnormal (Farrant, 1985, p. 113).

There are many difficulties put in the way of the handicapped and their parents. As Rothman (1984 and 1985) argues, we have designed our way of life for the fit, well and striving. Because they do not fit, because they lack the appropriate body image or a sufficiently high IQ (whatever that implies), the handicapped are stigmatized. The woman who decides to carry to term a less than perfect foetus and bears a handicapped child is, because of the choice she had, likely to have condemnation of her act added to the burdens that caring for the handicapped already imposes.

The normative expectations that some children will be born handicapped are being changed to the expectation that a woman is responsible for having tests to establish the fitness of the foetus and to abort a damaged foetus (Farrant, 1985). Rothman (1985, p. 189) reports that over 80 per cent US respondents approve of abortion in such circumstances. Raynor Rapp (1984, p. 320) cites reports which suggest that 95 per cent of prenatally diagnosed Down's syndrome pregnancies are terminated after prenatal diagnosis. All the dangers of the eugenicist approach present themselves. The misuse of such ideas in the Nazi holocaust should constantly be remembered to alert us to the dangers.

What are the meanings for those already living, who deviate from the fully fit and able, of this concentration of resources upon the attempt to produce the 'perfect child'? Gene therapy, even if more advanced than at present, cannot prevent all handicap. Some children will be disabled later in life through illness or accident, as will some adults. A humane society will continue to help and care for the handicapped, to ensure by all means that they are recognized as fully social beings. Concentrating on removing handicap may well make it harder for inevitable handicap to be accepted, not least by the handicapped themselves. To think increasingly of mothers as vessels for the production of 'perfect children' will add to the problems for those who will still bear handicapped children.

These arguments do not necessarily suggest that the geneticists' efforts are entirely misplaced, but that at least as much research and attention should be paid to the social aspects of their well-meaning efforts as to the development of the genetic manipulations themselves.

If attempts to reduce handicap in some children may unintentionally make life harder for others and also for their parents, what are we to say? How can we conclude about NRT and gene therapy? Is the Luddite approach correct after all? There is another approach – one that does not concentrate entirely on the foetus and its genetic composition, but pays as much attention to the features in societies which lead one group to despise another or oppress another, which withhold resources from those needing help. Such an approach would attempt to make our society more humane rather than concentrating most effort on improving the quality of biological life. It would be consistent with one of the themes of this book that the importance of the biological base should be recognized, but that the social is as important; furthermore, that the one cannot be isolated from the other. Our destinies are not entirely in our genes. But before jumping to conclusions perhaps we should try to draw the threads together.

CONCLUSION

This last chapter has attempted to analyse, in the terms of the framework that has been used throughout this book, the critical developments which have been taking place in this last quarter of the twentieth century in human reproduction. It has sought to set out the analysis in such a way as to help inform the decisions which have yet to be taken and which will set the pattern of reproduction for the twenty-first century.

In the history of the development of techniques for care in childbirth, for fertility control, both conception and contraception, and for genetic therapy, all the elements which were referred to in the theoretical introduction (Chapter 1), and which have guided analysis throughout, can be seen to be relevant.

Three assumptions were made. The first related to the social construction of all healing knowledge; the second was that the knowledge deployed was not merely cultural in origin, but related also to the social and economic structure of the society; the third, that the healing knowledge and practice would inevitably relate to the biological base. In the case of human reproduction these assumptions have guided the features that have been drawn out.

While noting and being impressed by the remarkable work of molecular biologists, endocrinologists and other scientists in uncovering the workings of the human body, we have also noted the selective nature of what is known. The problems to be solved were set by male scientists in a masculinist mode and related to problems they saw as interesting, exciting and relevant. Attention to the biological to the exclusion, it seems, of the social, and also to particular facets of the biological, has led to knowledge which is more relevant to some human problems than to others. In application of the knowledge, assumptions are made by practitioners about what couples, and especially women, want. The relevance of the assumption which was made (page 2), that no simple judgement of what is efficacious can be made in healing practice, has emerged clearly. Asking the supplementary question of the NRT, 'Efficacious in whose terms?' has revealed how complicated that answer can be (cf. Rose, 1987).

The way in which the knowledge has developed is socially situated in a wider structure than that provided by biology laboratories. Ultrasound, now so widely used in antenatal care, was developed, almost accidentally, from the imaging techniques used to detect submarines in the Second World War (Oakley, 1984 and 1987). AID was developed from the application to humans of practices developed in animal husbandry which were designed to improve the stock and were in line with many hundreds of years of controlled breeding in farm animals and plants.

So far as the importance of taking the biological base into account is concerned, in the case of human reproduction the relationship of the healing arts to that base is sharply revealed. It is not so much the biological given of itself which transpires to be most important; the very conscious and deliberate attempts to modify that base are the most obvious feature.

At the outset we noted that three aspects of the social structure were relevant to an understanding of illness, health and healing: the family and kin and more widely the gender order; the mode of production and the class order; and the structure of the state. The relevance of all of these has become clear in the analysis of human reproduction and also of the way in which established healing practices interact with these other facets of the social structure to reinforce existing tendencies or to modify the structures themselves. In the course of the book we have seen that this can happen in a variety of areas of healing knowledge and practice, but perhaps never more clearly than in the case of human reproduction, where NRT has made possible new family forms and thrown into disarray long-standing assumptions about kinship relations.

Insisting on taking the historical dimension into account has revealed what is radically innovatory about the new technologies and practice and to what a large extent both the biotechnology and the social responses to it have deep historical roots. The viewing of the interior of the body began with the new clinical medicine itself at the end of the eighteenth century. To see inside women's reproductive organs was one of the early obstetric developments, which gave men a view of their insides that women had never had. The new imaging, derived from ultrasound, is the natural successor to those early developments. It has provided images which women can share but which are used in particular ways to support images of birth and the foetus of a particular kind – for example, of the 'foetus-as-spaceman' (Petchesky, 1987, p. 64; see also Rothman, 1986, p. 114), an image quite different from that which women formerly had of the child developing inside us, which was essentially tactile rather than visual. The responses to IVF are similar to those to AID, which in their turn echoed debates about the legalization of adoption. These responses have their origins, further-more, in the ground rules which were laid down for the aristocratic patrilineal system of much earlier times. The latter may have not had so much effect on the lives of ordinary people, whose arrangements were less trammelled by inherit-ance and more immediately adaptable to the exigencies of daily life.

A focus on the division of labour has also helped the analysis of human reproduction. Perhaps more important has been the analysis of what health work is, which led to the clear need to include the unpaid labourers in the division of health labour. In the case of a parturient woman, it is much easier than in some patient categories to see the distinction between the active and passive participant, between the woman as subject but also as object. The labouring woman is clearly a worker, but in the relationship with her carers she may be permitted to take or insist upon a more or less active role, to play a greater or lesser part in the decisions surrounding the manner of her delivery. The woman who has a caesarean section, when undoubtedly it was the only way to save her life as well as that of her child, has every reason to be grateful to the high skill of obstetric surgeons. The woman who has a caesarian as a conse-quence of interventions made in the name of the active management of labour, interventions about which she was in the first place neither fully informed nor consulted, is likely to take a different view of that same surgery.

There is clear and active involvement of many actors in the reproductive process. Whereas for men this involvement is ordinarily limited to the act of copulation, quite an amount of health work may nowadays be required of men in the investigation and treatment of infertility. It remains less than that of a woman; for she has not only the labour of the birth, but also many other procedures to go through, even in a physiologically normal pregnancy. Where technologies such as amniocentesis or IVF are involved, her work is again heavier than that of a man. This work of both husband and wife is not only unpaid, but increasingly has to be paid for, a somewhat unusual economic relationship. The question of the labour of a carrymother, as to whether, how and what she should be paid, raised these issues in an acute form.

Human reproduction also brings sharply into view all the hazards in 'people work' where doing things *for* can easily turn into doing things *to* people (Hughes, 1971, p. 305). NRT, in sharp contrast to a physiological birth, shows how many things may be done to, rather than for, a mother in the course of assisting her birth. Some of the procedures appear to be done for the foetus rather than the mother, some for the ease or satisfaction of professionals. The power relations in 'people work' are brought sharply into focus, power relations which derive in part from those which lie between the professional and the client, and in part from the general domination of men over women in the society, which may mean that the mother's goals in the process of birth and procreation are superseded by those of others, whether in her name or in the name of her unborn child. (See, for example, Farrant's finding that 80 per cent of consultants interviewed thought that doctors should have the final say in whether or not a woman should have an abortion: 1985, p. 106.)

Looking at the division of labour has revealed, as indeed has been plain throughout, the continuing male domination of the professions at the most senior levels: the maleness of the science which lies behind those professions, of those who implement the knowledge and who make decisions about its use. In historical context our loss of power as women in superintending the reproductive processes has become clear. We have noted above the increased and increasing tendency to treat the parturient woman herself as an object, the vessel for the production of the child, rather than as a woman in her own right. The rapid development of high-tech has meant that mothers no longer have experience relevant for their daughters, who are forced to pay attention to the professionals and to their peers. In this way the use of the new technologies has brought about changes in the generational order. These are changes which, as we saw, were instituted deliberately, early in the century, by Medical Officers of Health through the agency of health visitors in an attempt to educate working-class mothers to particular modes of child rearing in the name of the health of their children. The obstetricians have replaced midwives as the prime authority on the birth process – first, in terms of their legal status, which, while practitioners in their own right, is clearly subservient, in that they must call a doctor in all cases of possible abnormality. Secondly, the obstetric definition of all births as potentially abnormal has reduced the midwives' *de facto* status in the hospital situation even further.

Throughout I have argued that the health-care system not only reflects, but actively plays a part in forming, the social structure. Mention has just been made of its impact on the generational order, rendering obsolete parts of the received wisdom of our foremothers and thereby demeaning their total experience and status. Health care has not been the only activity which has had this effect, but it has contributed. We have seen also how the mode of delivery of health care has not helped to reduce class inequalities in health experiences, albeit that these may have their prime origin in the economic structure of the society. This again has been seen to be the case in reproduction, where services are unequally distributed nationwide and the most advanced services are available only to those who can pay – some, like IVF, only to the very well off. In this way new kinds of privileged classes are being created. This occurs because of the way in which health care is locked into a profit-oriented society, but it plays its own part in supporting privilege and class oppression. We have also seen, in the discussion above, that the part that medicine has played over the last two centuries in helping to create a new form of the male-dominated gender order is continuing, and that a prime site for that lies in the reproductive services.

The interests of the state in controlling facets of health care are something which has come up time and again in this book; it is very clear in the case of reproduction, with control through legislative and judicial channels of the uses of NRT and rulings about the consequent new sets of relationships – the rights, duties and status of the carrymother being the most striking. Here again the male-dominated nature of the state structures has to be underlined. Not only are there still a majority of men in positions of political power, but there are still a majority of men among the administrators and the lawyers. These two sets of people will be strongly influenced by their biomedical advisers, where again the majority are men. Women in these positions work in a male-dominated environment.

The arguments of this book suggest that women lack the power for the literal homicide (as opposed to femicide) which Harris (1985) foresaw as a possible consequence of NRT. However, it is not the case that they are powerless to counteract the tendencies in the application and control of NRT, which seem at present too often to undermine our interests. There are increasing numbers of women in the public domain; not all women have been prepared to leave science to the men, nor have all of those who have gone into science taken up a masculinist stance. As Hilary Rose (1987) has said, science and technology are too important to be left to men. Already there are well-marshalled critical analyses, a number of which have been cited in this book. Clear heads must be kept, not always easy in this area which is not only emotive but difficult to analyse with clarity, especially in the face of the received wisdom. The diversity of interests among women in reproduction is perhaps not equalled by the diversity of interests among men, but there is diversity among them too as to what they want from reproduction and what they want their relationship with their offspring or inspring to be. There are diverse interests among the children too: more diverse than the frequent use of the phrase 'the best interests of the child' in the justification of procedures would lead one to believe. What seems to me to be essential if we are to have a satisfactory system of reproduction and child care in the twenty-first century is that the debate should be opened up beyond its present limits and that items such as those discussed here should be put on the agenda.

In this debate, as a woman, I would want to see items on the agenda which discuss the impact of the technologies on us as women, which open for discussion the conventional assumptions about what women are and want in relation to motherhood. As a person I am aware that the problems in the use and control of NRT affect, and may affect adversely, others than women. In particular I have drawn attention to the less-than-clear implications of gene therapy for children and the implications of the wish for the 'perfect child' for our values about the humanness of the handicapped.

At the beginning of this book I argued that the ways in which a society copes with the major events of birth, illness and death are central to the beliefs and practices of that society; in particular that the treatment of those who are temporarily or permanently dependent on others is a revealing indicator of the social values lying behind the allocation of material and non-material resources. I have not here dealt with the ways in which death is handled in the UK, but the evidence from the way birth is handled has revealed many important values by which we run our lives in this country, or permit them to be run. Reproduction is a crucial area which reveals starkly the relations between health care and the dominant societal values. For my part, as the reader will have realized, I am personally not happy with some of them, notably the increasing tendency to permit, and indeed encourage, profit to be made out of suffering and the failure to offer services for the relief of suffering even-handedly to persons in all social situations. Readers will make their own judgements.

Modern science and modern biomedicine in the hands of sensitive and dedicated practitioners have given us immense gifts of comfort, life and health. The technologies have also made possible the perpetration of hideous monstrosities; the threat of nuclear war has not yet receded. The unintended consequences of the NRTs may be, as we have seen, less than benign. Much remains unknowable at present, but it is possible to put ourselves in a much better position to know – to know, for example, how the technologies are now being used, to find out what problems are being created for others by the solutions of the problems of some.

As a sociologist I would want to argue strongly for research funding into the social implications of NRTs to be increased to match the expenditures on the technologies. Without adequate knowledge about the social implications, we cannot know how to decide which way NRTs should be used and controlled. To gain the knowledge is, of course, largely a matter of resource allocation. To collect the right data and make proper use of them requires courage, initiative and the vision to see beyond the frontiers of our present society. As the prophet said, without vision the people perish. I hope the vision will not be one which lets some of us survive at the expense of others; that the technologies will be deliberately used cautiously and for the good of society as a whole, not just for some groups within it.

Notes

1 Since the AIDS epidemic developed, however, women may prefer that the semen be frozen for some months in order that it may be tested to see if HIV/AIDS is present. This inserts third party high-tech intervention into an otherwise low-tech procedure.
2 See the discussion on surrogacy in the White Paper *Human Fertilisation and Embryology: A Framework for Legislation* (HMSO, 1987, paras 64–71). The 1985 Surrogacy Arrangements Act has already outlawed third party involvement in commercial surrogacy.
3. The White Paper (HMSO, 1987) reinforces this tendency. It proposes to make criminal the use of gametes donated by a third party to create an embryo inside the body without an appropriate licence from the proposed Statutory Licensing Authority. Only 'couples' (presumably heterosexual) are referred to in the section (para. 78) which discusses 'suitability' for infertility treatment; it is proposed that controls on suitability should be indirect and not by legislation.

References and Bibliography

Abel-Smith, B. (1960), *A History of the Nursing Profession* (London: Heinemann).

Abel-Smith, B. (1964), *The Hospitals 1800–1948* (London: Heinemann).

Abel-Smith, B. (1976), *Value for Money in Health Services* (London: Heinemann).

Abel-Smith, B. (1978), *National Health Service: The First Thirty Years* (London: HMSO).

Abrams, P., Abrams, S., Humphrey, R., and Snaith, R. (1986), *Creating Care in the Neighbourhood*, ed. D. Leat (London: Neighbourhood Care Action Programme).

Ackernecht, E. M. (1948), 'Anticontagionism between 1821–1867', *Bulletin of the History of Medicine*, 22, pp. 562–93.

Acton, W. MRCS (1862), 'The functions and disorders of the reproductive organs', 3rd edn (London: John Churchill), pp. 75, 88–9, 101–3, in Bauer and Ritt, op. cit., pp. 45–7.

Ahern, E. M. (1987), 'Chinese-style and Western-style doctors in Northern Taiwan', in J. D. Stoeckle (ed.), *Encounters between Patients and Doctors* (London: and Cambridge, Mass.: MIT Press).

Aitken-Swan, J. (1977), *Fertility Control and the Medical Profession* (London: Croom Helm).

Alaszewski, A. W. (1977), 'Doctors and paramedical workers: the changing pattern of interprofessional relations', *Health and Social Services Journal*, Centre 8 Paper, pp. B1–4.

Allsop, J. (1984), *Health Policy and the National Health Service* (London and New York: Longman).

Arditti, R., Klein, R. D., and Minden, S. (1984), *Test-Tube Women: What Future for Motherhood?* (London and Boston: Pandora).

Armstrong, D. (1976), 'The decline of the medical hegemony: a review of government reports during the NHS', *Social Science and Medicine*, 10, 3/4, pp. 157–63.

Armstrong, D. (1979), 'Child development and medical ontology', *Social Science and Medicine*, 13 A, 1, p. 9.

Armstrong, D. (1980), *An Outline of Sociology as Applied to Medicine* (Bristol: John Wright & Son).

Armstrong, D. (1983a), *An Outline of Sociology as Applied to Medicine*, 2nd edn (Bristol: John Wright & Son).

Armstrong, D. (1983b), *Political Anatomy of the Body: Medical Knowledge in Britain in the Twentieth Century* (Cambridge: Cambridge University Press).

Armstrong, D. (1985), 'Space and time in British general practice', *Social Science and Medicine*, 20, 7, pp. 659–66.

Arney, W. R. (1982), *Power and the Profession of Obstetrics* (Chicago and London: University of Chicago Press).

Aronovitch, B. (1974), *Give it Time: An Experience of Hospital 1928–32* (London: Deutsch).

Atkinson, P. (1981), *The Clinical Experience: the construction and reconstruction of medical reality* (Farnborough, Hants: Gower).

Austin, R. (1977), 'Sex and gender in the future of nursing', 1 and 2, *Nursing Times*, 73, 35, 25 August, pp. 113–16, and 1 September, pp. 117–19.

Baer, H. A. (1981), 'The organizational rejuvenation of osteopathy: a reflection of the decline of professional dominance in medicine', *Social Science and Medicine*, 15A, 5, pp. 701–11.

Balasubrahmanyan, V. (1984), 'Women as targets in India's family planning policy', in Arditti, Klein and Minden, op. cit.

Balint, M. (1956), *The Doctor, His Patient and the Illness* (London: Pitman).

Banks, J. A. (1954), *Prosperity and Parenthood* (London: Routledge & Kegan Paul).

Banks, J. A. (1981), *Victorian Values: Secularism and the Size of Families* (London and Boston: Routledge & Kegan Paul).

Banks, J. A., and Banks, O. (1964), *Feminism and Family Planning* (Liverpool: Liverpool University Press).

Banks, O. (1981), *Faces of Feminism: A Study of Feminism as a Social Movement* (Oxford: Martin Robertson).

Barrett, M. (1980), *Women's Oppression Today: Problems in Marxist Feminist Analysis* (London: Verso).

Barrett, M. (1981), 'Timpanaro: materialism and the question of biology', *Sociology of Health and Illness*, 3, 3, pp. 337–45.

Bauer, C., and Ritt, L. (1979) *Free and Ennobled: Source Readings in the Development of Victorian Feminism* (Oxford: Pergamon).

Beier, L. McC. (1981), 'The creation of the medical fringe 1500–1700', *Bulletin of the Society for the Social History of Medicine*, 29 December, pp. 29–31.

Bell, C., and Newby, H. (1976), 'Husbands and wives: the dynamics of the deferential dialectic' in D. L. Barker and S. Allen (eds), *Dependence and Exploitation in Work and Marriage* (London: Longman).

Berer, M. (1986), 'Breeding conspiracies: feminism and the new technologies', *Trouble and Strife*, 9, Summer, p. 29.

Berg, O. (1975), 'Health and quality of life', *Acta Sociologia*, 18, 1, pp. 3–22.

Berliner, H. (1984), 'Scientific medicine since Flexner', in Salmon (1984a), op. cit.

Blackwell, E. (1977) *Pioneer Work in Opening the Medical Profession to Women*, (New York: Schocken).

Blanpain, J. (1978), *National Insurance and Health Resources: The European Experience* (Cambridge, Mass., and London: Harvard University Press).

Blaxter, M. (1981), *The Health of the Children: A Review of Research on the Place of Health in Cycles of Disadvantage* (London: Heinemann Educational Books).

Blaxter, M. (1983), 'The causes of disease. Women talking', *Social Science and Medicine*, 17, 2, pp. 59–69.

Blaxter, M. (1987a), 'Self-reported health' in Cox *et al.*, op. cit.

Blaxter, M. (1987b) 'Attitudes to health', in Cox *et al.*, op. cit.

Blaxter, M., Fenner, N., and Whichelow, M. J. (1987) '"Healthy" behaviour', in Cox *et al.*, op. cit.

Blaxter, M., and Patterson, E. (1982), *Mothers and Daughters: A Three Generational Study of Health Attitudes and Behaviour*, SSRC/DHSS Studies in Deprivation and Disadvantage 5 (London: Heinemann Educational Books).

Bloor, M. (1976a), 'Bishop Berkeley and the adenotonsillectomy enigma: an exploration of variation in the social construction of medical disposals', *Sociology*, 10, p. 45.

Bloor, M. J. (1976b), 'Professional autonomy and client exclusion: a case study in ENT clinics', in M. Wadsworth and D. Robinson (eds.), *Studies in Everyday Medical Life* (London: Martin Robertson).

Blum, R., with Kreitman, K. (1981), 'Factors affecting individual use of medicines', in Blum *et al.*, op. cit.

Blum, R., Herxheimer, A., Stenzl, C., and Woodcock, J. (eds.) (1981), *Pharmaceuticals and Health Policy: International Perspectives on Provision and Control of Medicines* (London: Croom Helm).

Bodenheimer, T. S. (1984), 'The transnational pharmaceutical industry and the health of the world's people', in J. B. McKinlay (ed.), *Issues in the Political Economy of Health Care* (New York and London: Tavistock).

Boulton, M. G. (1983), *On being a Mother* (London: Tavistock).

Branca, P. (1975), *Silent Sisterhood: Middle Class Women in the Victorian Home* (London: Croom Helm).

British Medical Association (1977), *Evidence to the Royal Commission on the National Health Service* (London: BMA).

British Medical Journal (1986), 292, 24 May, pp. 1407–8.

Brockbank, W., and Kenworthy, F. (eds.) (1968), *The Diary of Richard Kay, a Lancashire Doctor, 1716–51* (Manchester: Chetham Society).

Brockington, C. F. (1965), *Public Health in the Nineteenth Century* (Edinburgh and London: C. & S. Livingstone).

Brown, A. (1981), 'Fathers in the labour ward: medical and lay accounts', L. McKee and M. O'Brien (eds.), in *The Father Figure* (London and New York: Tavistock).

Brown, B. (1979), 'Beyond separation: some new evidence on the impact of brief hospitalisation on young children', in Hall and Stacey, op. cit.

Brown, E. R. (1979), *Rockefeller Medicine Men: Capitalism and Medical Care in America* (Berkeley, Calif.: University of California Press).

Brown, G., and Harris, T. (1978), *Social Origins of Depression: A Study of Psychiatric Disorder in Women* (London: Tavistock).

Bucher, R., and Stelling, J. (1969), 'Characteristics of professional organizations', *Journal of Health and Social Behavior*, 10, pp. 3–15.

Bulmer, M. (1986), *Neighbours: The Work of Philip Abrams* (Cambridge: Cambridge University Press).

Burgess, R. G. (ed.) (1982), *Field Research: A Sourcebook and Field Manual* (London: Allen & Unwin).

Busfield, J. (1986), *Managing Madness* (London: Hutchinson).

Buswell, C. (1980a), Mothers' perceptions of professionals in child health care', Child Health Project Working Papers, mimeo (Coventry: University of Warwick).

Buswell, C. (1980b), 'Mothers as unpaid health workers', Child Health Project Working Papers, mimeo (Coventry: University of Warwick).

Buswell, C. (1981), 'The "mother's friend": contemporary perspectives on health visiting from some mothers' viewpoints', Child Health Project Working Papers, MS (Coventry: University of Warwick).

Butler, A. S. G. (1954), *Portrait of Josephine Butler* (London: Faber).

Butler, J. E. (1910), *Personal Reminiscences of a Great Crusade* (London: Horace Marshall); a new and posthumous edition of the second edition of 1898; the first was published in 1896.

Butler, J. R., and Vaile, M. S. B. (1984), *Health and Health Services: An Introduction to Health Care in Britain* (London and Boston: Routledge & Kegan Paul).

Byrne, P. S., and Long, B. E. L. (1976), *Doctors Talking to Patients: A Study of the Verbal Behaviour of General Practitioners Consulting in their Surgeries* (London: HMSO).

Caplan, R. L. (1984), 'Chiropractic', in Salmon (1984a), op. cit.

Carpenter, E. S. (1977), 'Women in male-dominated health professions', *International Journal of Health Services*, 7, 2, pp. 191–207.

Carpenter, M. (1977), 'The new managerialism and professionalism in nursing', in M. Stacey, M. Reid, C. Heath and R. Dingwall (eds), *Health and the Division of Labour* (London: Croom Helm; New York: Prodist).

Carpenter, M. (1980), *All for One: Campaigns and Pioneers in the Making of COHSE* (London: Confederation of Health Service Employees).

Carstairs, G. M. (1955), 'Medicine and faith in rural Rajasthan', in B. D. Paul (ed.), *Health, Culture and Community* (New York: Russell Sage).

Cartwright, A. (1967), *Patients and Their Doctors – A Study of General Practice* (London: Routledge & Kegan Paul).

Cartwright, A. (1979), *The Dignity of Labour?* (London: Tavistock).

Cartwright, A. (1983), *Health Surveys in Practice and in Potential* (London: King Edward's Hospital Fund for London, Oxford University Press).

Cartwright, A., and Anderson, R. (1981), *General Practice Revisited: A Second Study of Patients and Their Doctors* (London: Tavistock).

Cassel, J. (1955), 'A comprehensive health program among the Zulus', in B. D. Paul (ed.) *Health Culture and Community* (New York: Russel Sage).

Central Health Services Council (1962) *Relieving Nurses of Non-Nursing Duties in General and Maternity Hospitals*, Report of a Subcommittee of the Standing Nurse Advisory Committee (Farrer Report) (London: HMSO).

Chard, T., and Richards, M. (eds.), (1977), *Benefits and Hazards of the New Obstetrics* (London: Spastics International Medical Publications).

Chng, P. K., Hall, M. H., and MacGillivray, I. (1980), 'An audit of antenatal care: the value of the first antenatal visit', *British Medical Journal*, 281, 6249, 1 November, pp. 1184–6.

Chow, E. P. Y. (1984), 'Traditional Chinese medicine: an holistic system', in Salmon (1984a), op. cit.

Clark, A. (1968), *Working Life of Women in the Seventeenth Century* (1st edn 1919) (London: Frank Cass).

Clarke, J. N. (1983), 'Sexism, feminism and medicalism: a decade review of literature on gender and illness', *Sociology of Health and Illness*, 5, 1, pp. 62–82.

Cleary, J., Grey, O. P., Hall, D. J., Rowlandson, P. H., Sainsbury, C P. Q., and Davies, M. M. (1986), 'Parental involvement in the lives of children in hospital', *Archives of Disease in Childhood*, 61, pp. 779–87.

Clough, F. (1979), 'The validation of meaning in illness–treatment situations', in Hall and Stacey op. cit.

Cochrane, A. L. (1972), *Effectiveness and Efficiency: Random Reflections on Health Services* (London: Nuffield Provincial Hospitals Trust).

Coe, R. M. (1970), *Sociology of Medicine* (New York: McGraw-Hill).

Cohen, G., (1964), *What's Wrong with Hospitals?* (Harmondsworth: Penguin).

Collier, J., and Foster, J. (1985), 'Management of a restricted drugs policy in hospital: the first five years' experience', *Lancet*, 1, 8424, 9 February, pp. 331–3.

Cooter, R. (1982), 'Anticongianism and history's medical record', in Peter Wright and Andrew Treacher (eds.), *The Problem of Medical Knowledge: Examining the Social Construction of Medicine* (Edinburgh: Edinburgh University Press).

Corea, G., Klein, R. D., Hanmer, J., Holmes, H. B., Hoskins, B., Kishwar, H., Raymond, J., Rowland, R., and Steinbacher, R. (1985), *Man-Made Women: How New Reproductive Technologies Affect Women* (London: Hutchinson).

Cornwell, J. (1984), *Hard Earned Lives* (London: Tavistock).

Coser, R. L. (1972), 'Authority and decision making in a hospital: a comparative analysis', in E. Freidson and J. Lorber (eds.), *Medical Men and Their Work* (Chicago: Aldine Atherton).

Coulter, H. L. (1984), 'Homeopathy', in Salmon (1984a), op. cit.

Council for Science and Society (1980), *Childbirth Today: Policy Making in the National Health Service – a Case Study* (London: CSS).

Council for Science and Society (1982), *Expensive Medical Techniques: Report of a Working Party* (London: CSS).

Cox, B. D., Blaxter, M., Buckle, A. L. J., Fenner, N. P., Golding, J. F., Gore, M., Huppert, F. A., Nickson, J., Roth, M., Stark, J., Wadsworth, M. E. J., and Whichelow, M. (1987), *The Health and Lifestyle Survey* (London: Health Promotion Trust).

Cox, C., and Mead, A. (eds.), (1975), *A Sociology of Medical Practice* (London: Collier-Macmillan).

Crawford, R. (1977), 'You are dangerous to your health: the ideology and politics of victim blaming', *International Journal of Health Services*, 7, 4, pp. 663–80.

Crawford, R. (1980), 'Healthism and the medicalization of everyday life', *International Journal of Health Services*, 10, 3, pp. 365–88.

Crawford, R. (1984), 'A cultural account of "health": control, release and the social body', in J. B. McKinley (ed.), *Issues in the Political Economy of Health Care* (New York and London: Tavistock)

Croog, S. H., and Ver Steeg, D. F. (1972), 'The hospital as a social system', in H. E. Freeman, S. Levine and L. G. Reeder (eds.), *Handbook of Medical Sociology* (Englewood Cliffs,: Prentice-Hall).

Crowther, M. A. (1981), *The Workhouse System 1834–1929* (London: Batsford).

Currer, C. (1986), 'Concepts of Mental Well- and Ill-being: the Case of Pathan Mothers in Britain', in Currer and Stacey, op. cit.

Currer, C., and Stacey, M. (eds.) (1986) *Concepts of Health, Illness and Disease: A Comparative Perspective* (Leamington Spa: Berg).

Davidoff, L. (1971), 'The English Victorian governess', unpublished paper.

Davidoff, L. (1973) *The Best Circles: Society, Etiquette and the Season* (London: Croom Helm).

Davidoff, L. (1976), 'The rationalization of housework', in D. L. Barker and S. Allen (eds.), *Dependence and Exploitation in Work and Marriage* (London and New York: Longman).

Davidoff, L. (1979), 'The separation of home and work? Landladies and lodgers in nineteenth and early twentieth century England', in S. Burman (ed.), *Fit Work for Women* (London: Croom Helm).

Davidoff, L., l'Esperance, J., and Newby, H. (1976), 'Landscape with figures: home and community in English society', in J. Mitchell and A. Oakley (eds.), *The Rights and Wrongs of Women* (Harmondsworth: Penguin).

Davidoff, L., and Hall, C. (1987), *Family Fortunes: Men and Women of the English Middle Class 1780–1850* (London: Hutchinson).

Davies, C. (1971), 'Professionals in organizations: observations on hospital consultants', *Sociological Review*, 20, 4, NS.

Davies, C. (1972), 'Professionals in organisations: some preliminary observations on hospital consultants', *Sociological Review*, 20, 4, NS, p. 553.

Davies, C. (1976), 'Experience of dependency and control in work: the case of nurses', *Journal of Advanced Nursing Studies*, 1, pp. 273–81.

Davies, C. (1977), 'Continuities in the development of hospital nursing', *Journal of Advanced Nursing Studies*, 2, pp. 479–93.

Davies, C. (1979), 'Hospital-centred health care: policies and politics in the NHS', in P. Atkinson, R. Dingwall and A. Murcott (eds.), *Prospects for the National Health* (London: Croom Helm).

Davies, C. (1980a), 'Making sense of the census in Britain and the USA: the changing occupational classification and position of nurses', *Sociological Review*, 28, pp. 581–609.

Davies, C. (ed.) (1980b), *Rewriting Nursing History* (London: Croom Helm; Totowa, NJ: Barnes & Noble).

Davies, C. (1982), 'The regulation of nursing work: an historical comparison of Britain and the USA', in J. Roth (ed.), *Research in the Sociology of Health Care*, Vol. 2, pp. 121–60.

Davies, C. (1983), 'Historical explanations of the contemporary division of labour in child health care', in M. Stacey and C. Davies *Division of Labour in Child Health Care: Final Report to the SSRC* (Coventry: University of Warwick).

Davies, C. (1987) 'Making history: the early days of the HVA', *Health Visitor*, 60, May, pp. 145–8.

Davies, C. (1988), 'The health visitor as mother's friend: a women's place in public health 1900–1914', *Journal of the Society for the Social History of Medicine*, 1, 1, pp. 39–57.

Davies, C., and Francis, A. (1976), 'Perceptions of structure in NHS hospitals', in M. Stacey (ed.), *The Sociology of the NHS*, Sociological Review Monograph No. 22 (Keele: University of Keele).

Davies, C., and Rosser, J. (1985), *Equal Opportunities for Women in the NHS*, Report on an ESRC/DHSS project grant no. RDB/1/19/2, mimeo (Coventry: University of Warwick).

Davies, C., and Rosser, J. (1986), 'Gendered jobs in the health service: a problem for labour process analysis', in D. Knights and H. Willmott (eds.), *Gender and the Labour Process* (Aldershot: Gower).

Dean, M., and Bolton, G. (1980), 'The administration of poverty and the development of nursing practice in nineteenth century England', in Davies, op. cit.

Debus, A. G. (1972), 'Guintherius, Libavius and Sennert: the chemical compromise in early modern medicine', A. G. Debus (ed.), in *Science, Medicine and Society in the Renaissance: Essays to Honor Walter Pagel*, Vol. 1 (London: Heinemann).

Delphy, C. (1977) *The Main Enemy: A Materialist Analysis of Women's Oppression* (London: Women's Research and Resources Centre).

Denzin, N. K. (1970), *The Research Act* (Chicago: Aldine).

Department of Employment (1986) *New Earnings Survey* (London: HMSO).

Derber, C. (1984), 'Physicians and their sponsors: the new medical relations of production', in J. B. McKinlay (ed.), *Issues in the Political Economy of Health Care* (New York and London: Tavistock).

DHSS (1969), *Report of the Working Party on Management Structure in Local Authority Nursing Services*, Mayston Report (London: HMSO).

DHSS (1970), *Domiciliary Midwifery and Maternity Bed Needs: Report of the Sub committee*, Peel Report, Standing Maternity and Midwifery Advisory Committee (London: HMSO).

DHSS (1971), *Better Services for the Mentally Handicapped*, Cmnd 4683 (London: HMSO).

DHSS (1972a), *Second Report of the Joint Working Party on the Organization of Medical Work in Hospitals* , Cogwheel II (London: HMSO).

DHSS (1972b), *Management Arrangements for the Reorganized Health Service* (London: HMSO).

DHSS (1976a), *Prevention and Health, Everybody's Business* (London: HMSO).

DHSS (1976b), *Priorities for Health and Personal Social Services in England* (London: HMSO).

DHSS (1980), *Report of the Working Group on Inequalities in Health*, Black Report, mimeo (London: DHSS); see also Townsend and Davidson, 1982.

DHSS (1983a), *Health Care and its Costs* (London: HMSO).

DHSS (1983b), *NHS Management Enquiry Report*, Griffiths Report, DA (83) 38.

Dingwall, R. (1976), *Aspects of Illness* (London: Martin Robertson).

Dingwall, R., Eekelaar, J. M., and Murray, T. (1983), *The Protection of Children: State Intervention and Family Life* (Oxford: Blackwell).

Dingwall, R., and McIntosh, J. (eds.) (1978), *Readings in the Sociology of Nursing* (Edinburgh: Churchill Livingstone).

Dohrenwend, B. S., and Dohrenwend, B. P. (1976) 'Sex differences in psychiatric disorders', *American Journal of Sociology*, 91, pp. 1447–59.

Doll, R., and Hill, A. B. (1950), 'Smoking and carcinoma of the lung: preliminary report', *British Medical Journal*, 2, 4682 pp. 739–48.

Doll, R., and Hill, A. B. (1952), 'A study of the aetiology of carcinoma of the lung', *British Medical Journal*, 2, 4749 pp. 1271–86.

Doll, R., and Hill, A. B. (1954), 'The mortality of doctors in relation to their smoking habits: a preliminary report', *British Medical Journal*, 1, 4877 pp. 1451–5.

Doll, R., and Hill, A. B. (1956), 'Lung cancer and other causes of death in relation to smoking: a second report on the mortality of British doctors', *British Medical Journal*, 2, 5001 pp. 1071–81.

Doll, R., and Hill, A. B. (1964), 'Mortality in relation to smoking: ten years' observation of British doctors', *British Medical Journal*, 1, 5395 pp. 1399–1410, 1460–7.

Donegan, J. B. (1978), '*Women and Men Midwives: Medicine, Morality and Misogyny in Early America*' (Westport, Conn.: Greenwood).

Donnison, J. (1977), *Midwives and Medical Men: A History of Inter-Professional Rivalries and Women's Rights* (London: Heinemann).

Donzelot, J. (1979), *Policing the Family*, trans. G. Delenze (London: Hutchinson).

Doyal, L. (1985), 'Women and the National Health Service', in E. Lewin and V. Olesen (eds.), *Women, Health and Healing* (New York and London: Tavistock).

Doyal, L. (1987), 'Infertility – a life sentence? Women and the National Health Service', in M. Stanworth (ed.), *Reproductive Technologies: Gender, Motherhood and Medicine* (Cambridge: Polity Press).

Doyal, L., Hunt, G., and Mellor, J. (1981), 'Your life in their hands: migrant workers in the National Health Service', *Critical Social Policy*, 1, 2, pp. 54–71.

Doyal, L., with Pennell, I. (1979), *The Political Economy of Health* (London: Pluto).

Drysdale, G. (1867), *The Elements of Social Science, or Physical, Sexual and Natural Religion*, 7th edn (London); cited in L'Esperance, 1977.

Dubos, R. (1979), *Mirage of Health* (New York: Harper).

Dubos, R. (1985), 'Mirage of health', in N. Black, D. Boswell, A. Gray, S. Murphy and J. Popay (eds.), *Health and Disease*, (Milton Keynes and Philadelphia: Open University Press), pp. 4–9.

Dunnell, K., and Cartwright, A. (1972), *Medicine Takers, Prescribers and Hoarders* (London and Boston: Routledge & Kegan Paul).

Earwicker, R. (1981a), 'The emergence of a medical strategy in the labour movement 1906–1919', *Bulletin of the Society for the Social History of Medicine*, 29, pp. 6–9.

Earwicker, R. (1981b), 'Miners' medical services before the First World War: the South Wales coalfield', *Llasur*, 3, 2, pp. 39–52 (Welsh Labour History Society).

Eccles, A. (1982), *Obstetrics and Gynaecology in Tudor and Stuart England* (London: Croom Helm).

Eckstein, H. (1958), *The English Health Service* (Cambridge, Mass.: Harvard University Press).

Eder, N. R. (1982) *National Health Insurance and the Medical Profession in Britain: 1913–1939* (New York and London: Garland).

Ehrenreich, B. and J. (1978), 'Medicine and social control', in Ehrenreich, *op. cit.*

Ehrenreich, B., and English, D. (1974a), *Complaints and Disorders: The Sexual Politics of Sickness*, Glass Mountain Pamphlet No. 2 (London: Compendium).

Ehrenreich, B., and English, D. (1974b), *Witches, Midwives and Nurses: A History of Women Healers*, Glass Mountain Pamphlet No. 1 (London: Compendium).

Ehrenreich, B., and English, D. (1979), *For Her Own Good: 150 Years of the Experts' Advice to Women* (London: Pluto).

Ehrenreich, J. (ed.) (1978), *The Cultural Crisis of Modern Medicine* (New York and London: Monthly Review Press).

Elston, M. A. (1977), *Women, Equal Opportunity and the NHS*, unpublished draft prepared for the Equal Opportunities Commission as evidence to the Royal Commission on the National Health Service.

Engels, F. (1971), *The Condition of the Working Class in England*, trans. and ed. W. O. Henderson and W. H. Chaloner (Oxford: Blackwell).

Equal Opportunities Commission (1979), *EOC Response to the DHSS Discussion Document 'A Happier Old Age'* (Manchester: EOC).

Equal Opportunities Commission (1982), *Caring for the Elderly and Handicapped: Community Care Policies and Women's Lives* (Manchester: EOC).

Etzioni, A. (1969), *The Semi-Professions and Their Organization* (New York: Free Press; London: Collier-Macmillan).

Etzioni, A. (1973), *Genetic Fix* (New York: Macmillan; London: Collier-Macmillan).

Evers, H. (1981a), 'Care or custody? The experiences of women patients in long-stay geriatric wards', in B. Hutter and G. Williams (eds.), *Controlling Women: The Normal and the Deviant* (London: Croom Helm).

Evers, H. (1981b), 'Multi-disciplinary teamwork in geriatric wards: myth or reality?', *Journal of Advanced Nursing*, 6, pp. 205–14.

Evers, H. (1982), 'Professional practice and patient care: multi-disciplinary team work in geriatric wards, *Ageing and Society*, 2, pp. 57–76.

Evers H. (1985), 'The frail elderly woman: emergent questions in ageing and women's health', in E. Lewin and V. Olesen (eds.), *Women, Health and Healing* (New York and London: Tavistock).

Eyler, J. M. (1979), *Victorian Social Medicine: The Ideas and Methods of William Farr* (Baltimore, Md, and London: Johns Hopkins University Press).

Fabrega, H. (1973), *Disease and Social Behaviour* (Cambridge, Mass.: MIT Press).

Faderman, L. (c.1980), *Surpassing the Love of Men* (London: Junction Books).

Fagerhaugh, S. Y., and Strauss, A. (1977), *The Politics of Pain Management* (Nemlo-Park, Calif.: Addison-Wesley).

Farrant, W. (1985), 'Who's for amniocentesis? The politics of prenatal screening', in H. Homans (ed.), *The Sexual Politics of Reproduction*, (Aldershot: Gower).

Feierman, S. (1979), 'Change in African therapeutic systems', *Social Science and Medicine*, 13B, 4, pp. 277–84.

Field, D. (1976), 'The social definition of illness' in Tuckett, op. cit.

Field, M. (1967), *Soviet Socialized Medicine* (New York: Free Press).

Finch, J. (1983), *Married to the Job: Wives' Incorporation in Men's Work* (London: Allen & Unwin).

Finch, J., and Groves, D. (1980), 'Community care and the family: a case for equal opportunities?', *Journal of Social Policy*, 9, 4, 487–514.

Finch, J., and Groves, D. (eds.) (1983), *A Labour of Love: Women, Work and Caring* (London and Boston: Routledge & Kegan Paul).

Finlay, R. A. P. (1981), *Population and Metropolis: The Demography of London 1580–1650* (Cambridge: Cambridge University Press).

Fitton, F., and Achison, H. W. K. (1979), *The Doctor/Patient Relationship: A Study in General Practice* (London: HMSO).

Flint, C. (1986), 'A radical blueprint', *Nursing Times*, 82, 1, 1–7 January, p. 14; reprinted MIDIRS Information Pack No. 1, March 1986.

Forbes, T. R. (1979), 'By what disease or casualty: the changing face of death in London', in *Health Medicine and Mortality in the Sixteenth Century* (Cambridge: Cambridge University Press).

Fortune (1982), 'The 500 largest industrial corporations', 3 May, pp. 260–73.

Foucault, M. (1967), *Madness and Civilization: A History of Insanity in the Age of Reason*, trans. R. Howard (London: Tavistock).

Foucault, M. (1973), *The Birth of the Clinic: An Archaeology of Medical Perception*, trans. A. M. Sheridan Smith (London: Tavistock).

Foucault, M. (1979), *Discipline and Punish: The Birth of the Prison* (Harmondsworth: Peregrine).

Foucault, M. (1980), *Power/Knowledge: Selected Interviews and Other Writings 1972–77*, ed. C. Gordon, trans. C. Gordon, L. Marshall, J. Mepham and K. Soper (Brighton: Harvester).

Fox, R. C. (n.d.), 'Medical evolution', in *Explorations in General Theory in Social Science*, Vol. 2 (New York: Free Press).

Frankenberg, R. (1980), 'Medical anthropology and development: a theoretical perspective, *Social Science and Medicine*, 14B, 4, November, pp. 197–207.

Frankenberg, R. (1981), 'Allopathic medicine, profession and capitalist ideology in India', *Social Science and Medicine*, 15A, 2, March, pp. 115–25.

Freidson, E. (1961), *Patients' Views of Medical Practice* (New York: Russel Sage).

Freidson, E. (1970a), *Profession of Medicine: A Study in the Sociology of Applied Knowledge* (New York: Dodd Mead).

Freidson, E. (1970b), *Professional Dominance* (New York: Atherton).

Freidson, E. (1977), 'The futures of professionalisation', in M. Stacey, M. Reid, C. Heath and R. Dingwall (eds.) *Health and the Division of Labour* (London: Croom Helm; New York: Prodist).

Freidson, E. (1986), *Professional Powers: A Study of the Institutionalization of Formal*

Knowledge (Chicago and London: University of Chicago Press).

Fung, K. P., Chow, O. K. W., and So, S. Y. (1986) 'Attenuation of exercise-induced asthma by acupuncture', *Lancet*, 20–7 December, II, 8521–2, pp. 1419–22.

Gallagher, E. (1976), 'Lines of reconstruction and extension in the Parsonian sociology of illness', *Social Science and Medicine*, 10, 5, pp. 208–18.

Gamarnikow, E. (1978), 'Sexual divisions of labour: the case of nursing', in A. Kuhn and A. M. Wolpe (eds.), *Feminism and Materialism* (London: Routledge & Kegan Paul).

General Medical Council (1901) *The Medical Register* (London: GMC).

General Medical Council (1977), Minutes, 11 November, App. XIII, 'Evidence to the Royal Commission on the National Health Service', (London: GMC).

Gerhardt, U. (1979), 'The Parsonian paradigm and the identity of medical sociology', *Sociological Review*, 27, 2, p. 229.

Gill, D., and Horobin, G. (1972), 'Doctors, patients and the state: relationships and decision making', *Sociological Review*, 20, 4, NS, pp. 505–20.

Ginsberg, M. (1934), *Sociology* (London: Butterworth).

Godber, G. (1975), *The Health Service: Past, Present and Future* (London: Athlone).

Godber, G. (1983), 'The Domesday Book of British Hospitals', *Bulletin of the Society for the Social History of Medicine*, 32, pp. 4–13.

Goffman, E. (1961), *Asylums: Essays on the Social Situation of Mental Patients and other Inmates* (Garden City, NY: Anchor, Doubleday).

Goldie, N. (1977), 'The division of labour among mental health professionals', in M. Stacey, M. Reid, C. Heath and R. Dingwall (eds.), *Health and the Division of Labour* (London: Croom Helm).

Golombok, S., and Rust, J. (1986), The Warnock Report and single women: what about the children?' *Journal of Medical Ethics*, 12, 4, 182–6.

Golombok, S., Spencer, A., and Rutter, M. (1983), 'Children in lesbian and single-parent households: psycho-sexual and psychiatric appraisal', *Journal of Child Psychology and Psychiatry*, 24, pp. 551–72.

Gough, I. (1979), *The Political Economy of the Welfare State* (London and Basingstoke: Macmillan).

Gove, W. R., and Tudor, J. (1972–3) 'Adult sex roles and mental illness', *American Journal of Sociology*, 78, 4, pp. 812–35.

Graham, H. (1979), '"Prevention and health: every mother's business": a comment on child health policy in the seventies', in C. Harris (ed.), *The Sociology of the Family: New Directions for Britain*, Sociological Review Monograph 28 (Keele: University of Keele).

Graham, H. (1984), *Women, Health and the Family* (Brighton: Wheatsheaf Harvester).

Graham, H. (1985a), 'Caring for the family: a short report of the study of the organisation of health resources and responsibilities in 102 families with pre-school children, mimeo (Milton Keynes: Open University).

Graham, H. (1985b), 'Providers, negotiators and mediators: women as the hidden carers', in E. Lewin and V. Olesen (eds.) *Women, Health and Healing* (New York and London: Tavistock).

Graham, H., and McKee, L. (1980), *The First Months of Motherhood*, Research Monograph No. 3 (London: Health Education Council).

Graham, H., and Oakley, A. (1981), 'Competing ideologies of reproduction: medical and maternal perspectives on pregnancy', in H. Roberts (ed.) *Women, Health and Reproduction* (London: Routledge & Kegan Paul).

Graham, H., and Oakley, A. (1986), 'Competing ideologies of reproduction: medical and maternal perspectives on pregnancy', in Currer and Stacey, op. cit.

Grant, G. (1986), 'The structure on care networks in families with mentally handicapped adult dependants', mimeo (Bangor: Centre for Social Policy Research and Development, University College of North Wales).

Green, S. (1974), *The Hospital: An Organizational Analysis* (Glasgow: Blackie).

Greg, W. R. (1979), 'Prostitution', *Westminster Review*, LIII (1850), pp. 448–506, in Bauer and Ritt, op. cit., p. 45.

Grigg, J. (1979), 'Porters' problems, doctors' dilemmas', in P. Atkinson, R. Dingwall and A. Murcott (eds.) *Prospects for the National Health*, (London: Croom Helm).

Groves, D., and Finch, J. (1983), 'Natural selection: perspectives on entitlement to the invalid care allowance', in Finch and Groves, op. cit.

Guthrie, D. (1960) *A History of Medicine* (London: Nelson).

Hakim, C. (1979), 'Occupational segregation: a comparative study of the degree and pattern of the differentiation between men and women's work in Britain, the United States and other countries'. Research Paper no. 9 (London: Department of Employment).

Hall, D. (1977), *Social Relations and Innovation* (London: Routledge & Kegan Paul).

Hall, M. H., Chng, P. K., and MacGillivray, I. (1980), 'Is routine antenatal care worthwhile?', *Lancet*, 12 July, pp. 78–80.

Hall, D. and Stacey, M. (eds.) (1979), *Beyond Separation: Further Studies of Children in Hospital* (London: Routledge & Kegan Paul).

Hannay, D. R. (1979), *The Symptom Iceberg: A Study of Community Health* (London and Boston: Routledge & Kegan Paul).

Harley, D. N. (1981), 'Ignorant midwives – a persistent stereotype', *Bulletin of the Society for the Social History of Medicine*, 28, pp. 6–9.

Harris, J. (1985), *The Value of Life* (London: Routledge & Kegan Paul).

Harrison, B. (1981), 'Women's health and the women's movement in Britain 1840–1940', in Webster, op. cit.

Hart, J. T. (1973), 'Bevan and the doctors', *Lancet*, 3, 7839, 24 November, p. 1196–7.

Hawkes, J. (trans) (1982), *The London Journal of Flora Tristan 1842 or The Aristocracy and the Working Class of England* (London: Virago).

Helman, C. (1978), '"Feed a cold, starve a fever," – folk models of infection in an English suburban community and their relation to medical treatment', *Culture, Medicine and Psychiatry*, 2, pp. 107–37.

Helman, C. (1981), 'Disease versus illness in general practice', *Journal of the Royal College of General Practitioners*, 31, p. 548.

Helman, C. (1984), 'Feed a cold, starve a fever', in N. Black, D. Boswell, A. Gray, S. Murphy and J. Popay (eds.), *Health and Disease* (Milton Keynes and Philadelphia, Pa: Open University Press).

Helman, C. (1986), 'Feed a cold, starve a fever', in Currer and Stacey, op. cit.

Henry, S., and Robinson, D. (1979), 'The self-help way to health', in P. Atkinson, R. Dingwall and A. Murcott (eds.), *Prospects for the National Health* (London: Croom Helm).

Herxheimer, A., and Lionel, N. D. W. (1978), 'Minimum information needed by prescribers', *British Medical Journal*, 2, pp. 1129–32.

Herxheimer, A., and Stimson, G. V. (1981), 'The use of medicines for illness', in Blum *et al.*, op. cit.

Herzlich, C. (1973), *Health and Illness* (London and New York: Academic Press).

Herzlich, C., and Pierret, J. (1984) *Malades d'hier, malades d'aujourd'hui* (Paris: Payot).

Herzlich, C., and Pierret, J. (1985), 'The social construction of the patient: patients and illnesses in other ages', *Social Science and Medicine*, 20, 2, pp. 145–51.

Herzlich, C., and Pierret, J. (1986), 'Illness: from causes to meaning', in Currer and Stacey, op. cit.

Herzlich, C., and Pierret, J. (1987), (trans. E. Forster), *Illness and Self in Society* (Baltimore and London: The Johns Hopkins University Press).

Hill, A. Bradford (1962), *Statistical Methods in Clinical and Preventive Medicine* (London: Livingstone).

Hill, A. Bradford (1971), *Principles of Medical Statistics*, 8th edn (London: The Lancet).

HMSO (1949), *Report of the Working Party on Midwives* (London: HMSO).

HMSO (1951a), *Report of the Committee on Medical Auxiliaries* (London: HMSO).

HMSO (1951b), *Report of the Committee on Social Workers in the Mental Health Service* (London: HMSO).
HMSO (1952), *Report of the Inter-Departmental Committee on the Statutory Registration of Opticians* (London: HMSO).
HMSO (1955), *Report of the Working Party on the Training of District Nurses* (London: HMSO).
HMSO (1956), *Inquiry into Health Visiting* (London: HMSO).
HMSO (1959a), *Report of the Working Party on Social Workers in Local Authority Health and Welfare Services* (London: HMSO).
HMSO (1959b), *Report on the Maternity Services Committee* (London: HMSO).
HMSO (1968a), *Hospital Scientific and Technical Services* (London: HMSO).
HMSO (1968b), *Psychiatric Nursing: Today and Tomorrow* (London: HMSO).
HMSO (1968c), *Report of the Royal Commission on Medical Education*, Todd Report, Cmnd 3569 (London: HMSO).
HMSO (1970a), *Domiciliary Midwifery and Maternity Beds* (London: HMSO).
HMSO (1970b), *Report of the Working Party on the Hospital Pharmaceutical Services* (London: HMSO).
HMSO (1971), *Better Services for the Mentally Handicapped*, cmnd 4683 (London: HMSO).
HMSO (1972), *Report of the Committee on Nursing* (London: HMSO).
HMSO (1973), *The Remedial Professions* (London: HMSO).
HMSO (1979), *Report of the Royal Commission on the National Health Service*, Cmnd 7615 (London: HMSO).
HMSO (1984), *Human Fertilisation and Embryology*, Warnock Report, Cmnd 9314 (London: HMSO).
HMSO (1987), *Human Fertilisation and Embryology: a Framework for Legislation*, Cmnd 259 (London: HMSO).
Holland, W. W., Ipsen, J., and Kostrzewski, J. (eds.) (1979), *Measurement of Levels of Health* (Geneva: World Health Organization/International Epidemiological Association).
Holloway, S. W. F. (1964), 'Medical education in England, 1830–1858: a sociological analysis', *Medical History*, XLIX, pp. 299–324.
Holloway, S. W. F. (1966) 'The Apothecaries' Act, 1815: a reinterpretation', *Medical History*, X, Pt I, pp. 107–29; Pt II, pp. 221–35.
Holmes, B. B., and Hoskins, H. B. (1985), 'Prenatal and preconception sex choice technologies: a path to femicide?', in Corea, *et al.*, op. cit.
Homans, H. (1985) 'Discomforts in pregnancy: traditional remedies and medical prescriptions', in H. Homans (ed.), *The Sexual Politics of Reproduction* (Aldershot: Gower).
Honigsbaum, F. (1979), *The Division in British Medicine: A History of the Separation of General Practice from Hospital Care 1911–1968* (London: Kogan Page).
Hornstein, F. (1984), 'Children by donor insemination: a new choice for lesbians', in Arditti, Klein and Minden, op. cit.
Horton, R. (1970), 'African traditional thought and Western science', in M. Marwick (ed.), *Witchcraft, Sorcery and Magic* (Harmondsworth: Penguin), and in M. F. D. Young (ed.) (1971), *Knowledge and Control* (London: Collier-Macmillan).
Hoskins, H. B., and Holmes, B. B. (1984), 'Technology and prenatal femicide', in Arditti, Klein and Minden, op. cit.
Houd, S., and Oakley, A,. (1983), *Alternative Perinatal Services: Report on a Pilot Survey* (Copenhagen: World Health Organization, Regional Office for Europe).
d'Houtaud, A. (1976), 'La représentation de la santé: recherche dans un centre bilan de santé en Lorraine', *Revue Internationale d'Education pour la Santé*, 19, 2, pp. 99–118, and 3, pp. 173–88.
d'Houtaud, A. (1978), 'L'image de la santé dans une population Lorraine: approche

psychosociale des représentations de la santé', *Revue d'Epidémiologies et de Santé publique*, 26, pp. 299–320.

d'Houtaud, A. (1981), 'Nouvelles recherches sur les représentations de la santé, *Revue Internationale d'Education pour la Santé*, 24, 3, pp. 3–22.

d'Houtaud, A., and Field, M. (1984), 'The image of health: variations in perception by social class in a French population', *Sociology of Health and Illness*, 6, 1, pp. 30–60.

d'Houtaud, A., and Field, M. (1986), 'New research on the image of health', in Currer and Stacey, op. cit.

Hughes, E. (1971), *The Sociological Eye* (Chicago: Aldine).

Huntingdon, J. (1981), *Social Work and General Medical Practice: Collaboration or Conflict?* (London: Allen & Unwin).

Hutt, R. (1985), *Chief Officer Career Profiles: A Study of the Backgrounds, Training and Career Experience of Regional and District Nursing Officers* (Brighton: Institute of Manpower Studies, University of Sussex).

Iliffe, S. (1983), *The NHS: A Picture of Health* (London: Lawrence & Wishart).

Illich, I. (1975), *Medical Nemesis: The Expropriation of Health* (London: Calder & Boyars).

Illich, I. (1976), *Limits to Medicine* (London: Marion Boyars).

Illich, I. (1984), 'The epidemics of modern medicine', in N. Black, D. Boswell, A. Gray, S. Murphy and J. Popay (eds.) *Health and Disease* (Milton Keynes: Open University Press).

Inkster, I. (1977), 'Marginal men: aspects of the social role of the medical community in Sheffield 1790–1850', in J. Woodward and D. Richards (eds.) *Health Care and Popular Medicine in Nineteenth-Century England* (London: Croom Helm).

Jaco, E., and Gartley, E. (eds.) (1979), *Patients, Physicians and Illness: A Source Book in Behavioural Science and Health*, 3rd edn. (New York: Free Press; London: Collier-Macmillan).

Jago, J. D. (1975), '"Hal" – old word, new task: reflections on the words "health", and "medical",' *Social Science and Medicine*, 9, 1, pp. 1–6.

Jamous, H., and Peloille, B. (1970), 'Professions or self-perpetuating systems? Changes in the French university-hospital system', in J. A. Jackson (ed.) *Professions and Professionalization*, (Cambridge: Cambridge University Press).

Jeffery, R. (1977), 'Allopathic medicine in India: a case of deprofessionalization?', *Social Science and Medicine*, 11, 10, July, pp. 561–73.

Jefferys, M., and Sachs, H. (1983), *Rethinking General Practice* (London and New York: Tavistock).

Jewson, N. (1974), 'Medical knowledge and the patronage system in eighteenth century England', *Sociology*, 8, pp. 369–85.

Jewson, N. (1976), 'The disappearance of the sick man from the medical cosmology', *Sociology*, 10, pp. 225–44.

Jobst, K., Chen, J. H., McPherson, K., Arrowsmith, J., Brown, V., Efthimiou, J., Fletcher, H. J., Maciocia, G., Mole, P., Shifrin, K., and Lane, D. J. (1986), 'Controlled trial of acupuncture and breathlessness', *Lancet*, 2, 8521/2 20–27 December, pp. 1416–19.

Johnson, T. (1972), *Professions and Power* (London: Macmillan).

Johnson, T. (1977), 'The professions in the class structure', in R. Scase (ed.) *Industrial Society: Class, Cleavage and Control* (London: Allen & Unwin).

Johnson, T. (1982), 'The state and the professions: peculiarities of the British', in Giddens, A. and G. Mackenzie (eds.), *Social Class and the Division of Labour: Essays in Honour of Ilya Neustadt* (Cambridge: Cambridge University Press.)

Jordanova, L. J. (1979), 'Earth science and environmental medicine: the synthesis of the late enlightenment', in L. J. Jordanova and R. S. Porter (eds.) *Images of the Earth: Essays in the History of the Environmental Sciences* (Chalfont St Giles: British Society for the History of Science).

Jordanova, L. J. (1981), 'Policing public health in France 1780–1815', in T. Ogawa (ed.), *Public Health* (Tokyo: Saikon).

Jordanova, L. J. (1985), 'Gender, generation and science: William Hunter's Obstetrical atlas', in W. F. Bynum and R. Porter (eds.), *William Hunter and the Eighteenth Century Medical World* (Cambridge: Cambridge University Press).

Keller, A. G. (1972), 'Mathematical technologies and the growth of the idea of technical progress in the sixteenth century', in A. G. Debus (ed.), *Science, Medicine and Society in the Renaissance*, Vol. 1 (London: Heinemann).

Kennedy, I. (1983), *The Unmasking of Medicine: A Searching Look at Health Care Today* (London: Granada).

Kishwar, M. (1985), 'The continuing deficit of women in India and the impact of amniocentesis', in Corea *et al.*, op. cit.

Kitzinger, S. (1962), *The Experience of Childbirth* (London: Gollancz).

Kitzinger, S. (1971), *Giving Birth – The Parents' Emotions in Childbirth* (London: Gollancz).

Kitzinger, S., and Davis, J. A. (eds.) (1978), *The Place of Birth: A Study of the Environment in which Birth Takes Place with Special Reference to Home Confinements* (Oxford and New York: Oxford University Press).

Klein, R. (1983), *The Politics of the National Health Service* (London and New York: Longman).

Klein, R., and Lewis, J. (1976), *The Politics of Consumer Representation: A Study of Community Health Councils* (London: Centre for Studies in Social Policy).

Klein, R. D. (1984), 'Doing it ourselves: self-insemination', in Arditti, Klein and Minden, op. cit.

Klein, R. D. (1985), 'What's "new" about the "new" reproductive technologies?' in Corea *et al.*, op. cit.

Kleinman, A. (1978), 'Concepts and a model for the comparison of medical systems as cultural systems', *Social Science and Medicine*, 12, 2B, pp. 85–93.

Kleinman, A. (1980), *Patients and Healers in the Context of Culture* (Berkeley, Calif.: University of California Press).

Kleinman, A. (1986) 'Concepts and a model for the comparison of medical symptoms as cultural systems', in Currer and Stacey, op. cit.

Kratz, C. R. (ed.) (1979), *The Nursing Process* (London: Ballière Tindall).

Kronus, C. L. (1976), 'The evolution of occupational power: an historical study of task boundaries between physicians and pharmacists', *Sociology of Work and Occupations*, 3, 1, pp. 3–35.

Laing, R. D. (1968), *The Politics of Experience and the Bird of Paradise* (Harmondsworth: Penguin).

Laing, R. D., and Esterson, A. (1973), *Sanity, Madness and the Family*, 2nd edn (Harmondsworth: Penguin).

Lall. S. (1981), 'Economic considerations in the provision and use of medicine', in Blum *et al.*, op. cit.

Land, H. (1976), 'Women: supporters or supported?' in D. L. Barker and S. Allen (eds.), *Sexual Divisions and Society: Process and Change* (London: Tavistock).

Land, H. (1978), 'Who cares for the family?' *Journal of Social Policy*, 7, 3, pp. 357–84.

Lane, J. (1981), 'The provincial practitioner and his services to the poor', *Bulletin of the Society for the Social History of Medicine*, 28, pp. 10–14.

Lang, R. W. (1974), *The Politics of Drugs* (Aldershot: Saxon House).

Langendonck, J. V. (1975), *Prelude to Harmony on a Community Theme: Health Care Insurance Policies in the Six and Britain*, introduced and ed. Gordon Forsyth (London: Nuffield Provincial Hospitals Trust; Oxford University Press).

Larkin, G. V. (1978), 'Medical dominance and control: radiographers in the division of labour', *Sociological Review*, 26, 4, pp. 843–58.

Larkin, G. V. (1980), 'Professionalism, dentistry and public health', *Social Science and Medicine*, 14A, pp. 223–9.

Larkin, G. V. (1981), 'Professional autonomy and the ophthalmic optician', *Sociology of Health and Illness*, 3, 1, pp. 15–30.

Larkin, G. (1983), *Occupational Monopoly and Modern Medicine* (London and New York: Tavistock).

Larson, M. S. (1977), *The Rise of Professionalism* (Berkeley, Calif.: University of California Press).

Lasker, J. (1981), 'Choosing among therapies: illness behaviour in the Ivory Coast', *Social Science and Medicine*, 15A, 2, pp. 157–168.

Laslett, P. (1971), *The World We Have Lost*, 2nd edn (London: Methuen).

Last, J. M. (1963), 'The illness iceberg', *Lancet*, 6 July, pp. 28–31.

Lawrence, C. J. (1981), 'Sanitary reformers and the medical profession in Victorian England', in T. Ogawa (ed.) *Public Health*, (Tokyo: Saikon).

L'Esperance, J. (1977), 'Doctors and women in nineteenth century society: sexuality and role', in J. Woodward and D. Richards (eds.), *Health Care and Popular Medicine in Nineteenth Century England* (London: Croom Helm).

Levitt, R. (1976), *The Reorganized National Health Service* (London: Croom Helm).

Levitt, R. (1979), *The Reorganized National Health Service*, 2nd edn (London: Croom Helm).

Lewin, E. (1985), 'By design: reproductive strategies and the meaning of motherhood', in H. Homans (ed.), *The Sexual Politics of Reproduction* (Aldershot: Gower).

Lewis, G. (1975), *Knowledge of Illness in a Sepik Society* (London: Athlone).

Lewis, G. (1976), 'A view of sickness in New Guinea', in J. B. Louden (ed.), *Social Anthropology and Medicine*, (London: Academic Press).

Lewis, G. (1980), *Day of Shining Red* (Cambridge: Cambridge University Press).

Lewis, G. (1986) 'Concepts of health and illness in a Sepik society', in Currer and Stacey, op. cit.

Lewis, J. (1980), *The Politics of Motherhood: Child and Maternal Welfare in England, 1900–1939* (London: Croom Helm; Montreal: McGill/Queen's University Press).

Lewis, J. (1984) *Women in England 1870–1950: Sexual Divisions and Social Change* (Brighton: Wheatsheaf/Harvester; Bloomington, Ind.: Indiana University Press).

Lewis, O. (1955), 'Medicine and politics in a Mexican village', in B. D. Paul (ed.), *Health, Culture and Community* (New York: Russell Sage).

Lhomond, B. (1986), 'Sapphists, tribades, female inverts and lesbians: medical discourses on female homosexuality 1880–1930', communication to the International Women's History Conference, Amsterdam, March 1986.

Llewelyn Davies, M. (ed.) (197), *Life as We Have Known it, by Co-operative Working Women* (London: Virago).

Llewellyn Davies, M. (ed.) (1978), *Maternity. Letters from Working Women Collected by the Women's Co-operative Guild* (London: Virago); 1st published 1915.

Locker, D. (1981), *Symptoms and Illness* (London: Tavistock).

Lodge, M. (1985), 'Friends or strangers: a commentary on pre-National Health Service general practitioners', Warwick Working Papers in Sociology (Coventry: University of Warwick).

Lodge, M. (n.d.), 'Women and welfare: an account of the development of infant welfare schemes in Coventry 1900–1940, with special reference to the work of the Coventry Women's Cooperative Guild', in Bill Lancaster and Tony Mason (eds.), *Life and Labour in a Twentieth Century City. The Experience of Coventry* (Coventry: University of Warwick).

Loney, M., Boswell, D., and Clarke, J. (eds.) (1983), *Social Policy and Social Welfare* (Milton Keynes: Open University Press).

Lopez, A. D. (1984), 'Sex differentials in mortality', *World Health Organization Chronicle*, 38, pp. 217–24.

Loudon, I. (1986), *Medical Care and the General Practitioner 1750–1850* (Oxford: Clarendon Press).

Lown, J. (1983), '"Not so much a factory; more a form of patriarchy": gender and class during industrialization', in E. Gamarnikow, D. Morgan, J. Purvis and D. Taylorson (eds.), *Gender, Class and Work* (London: Heinemann).

Lown, J. (1984), 'Gender and class during industrialization: a study of the Halstead silk industry in Essex, 1825–1900', PhD thesis, University of Essex.

Lu, G.-D., and Needham, J. (1980), *Celestial Lancets: A History and Rationale of Acupuncture and Moxa* (London: Cambridge University Press).

Lumbroso, A. (1981), 'The introduction of new drugs', in Blum *et al.*, op. cit.

Macfarlane, A. (1970), 'Witchcraft in Tudor and Stuart Essex', in M. Douglas (ed.), *Witchcraft Confessions and Accusations* (London: Tavistock).

Macfarlane, A., and Mugford, M. (1984), *Birth Counts: Statistics of Pregnancy and Childbirth*, Vols. 1 and 2 (London: HMSO).

McFarlane, J. K. (1976), 'A charter for caring', *Journal of Advanced Nursing*, 1, pp. 187–96.

Macintyre, S. (1976a), 'To have or have not – promotion and prevention of childbirth in gynaecological work', in Stacey, op. cit.

Macintyre, S. (1976b), ' "Who wants babies?" The social construction of "instincts" ', in D. L. Barker and S. Allen (eds.), *Sexual Divisions and Society: Process and Change* (London: Tavistock).

Macintyre, S. (1977), 'The myth of the golden age', *World Medicine*, 12, 18, pp. 17–22.

Macintyre, S. (1977), *Single and Pregnant* (London: Croom Helm).

Macintyre, S., and Oldman, D. (1977), 'Coping with migraine', in A. Davis and G. Horobin (eds.), *Medical Encounters: The Experience of Illness and Treatment* (London: Croom Helm).

McKee, L., and O'Brien, M. (1982), 'The father figure: some current orientations and historical perspectives', in L. McKee and M. O'Brien (eds.), *The Father Figure* (London and New York: Tavistock).

McKendrick, N. (1982), 'Commercialization of shaving', in N. McKendrick, J. Brewer and J. H. Plumb, *The Birth of a Consumer Society: The Commercialization of Eighteenth Century England* (London: Europa).

McKeown, T. (1965), *Medicine in Modern Society* (London: Allen & Unwin).

McKeown, T. (1971), 'A sociological approach to the history of medicine', in G. McLachlan and T. McKeown (eds.), *Medical History and Medical Care* (London: Nuffield Provincial Hospitals Trust/Oxford University Press).

McKeown, T. (1976), *The Role of Medicine: Dream, Mirage or Nemesis* (London: Nuffield Provincial Hospitals Trust).

McKeown, T., and Brown, R. G. (1955–6), 'Medical evidence related to English population changes in the eighteenth century', *Population Studies*, 9, pp. 119–41.

McKeown, T., and Record, R. G. (1962), 'Reasons for the decline of mortality in England and Wales during the nineteenth century', *Population Studies*, 16, pp. 94–122.

McKinlay, J. B. (1975), 'A case for refocussing upstream – the political economy of illness', in H. J. Enelow and J. B. Henderson (eds.), 'Applying Behavioral Science to Cardiovascular Risk' (Proceedings of American Heart Association Conference, Seattle, Washington, 1974), *Behavioural Science Research Data Review*, pp. 7–17.

McLaren, A. (1977), 'The early birth control movement: an example of medical self-help', in J. Woodward and D. Richards (eds.), *Health Care and Popular Medicine in Nineteenth Century England* (London: Croom Helm).

Maclean, M. U. (1969), 'Traditional healers and their female clients: an aspect of Nigerian sickness behaviour', *Journal of Health and Social Behavior*, 10, pp. 172–86.

Maclean, M. U. (1971), *Magical Medicine* (London: Allen Lane).

Maclean, M. U. (1976), 'Some aspects of sickness behaviour among the Yoruba', in J. B. Loudon (ed.), *Social Anthropology and Medicine*, ASA 13 (London and New York: Academic Press).

Maclean, U. (1974), *Nursing in Contemporary Society* (London: Routledge & Kegan Paul).

McNamara, J. A., and Wemple, S. (1974), 'The power of women through the family in medieval Europe: 500–1100' in M. Hartman and L. W. Banner (eds.), *Clio's Consciousness Raised* (New York: Harper Torchbacks).

McNeil, M. (1979), 'Medical theory and demographic concerns in early industrial England', *Bulletin of the Society for the Social History of Medicine*, 25, pp. 12–20.

Madge, N. (ed.) (1983), *Families at Risk* (London: Heinemann).

Maggs, C. J. (1983), *The Origins of General Nursing* (London: Croom Helm).

Mangold, T. (1983), 'Relationships between doctors and salesmen are lurching out of control', *Listener*, 20 January, pp. 2–4.

Manson, T. (1977), 'Management, the professions and the unions', in M. Stacey, M. Reid, C. Heath and R. Dingwall (eds.), *Health and the Division of Labour* (London: Croom Helm; New York: Prodist).

Marriott, M. McKim (1955), 'Western medicine in a village of North India', in B. D. Paul (ed.), *Health, Culture and Community* (New York: Russell Sage).

Maxwell, R. J. (1981), *Health and Wealth: An International Study of Health Care Spending* (Lexington: Heath & Co.).

Maykovich, M. K. (1980), *Medical Sociology* (Sherman Oaks, Calif.: Alfred Publishing Co.).

Mechanic, D. (1978), *Medical Sociology*, 2nd edn (New York: Free Press).

Melville, A., and Johnson, C. (1982), *Cured to Death: The Effects of Prescription Drugs* (London: Secker & Warburg).

Mernissi, F. (1975), *Beyond the Veil: Male–Female Dynamics in a Modern Muslim Society* (Cambridge, Mass.: Wiley, Schenkman).

Merton, R. (1957), *Social Theory and Social Structure* (London: Collier-Macmillan).

MIDIRS (1986), *Information Pack No. 1*, March (London: Midwives Information and Resource Service).

Ministry of Health (1955), *Committee of Enquiry into the cost of the National Health Service*, Guillebaud Report (London: HMSO).

Ministry of Health (1959), *Report of the Maternity Services Committee*, Cranbrook Report (London: HMSO).

Ministry of Health (and Scottish Home and Health Department) (1966), *Report of the Committee on Senior Nurse Staff Structure*, Salmon Report (London: HMSO).

Ministry of Health (1967), *First Report of the Joint Working Party on the Organization of Medical Work in Hospitals*, Cogwheel 1 (London: HMSO).

Morris, C. (1977), 'Plague in Britain', in *The Plague Reconsidered: A New Look at the Origins and Effects in Sixteenth and Seventeenth Century England*, Local Population Studies Supplement (Matlock, Derbyshire), pp. 37–48.

Morris, R. J. (1976), *Cholera 1832. The Social Response to an Epidemic* (London: Croom Helm).

Murcott, A. (1977), 'Blind alleys and blinkers: the scope of medical sociology', *Scottish Journal of Sociology*, 1, p. 2.

Murcott, A. (1981), 'On the typification of "bad" patients' in P. Atkinson and C. Heath (eds.), *Medical Work: Realities and Routines* (Aldershot: Gower).

Nathanson, C. (1975), 'Illness and the feminine role', *Social Science and Medicine*, 9, 2, pp. 57–62.

Nathanson, C. A. (1977), 'Sex, illness, and medical care: a review of data, theory and method', *Social Science and Medicine*, 11, 1, pp. 13–25.

National Council for Single Women and their Dependants (1979), *The Loving Trap* (London: National Council for Single Women and their Dependants).

Navarro, V. (1975), 'The industrialization of fetishism or the fetishism of industrialization: a critique of Ivan Illich', *Social Science and Medicine*, 9, 7, pp. 351–63.

Navarro, V. (1978), *Class Struggle, the State and Medicine: An Historical and Contemporary Analysis of the Medical Sector in Great Britain* (London: Martin Robertson).

Navarro, V. (1979), *Medicine under Capitalism* (London: Croom Helm).

Navarro, V. (ed.) (1982), *Imperialism, Health and Medicine* (London: Pluto).

Nelson, C. (1974), 'Private and public politics: women in the Middle Eastern World', *American Ethnologist*, 1, pp. 551–65.

Newman, C. (1957), *The Evolution of Medical Education in the Nineteenth Century* (Oxford: Oxford University Press).

Nursing Policy Studies Centre (1986), *First Annual Report*, mimeo (Coventry: University of Warwick).

Nursing Policy Studies Centre (1987), *Reports* (Coventry: University of Warwick).

Nuttall, P. D. (1983a), 'British nursing – beginning of a power struggle', *Nursing Outlook*, 31, p. 3.

Nuttall, P. (1983b), 'Male takeover or female giveaway?', *Nursing Times*, 79, 2, 12 January, pp. 10–11.

Oakley, A. (1972), *Sex, Gender and Society* (London: Temple Smith).

Oakley, A. (1976), 'Wisewoman and medicine man: changes in the management of childbirth', in J. Mitchell and A. Oakley (eds.), *The Rights and Wrongs of Women* (Harmondsworth: Penguin).

Oakley, A. (1984), *The Captured Womb: A History of the Medical Care of Pregnant Women* (Oxford and New York: Blackwell).

Oakley, A. (1987), 'From walking wombs to test tube babies', in M. Stanworth (ed.), *Reproductive Technologies: Gender, Motherhood and Medicine*, (Cambridge: Polity Press).

O'Brien, M. (1981), *The Politics of Reproduction* (Boston and London: Routledge and Kegan Paul).

O'Faolain, J., and Martines, L. (eds.), (1979), *Not in God's Image: Women in History* (London: Virago).

Office of Health Economics (1984), *Understanding the NHS in the 1980s* (London: OHE).

Office of Health Economics (1986), *Health Expenditure in the UK* (London: OHE).

Olesen, V., Schatzman, L., Droes, N., Hatton, D., Chico, N., and Chesla, K. (1985), 'Ordinary people, ordinary ailments: conceptual increments from a study of ethnocare', paper presented to the Ninth Social Science and Medicine Conference, Helsinki, Finland, mimeo (San Francisco: University of California).

Oliver, J. (1983), 'The caring wife', in Finch and Groves, op. cit.

Øvretveit, J. (1985), 'Medical dominance and the development of professional autonomy in physiotherapy', *Sociology of Health and Illness*, 7, 1, pp. 76–93.

Owens, D. (1982), 'The desire to father: reproductive ideologies and involuntarily childless men', in L. McKee and M. O'Brien (eds.), *The Father Figure* (London and New York: Tavistock).

Palmer, D. (1978), 'The protracted foundations of a national maternity service: the struggle to reduce maternal mortality in England and Wales, 1919–39', MA thesis, University of Warwick.

Palmer, D. (1987), 'Women, health and politics 1919–1939: professional and lay involement in the women's health campaign', PhD thesis. University of Warwick.

Parry, N., and Parry, J. (1976), *The Rise of the Medical Profession: A Study of Collective Social Mobility* (London: Croom Helm).

Parsons, T. (1951), *The Social System* (Glencoe, Ill.: Free Press).

Parsons, T. (1972), 'Definitions of health and illness in the light of American values and social structure', in Jaco and Gartley, op. cit.

Parsons, T. (1977), *The Evolution of Societies*, ed. T. Jackson (Englewood Cliffs, NJ: Prentice-Hall).

Pater, J. E. (1981), *The Making of the National Health Service* (London: King Edward's Hospital Fund for London).

Patrick, D. L., and Scambler, G. (eds.) (1982), *Sociology as Applied to Medicine* (London: Baillière Tindall).

Patterson, E. (1981), 'Food-work: maids in a hospital kitchen', in P. Atkinson and C. Heath (eds.), *Medical Work: Realities and Routines* (Aldershot: Gower).

Pearson, G. (1975), *The Deviant Imagination: Psychiatry, Social Work and Social Change* (London and Basingstoke: Macmillan).

Pelling, M. (1978a), 'Medical practice in Norwich 1550–1640', *Bulletin of the Society of the Social History of Medicine*, 23, pp. 30–1.

Pelling, M. (1978b), *Cholera, Fever and English Medicine 1825–1865* (Oxford: Oxford University Press).

Pelling, M. (1982), 'Occupational diversity: barber-surgeons and the trades of Norwich 1550–1640', *Bulletin of the History of Medicine*, 56, pp. 484–511.

Pelling, M. (1983), 'Medicine since 1500', in P. Corsi and P. Weindling (eds.), *Information Sources in the History of Science and Medicine* (London: Butterworth).

Pelling, M. (1985a), 'Medicine and sanitation', in J. F. Andrews (ed.), *William Shakespeare, His World, His Work, His Influence, Vol. 1 His World* (New York: Scribner's).

Pelling, M. (1985b), 'Healing the sick poor: social policy and disability in Norwich 1550–1640', *Medical History*, 29, pp. 115–37.

Pelling, M. (1986), 'Appearance and reality: barber-surgeons, the body and disease', in A. Beier (ed.), *London 1500–1700: The Making of the Metropolis* (London and New York: Longman).

Pelling, M. (1987), 'Medical practice in the early modern period: trade or profession?', in W. Prest (ed.), *The Professions in Early Modern England* (London: Croom Helm).

Pelling, M., and Webster, C. (1979), 'Medical practitioners', in Webster, op. cit.

Perkin, H. (1969), *The Origins of Modern English Society 1780–1880* (London: Routledge & Kegan Paul).

Petchesky, R. P. (1985), 'Abortion in the 1980s: feminist morality and women's health', in E. Lewin and V. Olesen (eds.), *Women, Health and Healing: Toward a New Perspective* (London and New York: Tavistock).

Petchesky, R. P. (1987), 'Fetal images: the power of visual culture in the politics of reproduction', in M. Stanworth (ed.), *Reproductive Technologies: Gender, Motherhood and Medicine* (Cambridge: Polity Press).

Peters, G. (1981), 'Information and education about drugs', in Blum *et al.*, op. cit.

Peterson, M. J. (1978), *The Medical Profession in Mid-Victorian London* (Berkeley, Calif.: University of California Press).

Peterson, M. J. (1980), 'The Victorian governess: status incongruence in family and society, in M. Vicinus (ed.), *Suffer and Be Still: Women in the Victorian Age* (London: Methuen).

Pfeffer, N. (1985), 'The hidden pathology of the male reproductive system', in H. Homans (ed.), *The Sexual Politics of Reproduction* (Aldershot: Gower).

Pfeffer, N. (1987), 'Artificial insemination, *in vitro* fertilization and the stigma of infertility', in M. Stanworth (ed.), *Reproductive Technologies: Gender, Motherhood and Medicine* (Cambridge: Polity Press).

Pfeffer, N., and Woollett, A. (1983), *The Experience of Infertility* (London: Virago).

Phillips, A., and Rakusen, R. (eds.) (1978), *Our Bodies Ourselves: A Health Book by and for Women* (Harmondsworth: Penguin); US publication by the Boston Women's Health Book Collective.

Phillipson, C. (1981), 'Women in later life: patterns of control and subordination', in B. Hutter and G. Williams (eds.) *Controlling Women: The Normal and the Deviant*, (London: Croom Helm).

Pill, R. (1970), 'The sociological aspects of the case-study sample', in Stacey *et al.*, op. cit.,

Pill, R., and Stott, N. (1982), 'Concepts of illness causation and responsibility: some preliminary data from a sample of working class mothers', *Social Science and Medicine*, 16, pp. 43–52.

Pill, R., and Stott, N. (1986), 'Concepts of illness causation and responsibility: some preliminary data from a sample of working class mothers', in Currer and Stacey, op. cit., ch. 13.

Pinker, R. (1966), *English Hospital Statistics 1861–1938* (London: Heinemann).

Pollock, K. (1984), 'Mind and matter: a study of conceptions of health and illness among three groups of English families with particular reference to multiple sclerosis, schizophrenia and "nervous breakdown",' PhD thesis, University of Cambridge.

Porter, R. (1979), 'Medicine and the enlightenment in eighteenth century England', *Bulletin of the Society for the Social History of Medicine*, 25, pp. 27–40.

Porter, R. (1983), 'The language of quackery', *Bulletin of the Society for the Social History of the Medicine*, 33, p. 68; reference here is also to the longer mimeo version (London: Welcome Institute for the History of Medicine).

Power, R. (1984), 'A natural profession?', MA thesis, South Bank Polytechnic.

Powles, J. (1973), 'On the limitations of modern medicine', *Science, Medicine and Man*, 1, pp. 1–30.

Poynter, F. N. L., and Keele, K. D. (eds.) (1961), *A Short History of Medicine* (London: Scientific Book Club).

Raach, J. H. (1962), *A Directory of English Country Physicians 1603–43* (London: Dawsons).

Radical Statistics Health Group (1976), *Whose Priorities?* (London: RSHG).

Radical Statistics Health Group (1978), 'A critique of *Priorities for Health and Personal Social Services in England*', *International Journal of Health Services*, 8, 2, pp. 367–400.

Rakusen, J. (1981), 'Depoprovera: the extent of the problem: a case study in the politics of birth control', in H. Roberts (ed.), *Women, Health and Reproduction* (London: Routledge & Kegan Paul).

Randall, V. (1982), *Women and Politics* (London: St Martin).

Rapp, R. (1984), 'XYLO: a true story', in Arditti, Klein and Minden, op. cit.

Rawcliffe, C. (1983), 'The hospitals of later medieval London', *Bulletin of the Society for the Social History of Medicine*, 32, pp. 24–6.

Reidy, A. (1984), 'Marxist functionalism in medicine: a critique of the work of Vicente Navarro on health and medicine, *Social Science and Medicine*, 19, 9, pp. 897–910.

Reiter, R. R. (ed.) (1975), *Toward an Anthropology of Women* (New York and London: Monthly Review Press).

Rich, A. (1977), *Of Women Born: Motherhood as Experience and Institution* (London: Virago).

Richman, J. (1982), 'Men's experiences of pregnancy and childbirth', in L. McKee and M. O'Brien (eds.) *The Father Figure* (London and New York: Tavistock).

Richman., J., and Goldthorp, W. O. (1978), 'Fatherhood: the social construction of pregnancy and birth', in Kitzinger and Davis.

Ringen, K. (1979), 'Edwin Chadwick, the market ideology, and sanitary reform: on the nature of the nineteenth century public health movement', *International Journal of Health Services*, 9, 1, 107–20.

Roberts, D. F. (1976), 'Sex differences in disease and mortality', in L. O. Carter and J. Peel (eds.), *Equalities and Inequalities in Health* (London and New York: Academic Press).

Roberts, H. (1981), 'Male hegemony in family planning', in H. Roberts (eds.), *Women, Health and Reproduction* (London and Boston: Routledge & Kegan Paul).

Roberts, R. S. (1962), 'The personnel and practice of medicine in Tudor and Stuart England, part I: The Provinces', *Medical History*, 6, pp. 363–82.

Roberts, R. S. (1964), 'The personnel and practice of medicine in Tudor and Stuart England, part II: London', *Medical History*, 8, pp. 217–34.

Robinson, D. (1971), *The Process of Becoming Ill* (London: Routledge & Kegan Paul).

Robinson, J. (1985), personal communication; but see also Nursing Policy Studies Centre, 1986.

Robinson, S., Golden, J. and Bradley, S. (1983), *A Study of the Role and Responsibility of the Midwife* (London: Chelsea College).

Roemer, M. I. (1977), *Comparative National Policies on Health Care* (New York: Dekker).

Roggencamp, V. (1984), 'Abortion of a special kind: male sex selection in India', in Arditti, Klein and Minden, op. cit.

Rosaldo, M. S. (1980), 'The use and abuse of anthropology: reflections on feminism and cross cultural understanding', *Signs: A Journal of Women in Culture and Society*, 5, 3, pp. 389–417.

Rosaldo, M. S., and Lamphere, L. (1974), *Women, Culture and Society* (Stanford, Calif.: Stanford University Press).

Rose, H. (1982), 'Making science feminist', in E. Whitelegg, M. Arnot, E. Bartels, V. Beechey, L. Birke, S. Himmelweit, D. Leonard, S. Ruehl and M. A. Speakman (eds.), *The Changing Experience of Women* (Oxford: Martin Robertson Open University).

Rose, H. (1983), 'Hand, heart and brain: towards a feminist epistemology of the natural sciences', *Signs: A Journal of Women in Culture and Society*, 9, 1, pp. 73–90.

Rose, H. (1987), 'Victorian values in the test-tube: the politics of reproductive science and technology', in M. Stanworth (ed.), *Reproductive Technologies: Gender, Motherhood and Medicine* (Cambridge: Polity Press).

Rose, H., and Hanmer, J. (1976), 'Women's liberation, reproduction and the technological fix', in D. L. Barker and S. Allen (eds.), *Sexual Divisions and Society: Process and Change* (London: Tavistock), pp. 199–223.

Rose, S., Lewontin, R. C., and Kamin, L. J. (1984), *Not in Our Genes: Biology, Ideology and Human Nature* (Harmondsworth: Penguin).

Rosen, G. (1958), *A History of Public Health* (New York: MD Publications).

Rosengren, W. R., and Lefton, M. (1969), *Hospitals and Patients* (New York: Atherton).

Rosser, J., and Davies, C. (1984a), *Equal Opportunities for Women*, Warwick Working Papers in Sociology (Coventry: University of Warwick).

Rosser, J., and Davies, C. (1984b), 'Gendered jobs and professional work: the case of health service administration (or visible women, invisible work: "what would we do with her?")', mimeo (Coventry: Department of Sociology, University of Warwick).

Roth, J. A. (1963), *Timetables: Structuring the Passage of Time in Hospital Treatment and Other Careers* (Indianapolis, Ind., and New York: Bobbs-Merrill.

Roth, J. (1974), 'Professionalism: the sociologist's decoy', *Sociology of Work and Occupations*, 12, pp. 6–23.

Rothman, B. K. (1984), 'The meanings of choice in reproductive technology', in Arditti, Klein and Minden, op. cit.

Rothman, B. K. (1985), 'The products of conception: the social context of reproductive choices', *Journal of Medical Ethics*, 11, 4, pp. 188–93.

Rothman, B. K. (1986), *The Tentative Pregnancy* (New York: Viking).

Rowbotham, S. (1974a), *Hidden From History: 300 Years of Women's Oppression and the Fight against It* (London: Pluto).

Rowbotham, S. (1974b), *Women, Resistance and Revolution* (Harmondsworth: Penguin).

Rowbotham, S. (1979), 'The trouble with "patriarchy"', *New Statesman*, 98, 2544/5, pp. 970–1.

Rowbottom, R. W. (1978), 'Professionals in health and social service organisations', in E. Jaques (ed.), *Health Services: The Nature and Organisation and the Role of Patients, Doctors and the Health Professions* (London: Heinemann).

Rowland, R. (1984), 'Reproductive technologies: the final solution to the woman question?', in Arditti, Klein and Minden, op. cit.

Royal College of Obstetricians and Gynaecologists (1983), *Report of the RCOG Ethics Committee on In-Vitro Fertilization and Embryo Replacement or Transfer* (London: RCOG).

Rubin, L. S. (1979) 'Biofeedback: medicine's newest cure-all?' *Family Health*, 11, pp. 50–3.

Ruzek, S. B. (1978), *The Women's Health Movement: Feminist Alternatives to Medical Control* (New York: Praeger).

Sachs, A., and Wilson, J. H. (1978), *Sexism and the Law: A Study of Male Beliefs and Legal Bias in Britain and the United States* (Oxford: Martin Robertson).

Salmon, J. W. (ed.) (1984a), *Alternative Medicines: Popular and Policy Perspectives* (New York and London: Tavistock).

Salmon, J. W. (1984b), 'Organizing medical care for profit', in J. B. McKinlay (ed.), *Issues in the Political Economy of Health Care* (New York and London: Tavistock).

Sangari, K. (1984), 'If you would be the mother of a son', in Arditti, Klein and Minden, op. cit.

Saunders, L. (1954), *Cultural Differences in Medical Care: The Case of the Spanish-speaking People of the Southwest* (New York: Russell Sage).

Savage, W. (1986) *A Savage Enquiry: Who Controls Childbirth?* (London: Virago).

Saville, J. (1983), 'The origins of the welfare state', in M. Loney, D. Boswell and J. Clarke (eds.), *Social Policy and Social Welfare* (Milton Keynes: Open University Press).

Sawyer, R. C. (1983), 'Ordinary medicine for ordinary people: illness and its treatment in the East Midlands 1600–1630', *Bulletin of the Society for the Social History of Medicine*, 33, pp. 20–3.

Schofield, R. S., and Wrigley, E. A. (1981), *The Population History of England 1541–1871: A Reconstruction* (London: Edward Arnold).

Schwartz, L. R. (1969), 'The hierarchy of resort in curative practices: the Admiralty Islands, Melanesia', *Journal of Health and Social Behaviour*, 10, pp. 201–9.

Seabrook, J. (1973), *The Unprivileged: A Hundred Years of Family Life and Tradition in a Working-Class Street* (Harmondsworth: Penguin).

Seabrook, J. (1986) 'The unprivileged: a hundred years of their ideas about health and illness', in Currer and Stacey, op. cit.

Sharma, V. M. (1980), *Women, Work and Property in North-West India* (London: Tavistock).

Sheppard, H. J. (1972), 'The mythological tradition and seventeenth century alchemy', in A. G. Debus (ed.), *Science, Medicine and Society in the Renaissance*, Vol. 1 (London: Heinemann).

Silverman, D. (1970), *The Theory of Organisation* (London: Heinemann).

Silverman, M. (1977), 'The epidemiology of drug promotion', *International Journal of Health Services*, 7, p. 157.

Silverman, M., and Lee, P. R. (1974), *Pills, Profits and Politics* (Berkeley, Calif.: University of California Press).

Silverman, M., and Lydecker, M. (1981), 'The promotion of prescription drugs and other puzzles', in Blum *et al.*, op. cit.

Silverman, W. A. (1980), *Retrolental Fibroplasia: A Modern Parable* (London: Academic Press).

Simms, M. (1985), 'Legal abortion in Great Britain', in H. Homans (ed.), *The Sexual Politics of Reproduction* (Aldershot: Gower).

Simms, M., and Smith, C. (1982), 'Young fathers: attitudes to marriage and family life', in L. McKee and M. O'Brien (eds.), *The Father Figure* (London and New York: Tavistock).

Slack, P. A. (1976), 'Plague and public order in 16th and 17th century England', *Bulletin of the Society for the Social History of Medicine*, 19, p. 20.

Slack, P. A. (1979), 'Mortality crises and epidemic disease in England', in C. Webster (ed.), *Health, Medicine and Mortality in the Sixteenth Century* (Cambridge: Cambridge University Press).

Slack, P. A. (1980), 'Social policy and the constraints of government, 1547–58', in J. Loach and R. Tittler (eds.), *The Mid-Tudor Policy c. 1540–1560* (London: Macmillan).

Slack, P. A. (1985), *The Impact of Plague in Tudor and Stuart England* (London: Routledge & Kegan Paul).

Slack, P. A. (1986), 'Metropolitan government in crises: the response to plague', in A. Beier and R. Finlay (eds.), *London 1500–1700: The Making of the Metropolis* (London and New York: Longman).

Smart, C. (1987), ' "There is of course the distinction dictated by nature": law and the problem of paternity', in M. Stanworth (ed.), *Reproductive Technologies: Gender, Motherhood and Medicine* (Cambridge: Polity Press).

Smith, A. (1968), *The Science of Social Medicine* (London: Staples).

Smith, D. (1974a), 'Women, the family and corporate capitalism', in M. Stephenson (ed.), *Women in Canada* (Toronto: New Press).

Smith, D. (1974b), 'Women's perspective as a radical critique of sociology', *Sociological Inquiry*, 44, pp. 7–13.

Smith, D. (1975), 'Women and psychiatry', in D. E. Smith and S. J. David (eds.), *Women Look at Psychiatry* (Vancouver: Press Gang Publishers).

Smith, F. B. (1979), *The People's Health 1830–1910* (London: Croom Helm).

Smith, H. (1976), 'Gynaecology and ideology in seventeenth century England', in B. A. Carroll (ed.), *Liberating Women's History: Theoretical and Critical Essays* (Urbana, Ill.: University of Illinois Press), pp. 97–114.

Snowden, R., and Mitchell, G. D. (1983), *The Artificial Family: A Consideration of Artificial Insemination by Donor* (London: Unwin/Counterpoint).

Social Services Committee (1983), Session 1982–3, *Public Expenditure on the Social Services* (London: HMSO).

Sokolowska, M. (1974), 'Two basic types of medical orientation', in A. Podgorecki (ed.), *Socio-Technics Current Sociology*, 23, 1, pp. 163–74 reprinted in Currer and Stacey, op. cit., 1986.

Sokolowska, M., Ostrowska, A., and Titkow, A. (1975), 'The sociology of health of Polish society: trends and current state of research', in 'Problems of Current Sociological Research', *Current Sociology*, 23, pp. 1–3.

Spencer, N. J. (1984), 'Parents' recognition of the ill child', in J. A. Macfarlane (ed.), *Progress in Child Health* (Edinburgh: Churchill Livingstone).

Spring Rice, M. (1939), *Working Class Wives* (Harmondsworth: Penguin).

Stacey, M. (1960), *Tradition and Change* (London: Oxford University Press).

Stacey M. (1969), 'The myth of community studies', *British Journal of Sociology*, 20, 2, pp. 134–47.

Stacey, M. (1974), 'Consumer complaints procedure in the British NHS', *Social Science and Medicine*, 8, 8, pp. 429–35.

Stacey, M. (1976), 'The health service consumer: a sociological misconception', in *Sociology of the National Health Service*, Sociological Review Monograph 22 (Keele: University of Keele).

Stacey, M. (1979), 'New perspectives in clinical medicine: the sociologist', *Journal of Royal College of Physicians of London*, 13, 3, pp. 123–9.

Stacey, M. (1980), 'Charisma, power and altruism: a discussion of research in a child development centre', *Sociology of Health and Illness*, 2, 1, pp. 64–90.

Stacey, M. (1981), 'The division of labour revisited or overcoming the two Adams', in P. Abrams and R. Deem (eds.), *Practice and Progess: British Sociology 1950–1980*, (London: Allen & Unwin).

Stacey, M. (1984), 'Who are the health workers? Patients and other unpaid workers in health care', *Economic and Industrial Democracy*, 5, pp. 157–84 (London and Beverly Hills: Sage).

Stacey, M. (1985a), 'Women and health: the United States and the United Kingdom compared', in E. Lewin and V. Olesen (eds.), *Women, Health and Healing* (New York and London: Tavistock).

Stacey, M. (1985b), 'Commentary', *Journal of Medical Ethics*, 11, 4, pp. 193–5.

Stacey, M. (1986a), 'Establishing criteria for appropriate care: a dilemma for the profession', paper read to the Forum on Maternity and the Newborn, Royal Society of Medicine, 22 March.

Stacey, M. (1986b), 'Concepts of health and illness and the division of labour in health care', in Currer and Stacey, op. cit.

Stacey, M., and Davies, C. (1983), *Division of Labour in Child Health Care: Final Report to the SSRC*, mimeo (Coventry: University of Warwick).

Stacey, M., and Price, M. (1981), *Women, Power and Politics* (London: Tavistock).

Stacey, M. (ed.), Dearden, R., Pill, R., and Robinson, D. (1970), *Hospitals, Children and Their Families: The Report of a Pilot Study* (London: Routledge & Kegan Paul).

Stanway, A. (1982), *Alternative Medicine* (New York: Penguin).

Stanworth, M. (1987a), 'Introduction', in M. Stanworth (ed.), *Reproductive Technologies: Gender, Motherhood and Medicine* (Cambridge: Polity Press).

Stanworth, M. (1987b), 'Reproductive technologies and the deconstruction of motherhood', in M. Stanworth (ed.), *Reproductive Technologies: Gender, Motherhood and Medicine* (Cambridge: Polity Press).

Starr, P. (1982), *The Social Transformation of American Medicine* (New York: Basic Books).

Stevens, R. (1966), *Medical Practice in Modern England: The Impact of Specialization and State Medicine* (New Haven, Conn. and London: Yale University Press).

Stevenson, G. (1976), 'Social relations of production and consumption in the human service occupations', *Monthly Review*, 28, pp. 78–87.

Stevenson, J. (1977), *Social Conditions between the Wars* (Harmondsworth: Penguin).

Stimson, G. V. (1974), 'Obeying doctor's orders: a view from the other side', *Social Science and Medicine*, 8, 2, pp. 97–104.

Stimson, G., and Webb, B. (1975), *Going to See the Doctor: The Consultation Process in General Practice* (London and Boston: Routledge & Kegan Paul).

Stocking, B., and Morrison, S. L. (1978), *The Image and the Reality: A Case Study of the Impact of Medical Technology* (Oxford: Nuffield Provincial Hospitals Trust Oxford University Press).

Strauss, A., Schatzman, L., Ehrlich, D., Bucher, R., and Sabshin, M. (1963), 'The hospital and its negotiated order', in E. Freidson (ed.), *The Hospital in Modern Society* (New York: Free Press).

Strauss, A. L., Fagerhaugh, S., Suczek, B., and Wiener, C. (1982a), 'The work of hospitalized patients', *Social Science and Medicine*, 16, 9, pp. 977–86.

Strauss, A., Fagerhaugh, S., Suczek, B., and Wiener, C. (1982b), 'Sentimental work in the technological hospital', *Sociology of Health and Illness*, 4, 3, pp. 254–78.

Strong, P. (1979), 'Sociological imperialism and the profession of medicine: a critical examination of the thesis of medical imperialism', *Social Science and Medicine*, 13A, 2, pp. 199–215.

Strong, P. M. (1982), 'Materialism and microsociology – a reply to Michele Barrett', *Sociology of Health and Illness*, 4, 1, pp. 98–101.

Summers, A. (1979), 'A home from home – women's philanthropic work in the nineteenth century', in S. Burman (ed.), *Fit Work for Women* (London: Croom Helm).

Summers, A. (1983), 'Pride and prejudice: ladies and nurses in the Crimean War', *History Workshop*, 16, pp. 33–56.

Szasz, T. (1961), *The Myth of Mental Illness* (New York: Harper & Row).

Taylor, B. (1983), *Eve and the New Jerusalem* (London: Virago).

Taylor, J. (1979), 'Hidden labour in the National Health Service', in P. Atkinson, R. Dingwall and A. Murcott (eds.), *Prospects for the National Health* (London: Croom Helm).

Thomas, A. (reporter) (1978), 'Discussion on Arthur Kleinman's Paper', *Social Science and Medicine*, 12, 2B, p. 95.

Thomas, K. (1970), 'Anthropology and the study of English witchcraft', in M. Douglas (ed.), *Witchcraft Confessions and Accusations* (London: Tavistock).

Thomas, K. (1971), *Religion and the Decline of Magic* (London: Weidenfeld).

Thompson, E. P. (1963), *The Making of the English Working Class* (London: Gollancz).

Thompson, H. B. (1857), *Choice of a Profession: A Concise Account and Comparative Review of the English Professions* (London: Chapman & Hall).

Tillich, P. (1961), 'The meaning of health', *Perspective Biology and Medicine*, 5, p. 92.

Timpanaro, S. (1980), *On Materialism* (London: Verso).

Titmuss, R. H. (1973), *The Gift Relationship* (Harmondsworth: Penguin).

Tolliday, H. (1978), 'Clincial autonomy', in E. Jaques (ed.), *Health Services: The Nature and Organisation and the Role of Patients, Doctors and the Health Professions* (London: Heinemann).

Tomalin, C. (1985), *The Life and Death of Mary Wollstonecraft* (Harmondsworth: Penguin).

Towers, P. (1985), personal communication.

Towler, J., and Bramall, J. (1986), *Midwives in History and Society* (London: Croom Helm).

Townsend, P., and Davidson, N. (eds.) (1982), *Inequalities in Health: The Black Report* (Harmondsworth: Penguin).

Tuckett, D. (1976), *An Introduction to Medical Sociology* (London: Tavistock).

Twaddle, A. C. (1974), 'The concept of health status', *Social Science and Medicine*, 8, 1, pp. 29–38.

U 205 Open University Course Team (1985a), *Studying Health and Disease* (Milton Keynes: Open University Press).

U 205 Open University Course Team (1985b), *The Health of Nations* (Milton Keynes: Open University Press).

Uglow, J. (1983), 'Josephine Butler: from sympathy to theory, 1828–1906', in D. Spender (ed.), *Feminist Theorists: Three Centuries of Women's Intellectual Traditions* (London: Women's Press), pp. 46–164.

UKCC (1986), *Project 2000: A New Preparation for Practice* (London: UKCC).

Ungerson, C. (1983), 'Why do women care?' in Finch and Groves, op. cit.

Unschuld, P. (1978), 'Discussion on David McQueen's paper', *Social Science and Medicine*, 12, 2B, pp. 75–7.

Unschuld, P. (1979), 'Comparative systems of health care', *Social Science and Medicine*, 13A, 4, pp. 523–7.

Unschuld, P. (1980), 'The issue of the structured coexistence of scientific and alternative medical systems: a comparison of East and West German legislation', *Social Science and Medicine*, 14B, 1, pp. 15–24.

Unschuld, P. (1986), 'The conceptual determination (*Überformung*) of individual and collective experiences of illness', in Currer and Stacey, op. cit.

Vass, K. (1985), 'Misuse of antibiotics in the Third World', *Listener*, 19 September, p. 11–12.

Versluysen, M. C. (1977), 'Medical professionalism and maternity hospitals in eighteenth century London: a sociological interpretation', *Bulletin of the Society for the Social History of Medicine*, 21, p. 34–6.

Versluysen, M. C. (1980), 'Old wives' tales? Women healers in English history', in Davies, op. cit.

Versluysen, M. C. (1981), 'Midwives, medical men and "poor women labouring of child": lying-in hospitals in eighteenth century London', in H. Roberts (ed.), *Women, Health and Reproduction* (London and Boston: Routledge & Kegan Paul).

Vicinus, M. (1985), *Independent Women: Work and Community for Single Women, 1850–1920* (London: Virago).

Waddington, I. (1973a), 'The role of the hospital in the development of modern medicine: a sociological analysis', *Sociology*, 7, pp. 211–24.

Waddington, I. (1973b), 'The struggle to reform the Royal College of Physicians 1767–1771: a sociological analysis', *Medical History*, 17, pp. 107–26.

Waddington, I. (1977), 'General practitioners and consultants in early nineteenth century England: the sociology of intra-professional conflict', in J. Woodward and D. Richards (eds.), *Health Care and Popular Medicine in Nineteenth Century England* (London: Croom Helm).

Waddington, I. (1979), 'Competition and monopoly in a profession: the campaign for medical registration in Britain', *Amsterdams Sociologisch Jijdschrift*, 6, pp. 288–321.

Waddington, I. (1984), *The Medical Profession in the Industrial Revolution* (London: Gill & Macmillan), ch. 9, pp. 177–205.

Wadsworth, M. E. J., Butterfield, W. J. H., and Blaney, R. (1971), *Health and Sickness: The Choice of Treatment* (London: Tavistock).

Walkowitz, J. R., and Walkowitz, D. J. (1974), '"We are not beasts of the field":

prostitution and the poor in Plymouth and Southampton under the Contagious Diseases Acts', in M. S. Hartman and L. Banner (eds.), *Clio's Consciousness Raised: New Perspectives on the History of Women* (New York and London: Harper & Row).

Wallsgrove, R. (1980), 'The masculine face of science', in Brighton Women and Science Group (eds.), *Alice through the Microscope: The Power of Science over Women's Lives* (London: Virago).

Walsh, V. (1980), 'Contraception: the growth of a technology', in Brighton Women and Science Group (eds.), *Alice through the Microscope: The Power of Science over Women's Lives* (London: Virago).

Warner, J. H. (1980), 'Therapeutic explanation and the Edinburgh bloodletting controversy: two perspectives on the medical meaning of science in the mid-nineteenth century', *Medical History*, 24, pp. 241–58.

Watkins, D. (1985), 'What was social medicine: an historiographical essay. George Rosen revisited', paper presented to the Society for the Social History of Medicine.

Webster, C. (1975), *The Great Instauration: Science, Medicine and Reform 1626–1660* (London: Duckworth).

Webster, C. (1978), 'The crisis of the hospitals during the industrial revolution', in E. G. Forbes (ed.), *Human Implications of Scientific Advance*, Proceedings of the Fifteenth International Congress of the History of Science, Edinburgh, 10–15 August 1977 (Edinburgh).

Webster, C. (ed.) (1979), *Health, Medicine and Mortality in the Sixteenth Century* (Cambridge: Cambridge University Press).

Webster, C. (1980), 'Healthy or hungry thirties?' *Bulletin of the Society for the Social History of Medicine*, 27, pp. 22–3.

Webster, C. (ed.) (1981), *Biology, Medicine and Society 1840–1940* (Cambridge: Cambridge University Press).

Webster, C. (1982a), 'Healthy or hungry thirties?', *History Workshop Journal*, 13, pp. 110–29.

Webster, C. (1982b), 'Paracelsus and paracelsianism', *Bulletin of the Society for the Social History of Medicine*, 30–1, p. 47.

Webster, C. (1982c), 'Medicine as social history: changing ideas on doctors and patients in the age of Shakespeare', in L. G. Stevenson (ed.), *A Celebration of Medical History* (Baltimore, Md: Johns Hopkins University Press).

Webster, C. (1983), 'General practice under the panel', *Bulletin of the Society for the Social History of Medicine*, 32, pp. 20–3.

Webster, C. (1984), 'Health: historical issues', Discussion Paper No,. 5 (London: Centre for Economic Policy Research).

Webster, C. (1985), 'Health, welfare and unemployment during the depression', *Past and Present: A Journal of Historical Studies*, 109, pp. 204–30.

Webster, C. (forthcoming), 'Labour and the origins of the National Health Service', in N. Rupke (ed.), *Science, Politics and the Public Good* (London: Macmillan).

Weindling, P. (ed.) (1985), *The Social History of Occupational Health* (London: Croom Helm).

West, R. (1984), 'Alternative medicine: prospects and speculations', in N. Black, D. Boswell, A. Gray, S. Murphy and J. Popay (eds.), *Health and Disease* (Milton Keynes and Philadelphia, Pa: Open University Press).

Which? (1986), 'Magic or medicine?', October, pp. 443–7.

White, R. (1978), *Social Change and the Development of the Nursing Profession: A Study of the Poor Law Nursing Service 1848–1948* (London: Kimpton).

Whitehead, M. (1987), *The Health Divide: Inequalities in Health in the 1980s* (London: Health Education Council).

Willcocks, A. J. (1967), *The Creation of the National Health Service* (London: Routledge & Kegan Paul).

Williams, K. (1980), 'From Sarah Gamp to Florence Nightingale: a critical study of hospital nursing systems from 1840–1897', in Davies, op. cit.

Williams, R. G. A. (1981a), 'Logical analysis as a qualitative method, I: conflict of ideas and the topic of illness', *Sociology of Health and Illness*, 3, 2, pp. 140–164.

Williams, R. G. A. (1981b), 'Logical analysis as a qualitative method, II: conflict of ideas and the topic of illness', *Sociology of Health and Illness*, 3, 2, pp. 165–87.

Williams, R. G. A. (1983), 'Concepts of health: an analysis of lay logic', *Sociology*, 17, pp. 183–205.

Williamson, N. E. (1976), *Sons or Daughters: A Cross-Cultural Survey of Parental Preferences*, Sage Library of Social Sciences (London: Sage).

Wilson, E. (1977), *Women and the Welfare State* (London: Tavistock).

Wilson, E. (1980), *Only Halfway to Paradise: Women in Postwar Britain: 1945–1968* (London and New York: Tavistock).

Woodcock, J. (1981), 'Medicines – the interested parties', in Blum, *et al.*, op. cit.

Woodward, J. (1974), *To Do the Sick No Harm. A Study of the British Voluntary Hospital System to 1875* (London and Boston: Routledge & Kegan Paul).

Worsley, P. (1970), *The Trumpet Shall Sound: A Study of 'Cargo' Cults in Melanesia* (London: Paladin).

Young, A. (1976a), 'Internalising and externalising medical belief systems: an Ethiopian example', *Social Science and Medicine*, 10, 3/4, pp. 147–56.

Young, A. (1976b), 'Some implications of medical beliefs and practices for social anthropology', *American Anthropologist*, 78, pp. 5–24.

Young, A. (1978), 'Mode of production of medical knowledge', *Medical Anthropology*, V, 2, Spring, pp. 97–124.

Young, A. (1986), 'Internalising and externalising medical belief systems: an Ethiopian example' in Currer and Stacey, op. cit.

Young, G. (1981), 'A woman in medicine: reflections from the inside', in H. Roberts (ed.), *Women, Health and Reproduction* (London and Boston: Routledge & Kegan Paul).

Youngson, A. J. (1979), *The Scientific Revolution in Victorian Medicine* (London: Croom Helm).

Zipper, J., and Svenhuijsen, S. (1987), 'Surrogacy: feminist notions of motherhood reconsidered', in M. Stanworth (ed.), *Reproductive Technologies: Gender, Motherhood and Medicine* (Cambridge: Polity Press).

Zola, I. K. (1966), 'Culture and symptoms – an analysis of patients presenting complaints', *American Sociological Review*, 31, p. 615; reprinted in Cox and Mead, op. cit. (1975).

Index